The Greatest Killer

The Greatest Killer

Smallpox in History

with a new Introduction

Donald R. Hopkins

The University of Chicago Press • *Chicago and London*

DONALD R. HOPKINS participated in the World Health Organization's Smallpox Eradication Program in Asia and Africa. He is a former deputy director of the Centers for Disease Control and Prevention in Atlanta, Georgia and was named a MacArthur Fellow in 1995. He is associate executive director of the Carter Presidential Center.

The University of Chicago Press, Chicago 60637
The University of Chicago Press, Ltd., London
© 1983 by The University of Chicago
New Introduction © 2002 by The University of Chicago
All rights reserved. Published 2002
Printed in the United States of America

11 10 09 08 07 06 05 04 03   2 3 4 5

ISBN: 0-226-35166-1 (cloth)
ISBN: 0-226-35168-8 (paper)

This book was originally published as *Princes and Peasants: Smallpox in History* by The University of Chicago Press in 1983.

Library of Congress Cataloging-in-Publication Data

Hopkins, Donald R.
    [Princes and peasants]
    The greatest killer : smallpox in history, with a new introduction / Donald R. Hopkins.
        p. cm.
    Originally published as Princes and peasants, 1983.
    Includes bibliographical references and index.
    ISBN 0-226-35166-1 (cloth : alk. paper) — ISBN 0-226-35168-8 (pbk. : alk. paper)
    1. Smallpox—History. I. Title.

RC183.1 .H66   2002
614.5′21′09—dc21
                                                    2002023950

⊗ The paper used in this publication meets the minimum requirements of the American National Standard for Information Sciences—Permanence of Paper for Printed Library Materials, ANSI Z39.48-1992.

For my wife, Ernestine Mathis, my parents, Joseph Leonard and Iva Major, and in loving memory of Andy, and Inez Mathis

Mode of living or rank in society does not alter the susceptibility of a person. The prince and the peasant are alike subject to its influence.

K. C. Bose,
Indian Medical Gazette (1890)

Contents

Illustrations

Introduction

In 1806, President Thomas Jefferson wrote to Edward Jenner, the developer of smallpox vaccination, "Future generations will know by history only that the loathsome smallpox has existed."

I wrote this book twenty years ago to mark the conclusion of the successful program to eradicate smallpox worldwide. My colleagues and I had worked hard on the eradication program, and we expected that—as Jefferson suggested—the disease would become known only as a threat that had once existed in history, never as a threat to current and future generations. I quoted Jefferson's prediction at the end of the book, followed by my own fervent hope: "May it always be so."

Now, however, we face the prospect that this ancient virus may be resurrected, not as a naturally occurring disease but deliberately, for use as a biological weapon. This horrible possibility puts smallpox into the headlines once again. With its ability to spread easily and no cure available once its symptoms appear, smallpox is fatal to 25% or more of its victims and was rivaled only by plague as a source of terror in ancient times. Over three millennia, smallpox probably killed even more people than plague did.

Within months after smallpox was eradicated, we learned to fear a new disease, AIDS or HIV infection, which is now killing millions around the world. But AIDS/HIV is spread only by blood or direct sexual contact; the smallpox virus spreads through the air. In 1963, for example, twenty-five people in Sweden contracted smallpox by breathing air that carried the virus either in a hospital, in a previous victim's home, from a victim's laundry or corpse, or simply out-of-doors. Today there are even more opportunities for smallpox to spread—so many more people live in densely populated areas, routinely commute to work, work in larger buildings with central heating and air conditioning, and travel cross-country or internationally for business or pleasure. If smallpox were reintroduced as a biological weapon, we would all be potentially vulnerable—neither birthplace nor residence, wealth nor education would provide a safe haven.

As far as we know, the only remaining stocks of smallpox virus are stored in guarded laboratories in the United States and Russia. But even twenty years ago, I feared that someone somewhere might discover a forgotten vial of smallpox virus stored in a laboratory or hospital freezer. This is still a remote possibility. Could someone gain access to the known stocks of smallpox stored in the United States or Russia? This is also theoretically possible but less likely, in my opinion. A more likely potential danger today is that a rogue stock of the virus is being held elsewhere by someone willing to use it to kill.

So we are faced with a host of questions. Should the existing stocks of virus that we know of be destroyed or be used for research that might lead to better protection? Should we increase our supply of smallpox vaccine? Should we all be vaccinated, or only medical, military, and public safety personnel?

Since there is a vaccine against smallpox, why can't we simply protect ourselves now instead of vaccinating only if an outbreak occurs? It is true that resuming routine vaccination against smallpox would eliminate the threat of smallpox as a biological weapon. Routine vaccination was discontinued thirty years ago, when smallpox was eradicated, because the need for vaccination apparently no longer existed. Physicians were relieved because the available vaccine can produce rare but fatal complications. When smallpox vaccinations were routine, these complications killed scores of people. The risk of such complications today would be greater for healthy adults who were never vaccinated than it would be for unvaccinated infants—to say nothing of the even greater risk to millions of unsuspecting people whose immune systems have been compromised by age, previously unrecognized HIV infection, or other medications such as steroids. Would we be justified in causing the deaths of random individuals through an attempt to guard against something that may never happen?

Even if we could vaccinate everyone in the United States, could we get smallpox vaccine again to everyone who needs it worldwide? Those of us who worked in the World Health Organization's Smallpox Eradication Program did just that thirty-odd years ago, at immense effort and expense, in order to stop this terrible disease. It is heartbreaking to think that a killer disease we have already eradicated might be let loose once more upon the world.

Over time, smallpox took many more lives than all the carnage of the twentieth century and left many who survived disfigured and distraught. And, as you will read in this book, smallpox not only destroyed individuals and families, it changed the course of history many times. Let us hope that smallpox will remain a part of our history rather than a threat to our future.

Donald R. Hopkins, M.D., M.P.H.
Chicago, Illinois
January 2002

Preface

MY INTEREST IN THE HISTORY of smallpox began during my first assignment to help fight the disease in Sierra Leone, West Africa, in 1967–69. Having read the section on history in Dixon's textbook, *Smallpox*, I encountered minor references to the disease from time to time while reading various books on African history. I began to wonder whether it really made any difference that the various European monarchs mentioned by Dixon had died of smallpox when they did; I also began to realize that there was almost certainly a larger story than that described in Dixon's chapter.

The active research that culminated in this book began in January 1976 in an attempt to satisfy my curiosity about the history of smallpox while preparing the introduction to a paper I was writing on the lessons of the World Health Organization's Smallpox Eradication Program. I was especially fortunate during the first two years of this work in having ready access to two of the best libraries in the country. At that time I lived in Cambridge only a few blocks from Harvard University's main library, Widener, while teaching and doing research in the Department of Tropical Public Health at Harvard School of Public Health in Boston, next door to the Countway Library of Medicine.

I spent many evenings, weekends, and holidays during the first year of research in Widener Library, going through the indexes of books in the stacks, one by one, in search of references to smallpox, beginning in the sections on Africa, Japan, and China. It soon became apparent that a lot of material about smallpox's history had not been brought together or examined systematically. During the summer of 1977, a grant from the William F. Milton Fund of Harvard University enabled me to spend three weeks in London conducting further research at the extraordinarily rich Wellcome Library of the History of Medicine and, to a lesser extent, at the libraries of the London School of Hygiene and Tropical Medicine and the British Museum. I also took the opportunity then, as in many trips elsewhere since, to visit sites associated with the events described in this book. I assumed my current position as assistant director for International Health at the Centers for Disease Control in January 1978.

This is not a history of the Smallpox Eradication Program, but rather the story of the disease itself. The definitive account of the global eradication campaign is being prepared under the auspices of the World Health Organization by Drs. Frank Fenner, D. A. Henderson, Isao Arita, and I. D. Ladnyi. When that volume is completed in the next two or three years, we shall have an authoritative account of a public health accomplishment, the eradication of smallpox, which is almost as remarkable as the story of the disease.

The ideal author of a book that overlaps the fields of medicine and history as this one does would combine the judgment and perspective of a good professional historian with the knowledge of a physician experienced in the diagnosis and control of smallpox. I can claim only the latter qualifications. I believe most readers will agree, however, that quite apart from my ability to describe it, the impact of smallpox through the ages has been extraordinary.

Some professional historians might object to the special attention given in the book to the illnesses and deaths of royal victims. In addition to the reasons outlined below, I have done so for a more personal reason. As one whose entire experience of this disease had been in witnessing and combatting its effects among villagers in often remote, poverty-stricken regions of Africa and Asia, I was fascinated to discover evidence of the same despair, tragedy, fear, bewilderment, and mistakes I had seen in African and Asian villages in European palaces, North American hospitals, and elsewhere in the not so distant past.

This is the story of how smallpox, which will be known to future generations as the first disease of man to be deliberately eradicated, exerted a singular influence on human history through the ages before its extinction—suddenly removing or temporarily indisposing leaders of nations, destroying armies, disrupting cities, and laying waste to ordinary citizens, devastating virgin populations, and influencing fateful decisions in many other ways. To a lesser extent, this is also the story of a complex struggle between knowledge and ignorance.

In revealing how smallpox has influenced history, I deliberately linger on the illnesses and deaths of prominent persons. First, because they were bound to be of more obvious consequence to history than the illnesses or deaths of numerous less influential folk. Habsburg emperor Joseph I's premature death from smallpox in 1711, for example, had a historical impact that was felt for generations, whereas we don't even know the names of ordinary Viennese who died of the same disease that spring, much less the consequences of their deaths. Second, we can often draw on detailed descriptions of the illness, treatment, and death or convalescence of well-known persons. Similar detailed reports were rarely made for less prominent victims. Such accounts allow us to observe smallpox in action close-up and to see the desperate measures taken to try to alter the disease's course. By reconstructing events leading up to the illnesses of a few important victims, it also has been possible, in the light of current scientific knowledge, to suggest how and when they were infected and, in one case, to "correct" a mistaken contemporary conclusion about the source of a royal infection. Thus the role of chance in human history is repeatedly revealed here. As lesser indications of smallpox's historical terror, we can trace curious beliefs that arose in futile attempts to save its victims. The idea that the color red was somehow beneficial in curing patients with smallpox dates at least to tenth-century Asia, was once widespread in Europe, and was the subject of clinical trials on three continents early in the twentieth century. Gods or goddesses of smallpox were beseeched for relief in Asia, Africa, and Latin America, and in Europe, St. Nicaise of Rheims was recognized as the patron saint of smallpox victims. These curiosa are also a part of the story of smallpox.

Acknowledgments

THE FOLLOWING KINDLY PERMITTED me to use material originally published by them.

The description in chapter 5 of tribal practices in Orissa State, from Verrier Elwin, *The Religion of an Indian Tribe* (London: Oxford University Press, 1955).

My article on Benjamin Waterhouse, adapted in chapter 7, from the *American Journal of Tropical Medicine and Hygiene* 26 (1977): 1060–64, Paul Beaver, editor.

The excerpt in chapter 4 from Ramsudar Prabhudas's *Sitala Calisa: Forty Verses in Praise of the Smallpox Goddess, Sitala*, from Ralph W. Nicholas.

The description of Mary II's death in chapter 2, from Thomas B. Macaulay, *The History of England*, vol. 5 (London: Macmillan and Co., 1914).

Lorene Lakin's account of the 1903 Oregon epidemic in chapter 7, from the *Oregon Health Bulletin* 50, no. 10 (Oct.):2, Sherman A. Washburn, editor.

The accounts of smallpox's effect on North American Indians quoted in chapter 7, from John Joseph Heagerty, *Four Centuries of Medical History in Canada* (Bristol: John Wright and Sons, 1928).

Accounts of inoculation's introduction into Europe and of eighteenth-century theories about smallpox quoted in chapters 1 and 2, from Genevieve Miller, *The Adoption of Inoculation for Smallpox in England and France* (Philadelphia: University of Pennsylvania Press, 1957).

The accounts of smallpox's devastation of South American Indians quoted in chapter 6, from John Hemming, *Red Gold* (Cambridge: Harvard University Press, 1978).

The accounts of epidemics quoted in chapters 2 and 7, from Hugh Thursfield, "Smallpox in the American War of Independence," *Annals of Medical History*, 3d series, 2 (1940) 312–18.

Reports and statistics from the Smallpox Eradication series, 1966–79, from the World Health Organization.

In addition to the very timely support of the Milton Fund, which is gratefully acknowledged, I must also thank the staffs of Harvard's Widener Library, the Countway Library of Medicine, the Harvard-Yenching

Library, and the Wellcome Library, and the libraries of the London School of Hygiene and Tropical Medicine, the British Museum, and Emory University.

Space will not permit me to acknowledge by name the many friends and colleagues who brought information or illustrations to my attention. Some especially difficult references on Africa were provided by the late Dr. Gerald W. Hartwig of Duke University, Dr. K. David Patterson of the University of North Carolina, and by Dr. P. J. Imperato; on Poland by the late Professor Jan Rogowski; on Sweden by Dr. Marianne Jonsson; on Japan by Professor Teizo Ogawa and Dr. Shizu Sakai; on China by Dr. Chen Zheng-ren and Dr. Ma Kan Wen; on several topics by David Preston, and on Abraham Lincoln by Mr. Oliver Orr of the Library of Congress. Others who kindly translated articles are acknowledged with the citation of the article they translated. I must also express my profound gratitude to Dr. Eli Chernin and the late Professor G. L. Chandler, who helped teach me to write clearly; to Drs. Mark Boyer, Joe Waner, and Stan Foster for providing valuable comments on early drafts of the manuscript; and especially to Dr. D. A. Henderson of Johns Hopkins University, and two anonymous readers for the University of Chicago Press who generously devoted much time to constructive criticism of the penultimate draft. However, I alone am responsible for any errors in fact or in interpretation in this book.

I also thank Marilyn Myers, who typed most of the first draft; Patsy Bellamy, who typed the final two drafts; Shirley Jones and Lisa Hopkins, who prepared the figures and preliminary sketches of smallpox gods and goddesses; and Drs. G. I. Lythcott, W. H. Foege, and J. D. Millar, who helped cheer me on during the ups and downs of writing and rewriting.

Most of all, I thank my dear wife Ernestine, who tolerated and abetted my obsession these past six and a half years, advised me on various parts of the manuscript, and who also translated some articles and typed more than one of the middle drafts.

Finally, I gratefully acknowledge my long-standing indebtedness to Drs. Henry C. McBay, Frederick Mapp, and the late James H. Birnie, all of Morehouse College, who many years ago encouraged me to read Hans Zinsser's *Rats, Lice, and History,* Paul de Kruif's *Microbe Hunters,* and Bernard Jaffe's *Crucibles: The Story of Chemistry,* thereby kindling my interest in the history of science.

One

Variola Rex

ELIZABETH I HAD BEEN at Hampton Court Palace southwest of London for nearly a month. Young, attractive, and confident, she had been queen of England for four years. Beyond her own peaceful realm, Europe was in turmoil:

> In France there was civil war, hateful persecution in Spain, and in Scotland, where Mary (Queen of Scots) had just returned after the death of her French husband, there was almost anarchy. The Netherlands were filled with deep discontent, ready at any moment to burst into flames. England alone was quiet and prosperous; Elizabeth lived a gay and merry life, always vigilant, alert and prepared for emergencies. (Sandwith 1910, 298)

Prepared for any emergency, that is, except one.

Feeling unwell, the queen took a bath and went for a walk among the autumn colors in her garden, expecting that would help her shake off a minor disturbance to her constitution. A day or two later she became feverish, faint, and began shivering. On 15 October 1562, she concluded a letter to Mary, queen of Scots, saying "The fever under which I am suffering forbids me to write further" (Sitwell 1962, 123–24).

Elizabeth's advisors summoned a highly respected German-born physician, Dr. Burcot, to the palace, and although the queen's skin was still clear, he told her, "My liege, thou shalt have the pox" (Halliday 1955, 543). Burcot's diagnosis angered the queen, who was probably frightened by the thought that she might have smallpox. Even if she were lucky enough to survive an attack of smallpox, she still stood a good chance of being left with a badly scarred face. The queen of England cared about her life and her appearance, especially since her rival, the queen of Scots, was reputed to be beautiful. "Have away the knave out of my sight," she ordered (ibid., 544). Insulted, Burcot went home.

Hours later the queen became incoherent and soon sank into a coma. Even before then, Elizabeth and her advisers believed she was dying— unmarried and without a designated heir. The lords of the Privy Council were summoned from London and met in an adjoining room to discuss "the momentous question of the succession" (Law 1885, 1: 289–90). Here was the grave crisis many Englishmen had feared since her accession. The queen was desperately ill, and England's fate depended on the outcome of her illness. As news of the queen's condition spread, her kingdom was "scared out of its wits" (Sandwith 1910, 298).

After about four hours, Elizabeth regained consciousness and begged the council to appoint Lord Robert Dudley Protector of the Realm, while swearing, on her expected deathbed, "that though she loved and had always loved Lord Robert dearly, nothing improper had ever passed between them" (Jenkins 1958, 100). (Elizabeth's liaison with Dudley, the earl of Leicester, had been the subject of speculation throughout her kingdom.) A rash appeared soon after midnight.

Two men from the court were sent on horseback to fetch Dr. Burcot again and told him the queen was very sick and had sent for him. Still upset from his earlier encounter, Burcot angrily replied, "By God's pestilence, if she be sick, there let her die! Call me a *knave* for my good will!" (Halliday 1955, 544). A faithful servant then threatened to kill Dr. Burcot on the spot if he didn't do all he could to save the queen. Speechlessly furious, the doctor mounted his horse and galloped off to the palace, arriving well ahead of the queen's messengers.

Escorted into the royal presence again, Burcot told her, "Almost too late, my liege." When she asked him what was the cause of the spots on her skin, he replied, "Tis the pox" (ibid.). Her fears confirmed, the young queen began to complain about how much she loathed the smallpox. In no mood for soothing niceties, Burcot asked her brusquely, "By God's pestilence, which is better, to have the pox in the hands, in the face . . . or have them in the heart and kill the whole body?" (ibid.). The doctor then ordered a mattress to be put by the fire, wrapped the queen in a "great length of scarlet cloth," and held a drink to her lips (Sitwell 1962, 123–24).

Much to the relieved surprise of her court and countrymen, Elizabeth recovered, gradually, but she remained in her private apartments until all signs of smallpox had disappeared. By 11 November she was able to move to Somerset Palace. Soon she was writing Mary, queen of Scots, again, informing her that the disease had not left many scars on her face. Nor did it leave her bald. The story that Elizabeth lost her hair during the attack of smallpox and wore a wig the rest of her life for that reason is not true (Jenkins 1958, 7–8).

The grateful monarch paid Dr. Burcot one hundred marks, gave him a plot of land in Cornwall, and presented him with a pair of gold spurs inherited from her grandfather, Henry VII. She went on to rule and watch over England for forty-one more years.

It is easy to imagine what effect the popular queen's seemingly miraculous cure must have had on her contemporaries. One need only consider the fates of two other ladies of Elizabeth's court who had smallpox that same autumn to appreciate how fortunate she was in her unmarked recovery. Lady Mary Sidney, who had helped care for the ill queen, recovered, but was so disfigured that she never appeared at court again without wearing a mask. Mrs. Sibell Penn, former nurse to Edward VI, died of smallpox on 6 November. Another lady of the court also recovered, apparently without severe scarring.

Elizabeth was also luckier than many other royal victims, and millions of commoners before and since, who were scarred, blinded, or slain by the disease that one of her countrymen later called "the most terrible of all the ministers of death." In the suddenness and unpredictability of its attack, the grotesque torture of its victims, the brutality of its lethal or disfiguring outcome, and the terror that it inspired, smallpox is unique among human diseases.

Even before Queen Elizabeth's illness, smallpox had already killed two Japanese emperors, kings of Burma and of Siam, an Egyptian pharaoh, the first caliph of the Abbasid dynasty, and perhaps the Roman emperor Marcus Aurelius. It had probably contributed to the downfall of Athens. Earlier in the sixteenth century the same disease had been the Spaniards' most fearsome ally in the New World, annihilating millions of native Americans, including the last Aztec emperor, and probably the last independent ruler of the Incas. Many more deaths were to follow with far-reaching consequences. Jenner would not discover vaccination to prevent smallpox for another two hundred and thirty-four years.

SMALLPOX AND SMALLPOX VIRUSES

The deadly cause of Queen Elizabeth's illness is now known to be a diminutive, brick-shaped virus, *Variola major*. A person ill with smallpox shed millions of infective viruses into his immediate environment from the rash on his skin and open sores in the throat. Each victim remained infectious from just before the rash appeared until the last scab dropped off about three weeks later, but was most highly contagious during the first several days of that period. Corpses of victims who died of the infection were also a dangerous source of virus. Sometimes clothing, shrouds, or blankets recently contaminated with pus or scabs served as a vehicle for the virus, whereby persons who were not in direct contact with a patient would become infected. Most victims, however, acquired the virus through droplet infection while in face-to-face contact with a patient by inhaling contaminated air. Only very rarely was airborne smallpox virus known to have infected another person beyond the immediate vicinity of the victim. Not all persons who were exposed to smallpox became infected. The chances of being infected were about fifty-fifty for other susceptible members of the same household, for example.

During the first week after infection, the virus quietly established itself in an infected person. There was no sign of illness, and the new victim had no way of knowing whether he was infected, even if he realized he might be. Around the ninth day, the first signs and symptoms appeared: headache, fever, chills, nausea, and backache, sometimes with convulsions or delirium. Some victims experienced terrifying dreams during this prodromal stage, which lasted up to three or four days. Victims with fair skin often developed a diffuse scarlet coloration in their faces, which sometimes extended over the entire body. At the end of the prodrome, the fever subsided and the victim temporarily felt better, just as the virus declared its presence by producing the characteristic rash. Typically, the flat reddish spots appeared first on the face, then spread rapidly over the arms, chest, back, and finally the legs. The rash was denser on the face, lower arms and legs than on the center of the body. Over the next several days the miserable, aching victim was transformed into a hideous, swollen monster as the flat spots of the rash became raised pimples, then blisters, and then pustules, after which the pustules dried up and turned into crusts or scabs (plate 1). At its height, the many pustules of a dense rash sometimes made the victim's skin appear yellow. In fair-skinned victims, vesicles and early pustules were each surrounded by a thin red halo; during the papular stage, the entire lesion was red. Many died in the first few days of the rash, others soon after the first week of the rash, and some were carried to their graves even before the rash appeared. Once a person was infected, there was no effective treatment.

Some patients appeared exactly as if they had been severely scalded or burned, and even less seriously affected victims said the skin felt as though it were on fire. In addition to the skin, which sometimes sloughed off in large pieces, the virus attacked the throat, lungs, heart, liver, intestines, and other internal organs, and that is how it killed. Victims reeked of a peculiarly sickening odor. In some, the disease caused hemorrhaging internally and externally, the so-called black smallpox, which was almost always fatal. Overall, about one out of every four victims died. Survivors were immune and usually could not get the infection again, but they often were left with pockmarked faces, or less commonly, blind in one or both eyes.

The reader is referred to Dixon's excellent book (1962) for a detailed modern discussion of the pathology of smallpox infections. Smallpox in humans is assumed to have developed similarly to experimental ectromelia infections in mice, as described by Fenner (1948). Ectromelia virus first multiplies at the site where it is introduced into the skin, then invades regional lymph glands before spreading via the blood stream to scavenger cells in the liver and spleen. There it replicates intensively, then reinvades the blood stream in larger amounts, and by that means reaches the skin where it produces a visible rash.

Within each infected human cell, the smallpox virus multiplied by forcing the cell's own reproductive apparatus to replicate smallpox virus instead, which then leaked out to infect other cells, or was released more dramatically when the infected cell became overly packed with virus and ruptured. According to Dixon, the first evidence of smallpox virus after infection in humans occurs "at the end of the incubation period [when] the virus is liberated from its final site of multiplication in the reticulo-endothelial system, as a result of the bursting of infected cells. The virus shower probably commences just before the sudden rise in temperature and onset of symptoms of the initial phase" (1962, 170). The amount of virus liberated and the victim's ability, whether "natural" or acquired from vaccination, to limit viral invasion or dissemination in the skin and to minimize the severity of those lesions that did occur determined the outcome of each infection.

In fulminating infections, death usually occurred within three to five days, often caused by overwhelming toxemia or massive hemorrhaging into the skin, throat, lung, intestine, or uterus. Such patients had no characteristic papular or vesicular eruption, only a nonspecific red or violet patchy, petechial, or morbilliform rash such as may be seen in many other severe infections where natural clotting mechanisms are thrown into chaos. In other malignant infections, the smallpox virus caused diffuse destruction in the dermis, or deeper layer of the skin, and patients died between ten and fourteen days after onset of symptoms, with pustular lesions that were sometimes confluent. Patients with benign infections usually had more superficial lesions limited to the epidermis, which were less liable to secondary bacterial infection.

Smallpox deaths attributable to complications other than hemorrhage usually occurred eighteen days or more after symptoms began. These other potentially life-threatening complications most often resulted from secondary bacterial infection of wounds in the skin originally cased by the virus. The virus itself was usually responsible for destroying sebaceous glands, which, because they are more numerous on the face, resulted in the characteristic permanent pockmarks' being most common on the most visible part of the body. A few patients developed encephalomyelitis, manifest by drowsiness and speech disorder, in the second week of illness. In about 1 percent of patients, the virus caused ulcerations of the cornea, usually starting around the fourteenth day of illness, and resulted in permanent blindness of the affected eye or eyes. Blindness and secondary septic infections were apparently more frequent in undernourished victims. Recently, evidence has also emerged that scars resulting from smallpox lesions in the epididymis may have been a significant cause of infertility in male survivors. Ironically, one of the disease's most characteristic features, namely, the tendency of the rash to be denser on the face, hands and feet than on the trunk, remains unexplained (Dixon 1962; Phadke et al. 1973).

Variola major was the only species of smallpox known until late in the nineteenth century, when a new type of mild smallpox, subsequently named *Variola minor*, was recognized in Southern Africa and the West Indies and later spread to Brazil, North America, and parts of Europe. The disease caused by *V. minor* looked and spread exactly like the familiar severe smallpox, but whereas *V. major* killed about 25 percent of its victims, *V. minor* killed only 1 percent or less. Each type bred true, and recovery from either conferred immunity to both. But because *V. minor* provoked less intensive control efforts than did *V. major*, the mild variety tended to displace severe smallpox in Brazil, North America, England, and parts of East Africa. It was reported in Asia only rarely. Exactly where, when, and how *V. minor* first appeared are still unknown.

Besides the marked difference in mortality rates, it has recently been confirmed that victims of *V. minor* were less likely to be scarred than those who survived an attack of *V. major*. Jezek and Hardjotanojo (1978) found permanent facial scarring (five or more pockmarks) to be ten times as common (75%) after recovery from *V. major* than after an attack of *V. minor* (7%).

V. major and *V. minor* were only reliably differentiated in the laboratory in the late 1950s. A related virus with similar, but distinct characteristics intermediate between *V. major* and *V. minor*, with a fatality rate of about 12 percent, was first distinguished by Bedson and his colleagues (1965) in East and West Africa in 1963 and labeled *V. intermedius*. All three viruses caused smallpox; *V. major* predominated until just before the disease was eradicated.

V. major, *V. minor*, and *V. intermedius* are but three members of the genus of orthopoxviruses. There are over a dozen other members, including cowpox, buffalopox, camelpox, whitepox, monkeypox, and vaccinia. Most of the other members, except vaccinia, rarely infect humans. Discovery of monkeypox infections in humans for the first time in September 1970 after the eradication campaign had eliminated smallpox from West Africa (Foster et al. 1972), added new urgency to contemporary studies of orthopoxviruses. Monkeypox infections of humans cannot be distinguished clinically from smallpox infections, but fortunately monkeypox virus does not spread readily from person to person. Most human victims of monkeypox infections are apparently infected through direct contact with the virus's natural reservoir, which is still unknown. By applying the most sophisticated tools available to modern researchers, however, investigators have uncovered fascinating new information about the orthopoxviruses, especially smallpox, whitepox, and monkeypox, and their relation to each other (Arita & Henderson 1976; Breman et. al. 1980; Breman & Arita 1980). Whitepox and monkeypox have been shown not to threaten the success of the Smallpox Eradication Program as had been feared.

The exact biological relationship of variola and cowpox viruses to the vaccinia viruses used in modern vaccines remains, and will remain, obscure. This interesting riddle has very recently been masterfully explained, but not solved, in Dr. Derrick Baxby's *Jenner's Smallpox Vaccine* (1981). In brief, the problem is that although Edward Jenner initiated the vaccination era, apparently by using cowpox virus to immunize a child against smallpox, soon after his discovery some strains of "vaccine" were contaminated with smallpox virus. Until early in this century, it was wondered whether the vaccines in use since Jenner's time were cowpox or derived from smallpox. In 1939, Allan Downie showed that the vaccinia viruses present in vaccines then were distinct from contemporary cowpox as well as from smallpox, and more recent studies have confirmed that conclusion. If samples of Jenner's original vaccine were available for analysis now, the problem likely could be solved, but they are not. Baxby presents evidence to support his plausible theory that Jenner's vaccine and our current strains of vaccinia virus are one and the same, and that they are derived neither from cowpox nor from smallpox but from a virus that later became extinct in its natural habitat: horsepox.

It is important to distinguish between *vaccination*, which was first introduced by Jenner in 1796, and *inoculation* (sometimes called variolation to help distinguish it from the Jennerian immunization), which had been employed in India, China, and probably Africa to protect persons against smallpox centuries before the practice was introduced into Europe and North America in 1721. Inoculation was accomplished by inserting pus or powdered scabs containing smallpox virus from a previous patient into the skin of a susceptible person in order to deliberately cause an infection. A person infected artificially in this manner—rather than by the normal route of inhalation—could transmit the infection to others just as if he had been infected in the usual way, but ordinarily developed an illness and rash milder than usual. In vaccination, cowpox (horsepox?) or vaccinia virus is inserted in the skin to cause an infection. Like inoculation, a successful vaccination protected the vaccinee against smallpox. But a freshly vaccinated person developed a rash only infrequently and in any event could not spread smallpox to others, unless he had been infected with smallpox just before the vaccination took effect. Whereas persons who recovered from natural smallpox or from inoculation were almost always immune to subsequent infection by smallpox for the rest of their lives, it was realized only a few years after the introduction of Jennerian vaccination that the immunity induced by that otherwise superior method was not lifelong and that it was necessary for persons to be revaccinated after a few years in order to maintain complete immunity. Jenner himself was never convinced of the need for revaccination, as we shall see.

Properly performed, vaccination only rarely caused the death of a vaccinee, whereas even under the most favorable circumstances, the risk of death in inoculated persons was around 1 to 3 percent, a risk made consistantly lower by improved inoculation techniques introduced in the 1760s. Obviously even a poorly performed inoculation, on the average, entailed less risk of death for the inoculee than did a naturally acquired infection with *V. major*. However, natural infections with *V. minor* usually carried a risk of personal death of less than 1 percent, and a similar relatively small risk to infected communities, and it is interesting to wonder how *V. minor* would have been welcomed if it had appeared before vaccination was discovered. Chinese inoculators assiduously selected mild cases of smallpox from which to collect virus for inoculation, and had it occurred in China, they might have exploited a strain as mild as *V. minor* to make inoculation much safer, long before Jenner's vaccination. Such a development, or even the displacement of *V. major* by naturally spread *V. minor* might have removed the need that Jenner's vaccine filled.

Since smallpox was spread from person to person and does not naturally infect animals, it could only exist in a community so long as susceptible persons were available to keep the disease going. In recent years, for example, it has been estimated that measles virus requires a minimum population of about 2-3 hundred thousand persons in order to ensure that enough new susceptible persons are born annually to sustain the chain of infection indefinitely (Black 1966; Bartlett 1960, 1957). The population required to sustain smallpox is probably less than that, since smallpox is less contagious than measles and persons with smallpox are potentially infectious for longer periods than measles victims. However, much higher infant mortality rates from other causes in years past would have tended to raise the base population needed to ensure an adequate number of susceptibles. During the smallpox eradication campaign in Mali, smallpox survived for almost a year in an isolated village of 1,363 persons while infecting only 65 people, but such slow spread was unusual (Imperato et al., 1973).

Smallpox caused large epidemics when it first arrived in a virgin community where everyone was susceptible, but after most of the susceptible persons had been infected and became immune or died, the disease died down. If the infection was reintroduced later, after enough new susceptibles had been born or moved into the area, another *epidemic*, characterized by a rapid rise in the number of victims, often resulted. After a while, the disease would reappear so frequently that only young children were liable to infection, older persons having already had it months or years before. In some larger communities, the virus never disappeared entirely, but was constantly present, or *endemic*, going from one susceptible person to another and erupting into epidemics every five to fifteen years or so, when enough susceptible persons had accumulated.

Whether endemic or epidemic, smallpox spread more rapidly during the winter months in temperate climates and during the dry season in tropical countries. This seasonal variation undoubtedly resulted from many factors, such as impaired mobility in tropical countries during the rainy season. It has also been demonstrated experimentally that vaccinia virus, which presumably reacted like variola virus, indeed survives significantly longer when sprayed into test chambers under cool, dry conditions than in warmer, more humid air (Harper 1961).

THEORIES OF CONTAGION

At the risk of overgeneralization, it will be helpful to consider at least an outline of the evolution of man's thinking about infectious diseases and their control in general, and about smallpox in particular. Without such a perspective, many of the actions described in the remainder of this narrative would seem irrational or absurd. In fact, they were often logical responses to a frightful but misunderstood adversary and reveal the pathetic price of ignorance.

Modern methods that allowed the world to effectively control smallpox in the twentieth century are based on knowledge of several facts that, although they may now be taken for granted, were acquired only after centuries of painstaking observation, bold experimentation, and deadly mistakes. Only a few centuries ago, neither the nature of the organism causing smallpox nor the fact that it had a specific cause, nor even that it was a discrete disease, was comprehended. Similarly, how it was transmitted, the existence of immunity after infection, of an incubation period between infection and the appearance of symptoms, and how the disease could be treated or prevented were long-lived mysteries. This veil of ignorance was withdrawn slowly and irregularly, as conflicting beliefs, observations, and false interpretations overlapped and obscured early opportunities to verify theories that we now know to be true.

Centuries before the beginning of the Christian era, ancient civilizations such as India and Egypt subscribed to theurgical beliefs, which held that pestilences were punishments unleashed on mankind by divine judgment as retribution for wicked behavior. Among early Christians, this view was expanded to include the belief that God "could also employ [disease] to purge and cleanse man of his sins (Silverstein & Bialasiewicz 1980, p. 154). During the Graeco-Roman period (c. 400 B.C. to A.D. 500), it came to be held by the Hippocratic school that diseases resulted not from God, but from imbalances of four basic humors: blood (sanguine), yellow bile (choleric), black bile (melancholic), and mucous (phlegmatic). As classical medicine was maintained during the European Middle Ages (c. 500 to 1500) by Moslem scholars, this "humoral theory" became the basis of Rhazes' enunciation of the "innate seed theory" during the tenth century, wherein it was held that smallpox resulted from an inherent tendency of the blood to ferment and expel consequent waste through the pores of the skin. During the Middle Ages, as in ancient Rome, some

Europeans also attributed sudden epidemics, including epidemics of smallpox, to changes in the atmosphere, which was said to have assumed an "epidemic constitution."

In 1546, Girolamo Fracastoro (1478–1553) of Verona published a classic treatise in which he clearly stated the doctrine of specific contagion in respect to smallpox and measles, which he attributed to specific seeds, or *seminaria*. Fracastoro recognized three fundamentally different modes of contagion: by direct contact from person to person; by intermediate agents, or fomites, such as clothes or wooden objects; and at a distance, for example, through the air. In Fracastoro's view, the air served merely as a medium for his disease-specific seminaria.

In direct opposition to Fracastoro's belief in specific contagion, others, including the great English physician Thomas Sydenham (1624–89), still believed the atmosphere itself was responsible for pestilences, which they attributed to noxious miasms arising from the earth. Belief in this "miasmatic theory," a variant of the "epidemic constitution," persisted in Europe and North America well into the nineteenth century. Sydenham's major contribution to the struggle against smallpox, as we shall see, was to help further distinguish smallpox from other similar illnesses and to radically improve treatment of smallpox patients by reversing Rhazes' ill-founded, but still widely applied "heat therapy" (Wilkinson 1979, 3). Though Fracastoro and Sydenham each contributed substantially to the newly growing fund of knowledge and useful practices pertaining to smallpox in their times, each remained oblivious to other truths: Sydenham's belief in an epidemic constitution was matched by Fracastoro's belief in the Moslem heat therapy.

Two other theories prominent in eighteenth-century Europe and North America attributed smallpox to animalculae, or to venomous corpuscles. The "animalcular theory" was a direct consequence of Anton van Leeuwenhoek's (1632–1723) invention of the microscope and demonstration of microorganisms. In North America, "Cotton Mather and his friend, Benjamin Colman, were both animalculists, thinking it more reasonable that if the minute particles causing infection were living 'animated atoms' they would more easily find their way into the pores" (Miller 1957, 251–52). Mather's views on this topic can be traced directly to Benjamin Marten, who published his *New Theory of Consumptions* in London in 1720 (Beall & Shryock 1954, 87). But although the animalculists' basic premise was incorrect, other aspects of their thinking were surprisingly modern:

> If one Hypothesis or other may be at all admitted, with this farther and most reasonable Thought upon them, that these venomous Particles or Animacules do also flow into our Nostrils, Throat and Blood, by our Breath; then may they not give us a Reason, why the Small Pox communicated by Incisions in the way of Inoculation, does not produce so many

Pock and such a Flame and Corruption in the Body, as in the common Way of Infection it ordinarily does? Because in this Way not so many enter, nor immediately into such Parts of Hazards and Distress, as in the Nostrils, Throat and Inwards? (Benjamin Colman 1722, quoted in Dixon 1962, 170)

J. J. Paulet, author of *Histoire de la petite vérole*, is said to have "revived and strengthened" the animalcular theory in eighteenth-century France (Miller 1957, 265).

Elsewhere in eighteenth-century Europe, Marten was joined by Thomas Fuller in suggesting the true mode of infection of smallpox: "The chief and commonest Way of taking contagious Fevers, Small-Pox, and Measles, is by Infections; that is by receiving with the Breath, or thro' the Pores." The same two authors also joined in establishing the principle of "specific causality." As Fuller wrote, "Therefore the Pestilence can never breed the Small-Pox, nor the Small-Pox the Measles . . . any more than a Hen can a Duck, a Wolf a Sheep, or a Thistle Figs." (Wilkinson 1979, 9).

Like Rhazes, both Fuller and Marten apparently still believed smallpox was inevitable. A generation later, Angelo Gatti (1724–98) marked the end of belief in the innate seed theory, stressing instead "his belief that the 'variolous matter' was introduced into the organism from the outside, and subsequently transmitted from human body to human body. Once introduced, it reproduced itself and multiplied indefinitely." (Wilkinson 1979, 11).

The "corpuscular theory" was much more popular than the animalcular theory in early eighteenth-century Europe. This theory likened the contagion of smallpox, which was envisioned as consisting of "tiny, solid particles of a specific size and shape and producing an identical reaction," to a poison in its effect on the body (Miller 1957, 252–53). One of the most prominent advocates of this view was Hermann Boerhaave (1668–1738) of Leyden. Boerhaave also was one of several eighteenth-century writers who suggested to their contemporaries in vain that "people who have smallpox must have something remaining in their body which overcomes subsequent contagious infection" (Silverstein & Bialasiewicz 1980, 161).

Each of the numerous theories about the nature of smallpox formed the basis for countermeasures undertaken in good faith to prevent or treat the disease by those who believed (or whose doctors believed) in them. Vestiges of some of these beliefs and remedies, even the oldest ones, were still evident in some countries as recently as the 1960s and 1970s. For theurgists, smallpox could be prevented by appeasing the deity who controlled the disease and by avoiding acts that earned his or her wrath. To Christians, this meant avoiding sin. Humoralists sought to restore the imbalance smallpox signified by bleeding or purging the body of excessive humors. Rhazes' "heat therapy" as well as the "red treatment" were rationalized on the basis of his belief in the innate seed. To eighteenth-century Europeans who believed that the "innate fermentation" the disease represented was triggered by luxurious living and an injudicious diet, it followed naturally that the diet of smallpox patients, including those who took the infection by inoculation, must be restricted to minimize the severity of the infection. Those who espoused the miasmatic theory sought to promote their health by cleaning up their environment or moving to a healthier one. Contagionists also fled epidemic environs, for their own reasons, but advocated isolation or quarantine of contaminated people and goods as a means of controlling smallpox.

Some of the specific advances made against other infections also contributed indirectly to the battle against smallpox, if only conceptually. Leprosy, which began to spread widely in Europe during the sixth and seventh centuries and peaked seven centuries later, made Europeans aware of the idea of isolating persons with communicable diseases. Similarly, reaction to the plague, which in Europe marked "the onset and the waning of the Middle Ages, namely the plague of Justinian (543) and the Black Death (1348)," contributed further to development of the principles of isolation hospitals and disinfection procedures (fumigation and airing of sick rooms and burning of effects of dead victims) (Rosen 1958, 59). Quarantine was first practiced to prevent spread of plague from infested ships in southern Europe in the fourteenth century. The introduction of cinchona bark into Europe from Peru in 1632 for treatment of malaria "upset current systems of humoral thought about disease," served as a prototype of specific drug therapy, and when introduced into England by Sydenham, helped separate malaria from other febrile illnesses (Rogers 1962, 41–42). Fracastoro had suggested mercury as a less dramatic, but equally specific cure for syphilis in 1530, only a generation after that disease began its epidemic course in Europe.

In Asia especially, some aspects of smallpox and its control were understood or practiced earlier than in Europe. This is most strikingly apparent with inoculation, which was not introduced into Europe and North America until the early eighteenth century although it had been practiced in India, China, and probably parts of Africa for centuries.

Jenner signalled the eventual end of smallpox, which was still incompletely understood, with his epochal discovery in 1796, and his demonstration of the principle of nearly harmless artificial immunization, which itself built on the earlier practice of inoculation, later contributed to the control of other diseases. The "germ theory," revived in the 1830s and 1840s, served as the theoretical basis for pioneering studies by Robert Koch (1843–1910) and Louis Pasteur (1822–95), who laid the foundations of modern bacteriology in the 1870s. "Filterable viruses" were first distinguished as a class of organisms distinct from larger bacteria and protozoa in the 1890s, although the term "virus" had been used in a more general sense to refer to the agent responsible for causing smallpox even in Jenner's time. John Buist detected microscopic traces of the variola virus for the first time in 1887, followed by Giuseppe Guarnieri in 1893, by Councilman and others in 1904, and by E. Paschen in 1906. The "inclusion bodies" described by Guarnieri were at first thought to be protozoan parasites, comparable to those that had just been discovered to cause malaria. According to Wilkinson, this misinterpretation of the nature of the viral inclusion bodies persisted "well into the 1920s in one form or another" (1979, 21). As late as 1935, the twelfth edition of Osler's *Principles and Practice of Medicine* still listed smallpox among diseases of uncertain cause. The smallpox virus itself was finally seen for the first time in 1947, by Canadian and United States scientists who used electron microscopes to reveal one of the final secrets of *Variola Rex* (Nagler & Rake 1948; Van Rooyen & Scott 1948).

Origins

No one knows when this mighty microbe first began to affect people, nor where. Smallpox probably evolved and adapted to man gradually, from one of the relatively harmless pox viruses of domesticated animals. Similar incidental infections of humans have been observed more recently with cowpox. Such a fateful adaptation of smallpox may have occurred after humans began living in agricultural settlements and brought their newly domesticated animals to live with them, often in the same house (McNeill 1976, 107; Cockburn 1963, 197). Smallpox also might have originated from contact with wild animals, much as monkeypox appears to infect people sporadically in Central Africa today.

If the pattern of adaptation of other diseases from animals to man may be presumed to have occurred in this instance, the earliest human victims may have suffered a very severe or a very mild illness, but spread from one person to another would have been rare at first, until the virus became well adapted to humans. Because of the virus's most likely source, and its eventual need to maintain itself in humans by passing from person to person in a continuous chain of transmission, the first human victim of smallpox probably lived in one of the earliest concentrated agricultural settlements in Asia or Africa, sometime after about 10,000 B.C. (ibid.).

In attempting to answer the question, When and where is there the first evidence of smallpox? several limitations must be considered. In the first place, smallpox's debut among humans probably was sporadic. The earliest infections may have gone unnoted for centuries except by the victims and their families. Even when epidemics began to attract attention, smallpox was not necessarily distinguished from other diseases causing a rash, and when it was distinguished from other diseases, the few scribes who kept records probably preferred to record wars and other events than describe the appearance of an illness. Finally, even when an ancient clinical description survives, there remain the uncertainties of translation, of knowing when the description was written, and the possibility that smallpox was in fact different then from the disease we recognize now. All these constraints notwithstanding, there is evidence that smallpox was a scourge in ancient Egypt, India, China, and Greece.

EGYPT

Among the most convincing evidence of smallpox in the ancient world are three Egyptian mummies from the Eighteenth and Twentieth Dynasties (1570 to 1085 B.C.). Here there are no problems of translation. Modern observers have seen for themselves what these apparent victims of an illness with rash from three thousand years ago look like and have concluded that smallpox is the most likely diagnosis.

In 1910 a pioneering French paleopathologist, Sir Marc Armand Ruffer, and his collaborator, A. R. Ferguson, described a smallpoxlike eruption on the mummy of a middle-aged man who died during the Twentieth Dynasty. They reported that "the body was the seat of a peculiar vesicular or bullous eruption which in form and general distribution bore a striking resemblance to that of smallpox (1)." The same authors published an impressive, color drawing of the rash seen on a piece of skin removed from the mummy's thigh. When they examined the piece of skin microscopically, they found the "dome-shaped" vesicles were located in the middle prickle layer of the skin, where the eruption of smallpox is known to occur. Ruffer discovered a similar eruption on a mummy dating from the Eighteenth Dynasty, but apparently did not examine tissues from that mummy microscopically, nor did he publish a full description of the rash.

Most interesting of all is the mummy of Usermare-sekheperenre, Mighty Bull, Repulser of Millions, Golden Horus, King of Upper and Lower Egypt, Lord of the Two Lands, Pharaoh: Ramses V (plate 2). Ramses V ruled Egypt for about four years before he died in 1157 B.C. "from an acute illness" (Dixon 1962, ii). After carefully examining X-rays of Ramses V's head and teeth, Harris and Weeks (1973) reported that "there is little doubt that the King died in his early thirties" (167). It has long been assumed that Ramses V died of smallpox because of a "well-marked pustular eruption" on his mummy, which Ruffer said was "exactly similar" to the rash he and Ferguson described in another mummy from the same dynasty (1921, 175).

Little is known of Ramses V's reign except that he was on bad terms with his predecessor (Ramses IV) and his successor (Ramses VI), that there may have been a civil war during his reign in which "outsiders" attacked Egypt from the north, and that he was buried during the second year of his successor's reign. The latter was highly unusual, since pharaohs were ordinarily buried after a strictly prescribed seventy days of mummification, which would be well within the successor's first regnal year. Thus, Ramses V may have been deposed and imprisoned prior to his death, as Cerny (1975), an Egyptologist, theorized. From what we now know, however, an equally plausible explanation for the unusual timing of Ramses' burial is that if he died of smallpox, his embalmers would likely have suffered a fearsome epidemic about two weeks after starting to prepare his body, and the source of such a focal outbreak would surely have been suspected. In any other society the deceased would already have been buried or cremated by the time such an outbreak occurred, but not in the case of a pharaoh in ancient Egypt. Fear of the infection (if not an acute shortage of embalmers) could then have postponed the remaining preparation and burial. Serious deterioration of the corpse might also have caused authorities to deliberately prolong the mummification period.

By special permission of the late President Anwar el Sadat, I was allowed to examine the front upper half of Ramses V's unwrapped mummy in the Cairo Museum in 1979. It is one of the best preserved royal mummies in the museum. Inspection of the mummy revealed a rash of elevated "pustules," each about two to four millimeters in diameter, that was most distinct on the lower face, neck, and shoulders, but was also visible on the arms. Over the shoulders especially, these pustules were pale yellow against a dark brown-reddish background, the latter partly due to cosmetic compounds used in royal mummifications during that period. On his upper face, only smaller raised pimples (one to two millimeters) could be seen, which might have been shrunken more by tighter wrappings over the forehead. It was not possible to examine the palms or soles where the presence of pustules would be highly characteristic of smallpox, because his arms were folded across his chest with the palms down, and the shroud was stuck to his soles. No such rash could be seen on the chest or upper abdomen. Earlier photographs of this mummy published by G. Elliot Smith (1912), show that the rash is also prominent on the lower abdomen and scrotum. (An attempt to prove that this rash was caused by smallpox by electron-microscopic examination of tiny pieces of tissue that had fallen on the shroud was unsuccessful. I was not permitted to excise one of the pustules.) Three folds in the skin over the left cheek suggest that his face may have been swollen when he died. The appearance of the larger pustules and the apparent distribution of the rash are similar to smallpox rashes I have seen in more recent victims.

The Ebers Papyrus, which was written between 3730 and 1555 B.C., briefly describes an illness affecting the skin that Regoly-Merei (1966) feels bears some similarity to smallpox. Ebers believed he even found a specific word for smallpox in an Egyptian papyrus. But these and other alleged descriptions are far too vague to provide any reasonable written evidence of smallpox in ancient Egypt. However, the chronicles of Egypt's imperial rivals, the Hittites, tell of a mysterious, fatal, epidemic disease the Hittites said they caught from the Egyptians.

The Hittite Empire was at its peak in the area of modern Turkey during the reign of Suppiluliumas I (c. 1380–46 B.C.) when armies of the Hittite and Egyptian empires clashed several times in northern Syria.[1] Cuneiform Hittite tablets describe one of these wars around the middle of the fourteenth century B.C., after which the victorious Hittites were attacked by a pestilence. The disease originated among their Egyptian captives and spread to the Hittite army and civilian population, killing many ("Plagues and Fortunes," 1949). This epidemic raged among the Hittites for at least twenty years. Suppiluliumas I and his son Arnuwandas II, who succeeded him, both died of the disease within a year of each other. As a result, the early reign of Arnuwanda's inexperienced younger brother was marked by revolts and a series of invasions by neighboring states (Forrer 1937; Klengel & Klengel 1970). Order was eventually restored, and the Hittite Empire lasted another one-and-a-half centuries before it was overcome by the Assyrians and Phrygians. Of the illness, unfortunately, we know only that it was contagious, apparently spread from person to person, and was often fatal. It could well have been smallpox, as both Cooray (1965) and Hare (1954) believe. Recent discovery of a large library dating from the third milennium B.C. at Ebla, in present-day Syria, may provide more evidence about early epidemics in this part of the world.

Ancient Egyptians attributed epidemics, presumably including smallpox, to their goddess of pestilence, Sekhmet, who they believed "produced epidemics when aroused and abated them when she was mollified" (Rosen 1958, 29). There is no evidence that a more specialized deity concerned only with smallpox, or with all diseases that produced a rash, was ever differentiated in the Egyptian pantheon.

INDIA

Evidence of the long existence of smallpox in India derives primarily from clinical descriptions in ancient medical and religious texts. Wise translated some of the oldest Sanskrit medical writings, the *Charaka Samhita* and the *Susruta Samhita*. Part of the latter text is traditionally ascribed to the earliest known Hindu physician, Dhanwantari. Both texts were written some time before A.D. 400, and they may recount descriptions from as early as 1500 B.C. The *Susruta Samhita* includes a vivid description of smallpox:

> Before *Masurika* appears, fever occurs, with pain over the body, but particularly in the back. . . . When bile is deranged, in this disease, severe pain is felt in the large and small joints, with cough, shaking, listlessness

and languor; the palate, lips and tongue are dry with thirst and no appetite. The pustules are red, yellow, and white and they are accompanied with burning pain. This form soon ripens. . . . When air, bile and phlegm are deranged, in this disease the body has a blue colour, and the skin seems studded with rice. The pustules become black and flat, are depressed in the centre, with much pain. They ripen slowly . . . this form is cured with much difficulty, and it is called *Charmo* or fatal form. (Wise 1845, 234)

Dhanwantari is also alleged to be the source of an astonishing description of cowpox "vaccination" to prevent smallpox, some two thousand years before Jenner:

Take the fluid of the pock on the udder of the cow or on the arm between the shoulder and elbow of a human subject on the point of a lancet, and lance with it the arms between the shoulders and elbows until the blood appears. Then, mixing this fluid with the blood, the fever of the smallpox will be produced. (*History of Inoculation*, 13–14)

Since there is no other evidence of cowpox vaccination having been practiced in ancient India, the validity of this description seems doubtful. It is almost certain, however, that inoculation with smallpox virus was practiced in India in ancient times.

According to Holwell, an English surgeon who lived in India several years, the *Artharva Veda*, which was written sometime in the last millennium B.C., describes temple services and prayers used by Brahmin priests for worship of a smallpox diety, and inoculation for smallpox, from earliest times. Brahmin priests traveled the countryside in spring, the smallpox season, reciting prayers to the goddess of smallpox and inoculating susceptible persons—the world's first mobile inoculation teams (Kahn 1963, 600). Thus India was apparently the first ancient civilization to manifest a need for a specialized goddess of smallpox or of exanthematous diseases, a fact that may reflect an earlier appearance of smallpox in India.

As in imperial Egypt, the fate of a foreign army may inadvertently provide a clue to the existence of smallpox in ancient India. In 327 B.C., while camped on the lower Indus, Alexander the Great's army suffered from a fatal illness that included a rash. According to the Roman historian Rufus, "a scab attacked the bodies of the soldiers and spread by contagion" (Moore 1815, 58). No other description of this incident is known. Whether or not this was smallpox remains a mystery.

In sum, ancient Sanskrit medical texts, Brahmin traditions, sacred books, and Hindu mythology provide evidence that smallpox existed in India for a very long time, certainly before the birth of Christ. How long, we do not know.

CHINA

Nearly all of the earliest accounts of smallpox in China refer to the disease being introduced from outside that country. In contrast to the uncertain antiquity of smallpox in ancient Egypt and India, the most reasonable hypothesis from evidence now available is that smallpox was first introduced into historical China from the north around 250 B.C. It apparently arrived with the Huns only a few decades before the Chinese completed the Great Wall to keep them out. Anticipating a timeless human willingness to name new diseases after foreigners, the Chinese called the sickness "Hunpox."

In apparent corroboration of the presumed first appearance of smallpox in China at about this time, early Chinese texts refer to a disastrous "epidemic throughout the empire" in 243 B.C. (Cha 1976, 294). Additional evidence derives from an imperial dermatologist who reported that smallpox first appeared in China during the Han dynasty (206 B.C.–A.D. 220). Another source, the *Eastern (Korean) Precious Mirror of Medical Practice*, states that smallpox appeared in China at the close of the Chou dynasty (1122 B.C.–249 B.C.) and the beginning of the Han dynasty. In addition, Jesuit missionaries in Peking quoted a Chinese treatise based on the oldest writings of Chinese physicians and edited by the Imperial College of Physicians. According to the treatise, smallpox was unknown in China in very early ages and appeared for the first time during the Chou dynasty. This latter source has been widely quoted and often interpreted to mean that smallpox was already in China by 1122 B.C., i.e., at the beginning of the Chou dynasty. But almost all other evidence suggests the disease first arrived near the end of that dynasty, at least in historical times (Hirsch 1883; Thompson 1887; MacGowan 1884; Moore 1815).

As in India, the cult of a specific goddess of smallpox also arose among the Chinese as an early explanation of the origin and source of cure of this fearsome disease. But the fact that Chinese tradition dates the appearance of their smallpox goddess around the eleventh century A.D. suggests a relatively late appearance of smallpox in China, as compared to India.

According to Zinsser (1960), Paschen believed smallpox existed in China as early as 1700 B.C. Thorwald (1962) describes brief inscriptions on bones dating from the Shang period (16th–11th century B.C.) that allegedly refer to several infectious diseases, including smallpox, malaria, tuberculosis, leprosy, typhus, cholera, and plague. Chen (1969) refers to the same bone findings. As far as I have been able to discover, however, these findings, which are hard to believe, are the only evidence suggesting that smallpox may have been present in China before the Huns introduced, or reintroduced it, around 250 B.C. As we shall see, the first unmistakable clinical description of smallpox in China dates only from the fourth century A.D.

GREECE

After Egypt, India, and China, other important evidence of smallpox
before the birth of Christ is found in Greece. Hippocrates (c. 400 B.C.), in
describing different kinds of fevers, wrote of some that were "pustular,
dreadful to behold," which suggests the father of Western medicine may
well have seen smallpox (Baron 1827, 1: 179). But stronger evidence of
smallpox is found in the Athenian historian Thucydides' description of
the mysterious "Plague of Athens" that erupted during the Peloponnesian War. Various authors have attributed this disastrous epidemic to
measles, typhus, plague, or smallpox. Zinsser, Alivizatos, the Littmans
(1969), and others concluded it was most likely smallpox. The recent
analysis of this epidemic by Robert J. Littman and M. L. Littman, a
physician and a historian of the Greek language, is especially compelling.

The epidemic originated in "Ethiopia" and spread to Egypt and Libya
before descending on Athens via the port of Pireus in the spring of 430
B.C. It raged for two or three years, destroyed one-fourth of the Athenian
army and innumerable citizens, and spread eastward to Persia. The illness
was characterized, Thucydides (1977) says, by headache, malodorous
breath, cough, retching, convulsions, loss of memory, sleeplessness, diarrhea, and a rash of small "blisters" (or "pustules") and "sores." The rash
spread over the whole body, starting at the top, and some who recovered
were blind. The disease was lethal and contagious, but those who survived
it were immune. Most deaths occurred on the seventh or ninth day of the
illness. The only major sign of smallpox that Thucydides did not describe
is the pockmarks. That tantalizing omission may be consistent with the
Hippocratic school's emphasis on the prognosis rather than on the consequences of the disease, or may have occurred because the idea of a
consequent scar is implicit in the Greek word Thucydides used to describe
the sores (*ulcus*) (Littman & Littman 1969; Alivizatos 1950).

The devastation caused by the epidemic greatly weakened Athens
during the confrontation with its militaristic rival, Sparta, and contributed to Athens's defeat and subsequent decline. The city-state's premature demise had profound consequences for the Mediterranean world.
"It is the task of Athens," Sophocles had written, "to make life more
splendid." This pestilence shook the Athenians' faith in their ordered
world so profoundly that Thucydides reported:

> Athens owed to the plague the beginnings of a state of unprecedented
> lawlessness. . . . As for the gods, it seemed to be the same thing whether
> one worshipped them or not when one saw the good and the bad dying
> indiscriminately. (Thucydides 1977, 155)

An epidemic disease that may also have been smallpox appeared
among North African (Carthaginian) soldiers besieging Syracuse in 395
B.C. This epidemic, too, arrived from Libya. In this instance, Diodorus

described patients as having "pustules throughout the surface of the body as well as . . . spineaches and mental symptoms" (Alivizatos 1950, 348). Many died, and the siege had to be lifted. As a result of this epidemic, Carthage was unable to gain control of Sicily, which could have given it a decisive strategic advantage in its struggle with the fledgling Roman Empire during the Punic Wars less than a century later (Zinsser 1960, 92).

In ancient Egypt, India, and China, smallpox may have been introduced into local populations several times before it became permanently established and spread continually. Even after it became endemic in a population, later importations from the same or another source may still have been noticed and recorded. Thus a documented importation was not necessarily the first appearance of the disease in an area. By Roman times the Nile valley already had a population of about 7 million, China some 58 million, and India had more than 25 million—all populations large enough to sustain smallpox once it was introduced. Long before the birth of Christ, these ancient civilizations were in contact frequently enough to have allowed smallpox to be disseminated to each other, no matter where it arose.

In summary, smallpox probably first became adapted to humans as an endemic disease in Egypt or in India's Indus River valley sometime before 1000 B.C. From northeast Africa it could easily have spread to the Hittites in the fourteenth century B.C., to Athens and Persia in the fifth century B.C., and to Syracuse a generation later. A similar pattern of spread from northeast Africa to adjacent countries is also evident after

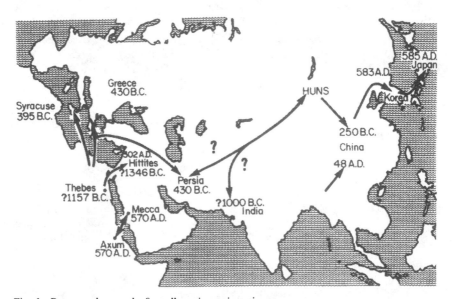

Fig. 1. Presumed spread of smallpox in ancient times

the birth of Christ. The disease may have passed to the Huns and other tribes in Central Asia from the Persians, or from northwest India, before the Huns carried it into China in the middle of the third century B.C. (fig. 1). During the last milennium B.C. as in later times, wars, the establishment and collapse of empires, and trade caravans probably all helped spread smallpox via infected people and their contaminated clothing once the disease became adapted to humans. Buddha, Christ, and Mohammed stimulated other movements that also spread smallpox. But by the beginning of the Christian era, smallpox appears to have been already endemic in northeast Africa, India, and probably China. It probably was not yet permanently established in thinly populated Europe.

Two

The Most Terrible of All the Ministers of Death

ALTHOUGH SMALLPOX WAS PROBABLY INTRODUCED into Europe from northeast Africa before the birth of Christ, it apparently did not become permanently established at that time, perhaps because Europe was too sparsely settled to permit the chain of infection to be sustained. Although the historian Hirsch (1883) accepts as smallpox a pestilence described in Rome at the time of Trajan (A.D. 98–117), the earliest substantive evidence of smallpox in Europe after the birth of Christ is the controversial "Plague of Antonius." This catastrophic epidemic struck the Roman Empire during the reign of Emperor Marcus Aurelius Antonius and was described by the emperor's Greek physician, Galen. Galen (130–200), who was the greatest physician of his age and the foremost proponent of the humoralist theory, dominated European medicine for centuries. His description of the Antonine plague, however, is uncharacteristically incomplete. Galen left Rome soon after the outbreak began; if he did so to avoid the epidemic, he was as smart as he was reputed to be. This may explain the brevity of his description.

The epidemic started in a Roman army fighting under General Avidius Cassius in Mesopotamia in 164 or 165, and forced Cassius to retreat. Returning soldiers brought the disease from Parthia (Persia) to Syria and Italy. It raged for fifteen years, reportedly claimed up to two thousand victims daily in Rome, and eventually killed Marcus Aurelius himself, at Vienna in 180. By the time it was over, the Littmans argue, the Plague of Antonius had "probably caused more deaths than any other epidemic during the [Roman] Empire before the mid-third century" (1973, 244). It claimed an estimated three and one half to seven million lives, which must have weakened the empire.

According to Galen, the Antonine plague was characterized by fever, inflamed mouth and throat, thirst, vomiting, diarrhea, a dry or pustular eruption, a "black exanthem covering an entire body and . . . many lesions which changed into ulcers" (Rosenthal 1959, 498). Referring to the rash, Galen wrote:

> Of some of these which had become ulcerated, that part of the surface called the scab fell away and then the remaining part nearby was healthy and after one or two days became scarred over. In those places where it

was not ulcerated, the exanthem was rough and scabby and fell away like some husk and hence all became healthy. (Littman & Littman 1973, 246)

Zinsser believed this epidemic may have been caused by several diseases occurring simultaneously, but that the most fatal one "was a condition which, if not smallpox, was closely related to it" (1960, 101). The Littmans argue convincingly that it was most likely smallpox. Galen himself said the illness was very similar to the "Plague of Athens" described by Thucydides; and Rhazes, the tenth-century Arabian physician who first distinguished smallpox and measles, believed Galen had described smallpox.

If smallpox was still not yet permanently established in Europe by the fourth century, it was not far away. In 302, Eusebius, bishop of Caesarea (Syria), described a disease characterized by "spreading ulcers, loss of sight, and many deaths" (Rosenthal 1959, 498). Further north, yet another potential source of smallpox appeared when the Huns, descendants of the same nomadic group accused of carrying smallpox into China around the middle of the third century B.C., began to push westward from eastern Europe in the second half of the fourth century A.D.

During their invasion of France in 451, the Huns beheaded the bishop of Rheims on the doorstep of his cathedral. Because the bishop was said to have recovered from smallpox the year before he was martyred, he became the patron saint of European smallpox victims, St. Nicaise (Maenchen-Helfen 1973). Since famine and epidemics of some sort are known to have forced Hun armies to retreat from Gaul and Italy in 447 and 452, this traditional account of St. Nicaise's martyrdom and patronate supports the possibility that smallpox caused the epidemics among the Huns in France at that time. If it was smallpox, it seems at least as likely that the disease was already in Europe when the Huns arrived as that they brought it with them.

Nearly a century after St. Nicaise's martyrdom, another epidemic began in Egypt and struck Byzantium, capital of the eastern half of the former Roman Empire. Unlike the western half of the empire, Byzantium had successfully resisted the Germanic tribes, but it was less successful against the Plague of Justinian (543), which, with the fall of Rome, marked the beginning of the European Middle Ages. From Procopius' description of feverish patients with buboes in the armpits and groin, there is little doubt that this epidemic, which claimed up to ten thousand lives per day, was bubonic plague. Yet some patients also "broke out with black blisters the size of a lentil" and Zinsser suspected that there were cases of severe smallpox occurring simultaneously with the bubonic plague (1960, 108). Indeed, at about the same time (541), Sigbent von Gemblours was describing a "pestilential illness with pustules and blisters" (*malae valetudines cum pustulis et vescicis*) in France (Jochman 1914, 799–800).

For almost a thousand years after the Plague of Justinian, medieval European medicine subsisted on the Graeco-Roman base laid down by Galen. Like much other classical knowledge, Galen's writings survived the Dark Ages via Arabic translations undertaken by Islamic scholars as a new empire emerged in West Asia and North Africa. Alongside persisting ancient theurgical beliefs, Galen's humoralist doctrine, and Greek-derived concepts that held that natural causes, especially climate and the physical environment, influenced the appearance of epidemic diseases, Christian thought contributed the idea that disease was a punishment for sin. Just as the early Christian Church obligingly accommodated converts seeking to escape what they believed to be wrathful epidemics sent by God, so in the later medieval period, Christian monasteries served increasingly as refuges for European girls and women whose beauty and hopes of worldly accomplishment had been destroyed by smallpox.

Bishop Gregory of Tours's eyewitness account of a mortal illness that spread across southern France and northern Italy in 580–81 dispels any lingering doubts of smallpox's presence in sixth-century Europe:

> The state of Tours was desolated by a severe pestilential sickness (Lue Valetudinaria)—such was the nature of the infirmity (languor) that a person, after being seized with a violent fever, was covered all over with vesicles and small pustules.... The vesicles were white, hard, unyielding, and very painful. If the patient survived to their maturation, they broke, and began to discharge, when the pain was greatly increased by the adhesion of the clothes to the body.... Among others, the Lady of Count Eborin, while laboring under this pest, was so covered with the vesicles, that neither her hands, nor feet, nor any part of the body, remained exempt, for even her eyes were wholly closed up by them. (Willan 1821, 91–92)

Although the lady of Count Eborin recovered, the Count d'Angouleme died in this epidemic, and his corpse "appeared black and burnt, as if it had been laid on a coal fire" (ibid., 89).

The Merovingian kings Chilperic and Guntram, who were brothers, each lost relatives during the epidemic described by Bishop Gregory. King Chilperic himself was infected, but recovered, but his two sons, Dogobert and Clodobert, did not. Bishop Gregory reported that when Chilperic's queen realized that Clodobert too was dying,

> she repented of her sins, rather late in the day, it is true, and said to the King: "God in his mercy has endured our evil goings-on long enough. Time and time again He has sent us warnings through high fevers and other dispositions, but we have never mended our ways.... We still lay up treasures, we who have no one to whom we can leave them.... Were our cellars not already over-flowing with wine? Were our graneries not stuffed to the roof with corn? Were our treasure houses not already full

enough with gold, silver, precious stones, necklaces and every regal adornment one could dream of? Now we are losing the most beautiful of our possessions! (Gregory of Tours 1977, 297)

The penitent queen persuaded the king to burn his tax files and to cease assessing his subjects. In addition, reported Gregory, "from this time onwards King Chilperic was lavish in giving alms to cathedrals and churches and to the poor, too" (ibid., 298).

King Guntram's wife, Austrigilde, also succumbed to the disease. Unlike her sister-in-law, however, she blamed her physicians, not God, for her predicament, asking the king:

Give me your solemn word . . . that you will cut their throats the moment that my eyes have closed in death. If I have really come to the end of my life, they must not be permitted to glory in my dying. When my friends grieve for me, let their friends grieve for them too. (Ibid.)

The two doctors were executed soon after the queen died.

This outbreak in southern Europe in 580–81 may have been related to the epidemic of smallpox that broke out among an Ethiopian army besieging Mecca in 569–70. The Ethiopian attack on Mecca was said to have been "connected with Justinian's (A.D. 565) attempt to divert the Chinese silk trade from the Persian land route to the Abyssinian sea route" (Parker 1907, 89). According to Sprengel (1794), the governor of a Greek enclave in Arabia sent Greek troops, at Emperor Justinian's behest, to fight alongside the Ethiopians against the Arabs. Greek soldiers infected by the Ethiopians purportedly carried smallpox to Italy on their return.

Around the same time that infected Greek soldiers would have been returning to Italy from Arabia, Bishop Marius of Avenches (near Lusaunne, Switzerland), a contemporary of Bishop Gregory of Tours, used the latin word *variola* (from *varius* = spotted, or *varus* = a pimple) for the first time to denote an epidemic illness then current in Italy and France. Five centuries later, Constantinus Africanus (1020–87), a widely traveled Carthagian scholar who began "the revival of medical learning in Italy" by translating Arabic works into Latin, first definitely limited use of the world *variola* to the disease we call smallpox. But since only a scant description of Bishop Marius's epidemic survives, we cannot be certain that the disease he referred to was smallpox and not bubonic plague (Moore 1815; Dixon 1962). However, the suggestion that Bishop Marius may well have been describing smallpox is interesting: In the short span of four decades we have Sigbent von Gemblours's description of a suspicious illness in France in 541, Marius's reference to an epidemic in France and Italy in 570—the same year smallpox supposedly was carried to Italy from Mecca—and ten years later, Gregory's clear description of epidemic smallpox in France and Italy.

After Gregory's unmistakable account in the sixth century, there is little mention of smallpox in Europe during the remainder of the Middle Ages except for importations by religious movements. Aaron, a physician, described an outbreak of smallpox at Alexandria in 622, after which Islamic armies spreading their new faith carried smallpox across north Africa and into Spain, Portugal and France before they were halted in 732. According to Kübler (1901), by the latter half of the tenth century smallpox was relatively common in many Arab-controlled areas, including Spain. The disease was so well known in Switzerland that the physician-monk Notkerus could confidently diagnose a case of smallpox before the rash appeared, which suggests that smallpox had been recognized in that part of tenth-century Europe for some time. The count of Flanders, Baldwin, is said to have died of smallpox in 961–62, and fifty-year-old Hugh Capet, king of France for nine years and founder of the dynasty, died "covered in spots," perhaps caused by smallpox, at the end of the tenth century (Law 1976; Paulet 1768).

The movement of numerous Christians to and from West Asia during the Crusades in the twelfth and thirteenth centuries apparently helped to reintroduce and spread smallpox in Europe, including Spain. "Pox houses" were erected along the routes traveled by the Crusaders, but may have sheltered diseases other than smallpox. Leprosy had become increasingly prevalent in Europe since the sixth and seventh centuries, and fear of this disease promoted development of the principle of isolation of patients with contagious diseases in Europe around this time. Edward I's Crusaders apparently brought smallpox to England when they returned from the Holy Land in 1300, and the disease appears to have been carried into "Germany" by Crusaders around the same time (Strickland 1885; Alivizatos 1950).

Smallpox apparently had reached England even before King Edward's Crusaders returned. Moore (1815) describes an Anglo-Saxon manuscript dating from the early tenth century containing prayers addressed to St. Nicaise on behalf of smallpox victims, and in 907, Alfreda, daughter of the Anglo-Saxon king Alfred the Great (and niece of Baldwin, count of Flanders) survived an attack of smallpox. Over two centuries before Alfreda's attack, Irish manuscripts began to mention epidemics of a disease called *Bolgach*, a word that came to be used for smallpox, but that might have meant leprosy or plague initially. Another native word that now means smallpox, *Galrabreac*, was also used in reference to some of these Irish epidemics between 675 and 778. (Edwardes 1902b; Dixon 1962). Shrewsbury (1949) believed a "yellow plague" that struck England about a decade before the first of the epidemics of *Bolgach* in Ireland was also smallpox.

On the opposite side of the continent, an intimate description of smallpox by a poet at Constantinople, Theodore Prodromos, dates from the end of the twelfth century. While most clinical descriptions of illnesses said to be smallpox during these centuries are vague when they exist at all, Prodromos leaves us assured that he had smallpox. After three days of fever and vomiting, he says,

> First my own body is showered with hailstones from the top of the head to the nails of the toes, which are unblessed. Yes, I do justly call them hail on account of their color being white and of the shape being spherical. The body is heated violently through and through with extraordinary torches from the fever . . . little by little [the pimples] gradually on the seventh day become murderous pustules. Have you ever seen a violent shower of rain coming down on a lake, how the entire surface of the lake swells up on account of the closely packed bubbles? Such at this time think of my wretched flesh to have become. (Codellas 1946, 213)

Prodromos became bald and had a "brandmarked and entirely variegated face" as a result of his attack.

Thus, by the end of the twelfth century, smallpox apparently was a well-known phenomenon in the center of western Europe, namely, in parts of France and Switzerland. It may have been only slightly less familiar in England, Spain, Italy, and Constantinople, where its occurrence may simply have been less well-documented than in the former area.

By far the most important event in the history of smallpox during the European Dark Ages emerged from the Moslem civilization flourishing on Europe's southern border. As Islamic influences diffused into Europe via the Middle East, Sicily, and Spain, Galen's European heirs came to revere the medical works of two pre-eminent Moslem physicians who were known in the West as Rhazes (850–925) and Avicenna (980–1037). Their origins and contributions are described more fully in chapter 5. Suffice it to note here that early in the tenth century, Rhazes, who was physician-in-chief of the hospital at Baghdad, published *A Treatise on the Small-pox and Measles*, in which he clearly distinguished smallpox and measles for the first time in the Western world. This was a major milestone in the diagnosis and history of the disease. In his *Treatise*, Rhazes also promulgated his "heat treatment," or "sweat therapy," which was designed to help smallpox victims expel superfluous fermented humors. The same work reveals that smallpox was a well-established, endemic disease of children in West Asia when Rhazes wrote. Rhazes' treatise was followed by works of several other Arabic physicians. These writings, with minor modifications, were incorporated into virtually all important European medical texts dealing with smallpox until Sydenham took a fresh view seven centuries later.

THIRTEENTH, FOURTEENTH, AND FIFTEENTH CENTURIES

According to Paschen (1924), Norman invaders brought smallpox to England in 1241–42, a half century before the return of King Edward I's infected Crusaders. But as we have seen, the disease almost certainly had reached England before either of those two events. Indeed, by the time the Normans are thought to have introduced smallpox, an Englishman, Gilbertus Anglicus, completed his *Compendium Medicinae* (C. 1240), which included a long description of causes and varieties of smallpox, thus strongly suggesting that the disease had been known in England for some time.

Garrison (1914) argues that Gilbertus's compendium refers to smallpox as a contagious disease for the first time. Gilbertus also advises use of red-colored items to treat patients with smallpox, making him the first known European author to do so (a Hispano-Arabic philosopher-physician, Averroes (1126–98), advocated the "red treatment" in his writings in the previous century). Only two generations later, another Englishman, John of Gaddesden, boasted about how he cured King Edward II's son John of smallpox by surrounding the prince with red blankets and red curtains, and by giving him red liquids to drink.

Smallpox was a "frequent" disease in France in the thirteenth century, according to Rolleston (1937). During the same century, a Danish ship carried the disease to Iceland for the first time, where it killed some twenty thousand persons in a small population in 1241. Other outbreaks were reported in Iceland in 1257 and 1291 as the disease spread over northern Europe (Edwardes 1902a, 1902b).

Perhaps because it was the century of the "Black Death," Medieval Europe's great pandemic of bubonic plague, the impact of which far exceeded the damage then being caused by smallpox, there are few references to smallpox in Europe during the fourteenth century. Lessons learned in the isolation of persons with leprosy, which also peaked in Europe during the thirteenth and fourteenth centuries, were applied to combat the plague. Effects of dead plague victims were burned, and their rooms aired and fumigated. Around the middle of the fourteenth century, the practice of quarantine, which later would also be used widely against smallpox, was employed for the first time, by French and Italian port cities, to prevent the spread of ship-borne plague.

Rolleston (1937) says smallpox was "well known" in fourteenth-century Germany, Spain, Italy, and France, but offers no details or evidence. We do know that the "red treatment" was used for smallpox victims in Italy and France at this time. When France's King Charles V caught smallpox, he was dressed in red shirt, red stockings, and red veils to aid his recovery. Irish manuscripts mention outbreaks of *Galrabraec* again in 1327 and 1368, and the latter outbreak is known to have affected the Irish nobility. Iceland reported at least four epidemics of smallpox in this century (Cumston 1925; Edwardes 1902b; Kübler 1901).

During the fifteenth century, as plague died out and leprosy started to wane, smallpox apparently began to slowly gather momentum in

Europe, although that perception may be due in part to greater availability of information. In Paris, smallpox was already a disease of children, suggesting that it was by now endemic in the city or that recent, frequent epidemics had "immunized" most surviving adults. According to Bonner (1964, xviii), an epidemic of smallpox that struck Paris around 1438 killed "some fifty thousand people, mostly children," an observation that if accurate, is remarkable, since a century before, Paris's population was only about two hundred thousand. Kübler (1901) and Gottfried (1978) record that during another Parisian epidemic seven years later, over six thousand small children were affected. These two epidemics appear to be the first specific evidence that smallpox was endemic in part of Europe. That this first indication of endemicity occurred in France, the most populous, densely settled European state, is not surprising.

Elsewhere, fifteenth-century epidemics affected entire populations, especially as the disease continued to spread into new areas. Sometime around 1430, smallpox spread from Iceland to a Norman colony on the west coast of Greenland. The repeated attacks of epidemic smallpox that followed this introduction "exterminated the colony, so that from the beginning of the fifteenth century Greenland was almost forgotten in Europe, and three hundred years later had to be discovered anew" (Immerman et. al. 1902, 16). Smallpox is not mentioned again in Greenland until 1734. Iceland itself suffered more epidemics in 1430–32, 1462–63 (1,600 deaths), and 1472.

Smallpox arrived in Sweden around the middle of the fifteenth century. Toward the end of the century, in 1493, Spanish soldiers of Emperor Maxmillian I carried the virus into "Germany" from Flanders, but it is unlikely that this was the first introduction of smallpox into Germany as has sometimes been assumed.

In 1494, the French king Charles VIII recovered from an attack of smallpox while leading his multinational army to the Siege of Naples. At Naples some of his men contracted venereal syphilis. That disease allegedly had just been imported into southern Europe from the New World by Christopher Columbus's crews. When Charles's soldiers carried syphilis into the heart of Europe after the Siege of Naples ended, the French began calling the new disease, which caused a rash similar to that caused by smallpox, *la grosse vérole*, to distinguish it from variola, which now became *la petite vérole*. Thus in English "pox" became "small-pox," and syphilis became known as the "great-pox" (Rosenthal 1959; Edwardes 1902b).

Sixteenth Century

Columbus's voyage and the dispersal of epidemic syphilis in Europe coincided with the renaissance of European civilization and medicine. In 1530 the Italian poet, physician, and scientist Fracastoro published his famous poem, *Syphilis sive morbus gallicus*, in which he recognized the venereal origin of the new epidemic disease in Europe, gave it its modern name of syphilis, and recommended mercury as a specific cure. Sixteen years later he published an even more important treatise, one of the greatest landmarks in the history of communicable diseases. In his *De contagione et contagionis morbis et eorum curatione*, Fracastoro attributed certain diseases, including smallpox and measles, to specific tiny seeds, or *seminaria*, and stated that such specific contagions could spread directly from person to person, indirectly via infected clothing, wooden objects, or other fomites, and even at a distance, for example, through the air. In remarking that fevers such as smallpox and measles "attack children especially, adults rarely, old men hardly ever," Fracastoro (1930,73) provides evidence that smallpox was endemic in Italy by the middle of the sixteenth century. He also described typhus fever clearly for the first time. During this same eventful generation, Rhazes' classic treatise on smallpox and measles was translated from Arabic into Latin, at Venice in 1498, and at Paris in 1528 and 1529. If Rhazes had been a beacon in the Dark Ages, Fracastoro signalled the dawn of a new age in European medicine, which in its early phases saw Italy in the vanguard.

By the sixteenth century, smallpox was well established over most of Europe, except possibly Russia. (Here again, it is difficult to distinguish lack of information about smallpox from true absence of smallpox.) It is not known exactly when the infection appeared in European Russia. According to Klein (1974), a sometimes fatal disease with "purulent eruption" was first mentioned in early fifteenth-century Russia, and there are similar descriptions, each of which might possibly refer to smallpox, dating from the sixteenth century.

As Europe's population increased and crowded into cities more and more, smallpox epidemics appeared with increasing frequency and intensity. As another indication of its growing influence, however, during epidemics in the 1560s smallpox reached out to reigning monarchs of France, Spain, and England. In the north, Denmark and Sweden had more smallpox, and Iceland suffered its first smallpox epidemic of the century in 1511, followed by others in 1555, 1574, 1580, and 1590. Epidemics were also reported in Italy at Mantua (1567), Naples (1577), and Brescia (1570, 1577, 1588). In the latter half of the century there were at least six severe epidemics in Italy, France, and Holland. Kübler describes an epidemic that began in Delft in October 1562 and lasted all winter and into the following summer.

England's Queen Elizabeth I was the most celebrated smallpox patient of sixteenth-century Europe. At the time of the queen's illness, smallpox had been especially prevalent in England during the preceding two or three years, and it had undoubtedly been endemic there for decades, if not centuries, before. The countess of Bedford and several other ladies of rank had died of it. In 1518, Elizabeth's father Henry VIII and his court were forced to leave Wallingford because of smallpox in that area. When Elizabeth's contemporary, Tsar Ivan IV, was seeking the hand of an English noblewoman, Lady Mary Hastings, several pretexts were found to delay the time when the tsar's emissary could actually see Lady Mary, because she had just recovered from smallpox and wanted to hide the scars on her face ("Medicine in Russia," 1897, 348). Greenwood considers the references to smallpox during Henry VIII's reign as the first unequivocal records of smallpox in England. While both Greenwood (1935) and Creighton (1894) refer to the case of a Mr. Richard Allington in 1561 as the first good clinical account of smallpox in English, Creighton accepts John of Gaddesden's famous patient as the sole case of variola described in English records before the sixteenth century.

In France, Charles d'Orleans, son of Francis I, was blinded in one eye by the disease, and four years after Queen Elizabeth's illness, Ambroise Paré (1510–90), the "father of modern surgery," treated several cases of smallpox during an epidemic in Paris, where many members of the nobility were affected. The French court returned to Paris from a two-year progress around the country during the latter outbreak, in time for the young king Charles IX and his sister Marguerite to get the infection. Both recovered, but the king had to be treated months later by Paré for a contracture that resulted from damage to a nerve when another physician bled the king for his smallpox. According to Packard (1926) the contracture had prevented Charles from bending or straightening his arm. Paré later published his observations on smallpox, plague, and measles at the urging of the Queen Mother.

Not even Paré could undo the damage wrought by smallpox on Charles's brother Alençon, who was one of Queen Elizabeth's frustrated suitors:

> When [Alençon] emerged from his chamber after a dangerous bout with smallpox, there was little left of the promising young prince. His appearance was totally changed: His face was deeply pitted, his eyes bloodshot, and rheumy, his voice thin and reedy, and his nose almost doubled in size. . . . His spirit too had undergone a profound change. . . . he found he no longer had a part to play in that world in which handsome faces and virile bodies were given first prize . . . (Mahoney 1975, 173)

Elizabeth cited Alençon's pockmarks as one of her excuses for not marrying him (ibid., 176).

Epidemics in Spanish ports, especially Cadiz, may have been the source of the first cases of smallpox in the New World in 1507 (see chapter 6). There were epidemics in Valencia in 1555, Seville in 1580 and 1597, and in Toledo in 1585–86. In Madrid, which in Bergamini's words grew from a "little-known town" of "a few thousand people" in 1556 to a population of one hundred and fifty thousand in 1700, over five thousand persons perished during an epidemic of smallpox in 1587. When Spain's King Philip II took Charles IX's sister, Elizabeth of Valois, as his third wife, the beautiful new queen of Spain was stricken with smallpox soon after she arrived from France in January 1560. Luckily, she had only a mild case, and recovered without severe scarring (Bergamini 1974; DeVillalba 1802; Merriman 1962).

SEVENTEENTH CENTURY

If smallpox began to reach alarming levels in Europe during the latter half of the sixteenth century, by the end of the seventeenth century, *V. major* had clearly succeeded plague, leprosy, and syphilis as the continent's foremost pestilence. Typhus, dysentery, and plague were still common killers of Europeans, but smallpox was now the most common. All four diseases flourished as a result of the wars and attendant turmoil prevalent in Europe in the seventeenth century. Vaughan (1923) records a contemporary German proverb that held "From love and smallpox but few remain free."

Not all the ferment in seventeenth-century Europe was martial. The burgeoning cities of Europe developed a new urban class, and "it was the intellectual activity of the urban groups, often encouraged and directed by royal patronage, which most profoundly influenced the growth of the secular culture that characterized the Renaissance and of which the new science was one of the most distinctive elements" (Rosen 1958, 83). Dissemination of results of the new scientific inquiries and clinical observations was facilitated by the appearance of academies and other learned bodies as well as medical journals. Leeuwenhoek's invention of the microscope was one of the most important accomplishments of this period, but even more relevant to the intensifying struggle against smallpox was the work of Thomas Sydenham in England.

Copious bleeding was still a mainstay of treatment for smallpox and many other illnesses in Sydenham's time, and while he did not do away with it altogether, he used it less. As Rosen (1958) tells us, by introducing cinchona bark as a specific treatment for malaria into England, Sydenham helped undermine belief in the humoral theory of disease. Some of Sydenham's contemporaries recommended a drink prepared from sheep's dung for treating smallpox victims (goat's dung for measles). Their rationale was that such "medicines" were effective in direct proportion to their repugnancy, since their purpose was to drive out the demon or other occult influence held responsible for the illness. Others still relied on the red treatment. Miller (1957) describes a quarrel in London over the usefulness of purgatives for treating smallpox that resulted in a duel in the quadrangle of Gresham College.

Sydenham changed many of the traditional treatments that European physicians employed to the detriment of their smallpox patients. "How is it," he asked at one point, "that so few of the common people die of this disease compared with the numbers that perish by it among the rich?" (Sandwith 1910, 301). Many agreed with his answer that the rich died in greater numbers because of the prevailing therapies, which only they could afford. In addition, many of the poor simply died unnoticed. A century before Sydenham, Forestus, a Dutchman, had begun changing earlier practices that called for opening the pustules after he noticed that persons whose scabs dropped off spontaneously did better (Moore 1815).

Sydenham's greatest contribution, as far as smallpox was concerned, was two-fold. Like Rhazes, he distinguished smallpox from measles clearly, but then he also distinguished patients with confluent smallpox from those with discrete smallpox rashes. Recognizing that the latter type of smallpox patients usually recovered, he recommended that no "treatment" was necessary for them, thus improving their chances of survival significantly. Second, he recommended a more appropriate "cooling treatment" for feverish victims, thus reversing the traditional heat treatment advanced by Rhazes. Sydenham's "cooling treatment" required open windows and lighter bed coverings. Even in the eighteenth century, smallpox patients from the same family were being crowded into one sickroom, with blankets nailed over the windows and bed curtains drawn to permit "hot" treatment, and patients slept on "stinking linen which it was thought dangerous to change" (Miller 1957, 39).

Sydenham's contributions were mainly clinical. As one of the foremost adherants of the miasmatic theory, he attributed the cause of smallpox to changes in the atmosphere, which assumed an "epidemic constitution." Even he did not act on the knowledge that smallpox was contagious and spread from person to person, if he was aware of it. The concept of smallpox's contagiousness finally took hold after it was recognized by Jean Baptiste van Helmont (1578–1644) of Belgium, and Hermann Boerhaave (1668–1738) of the Netherlands.

In addition to intellectual and medical-scientific ferment, Europe's new urban classes were also the source of a "new notion of [mercantile] wealth" based on trade and money instead of land (Rosen 1958, 83). The physician-economist William Petty (1623–87), a compatriot and almost exact contemporary of Thomas Sydenham, crystallized elements of the new mercantilist spirit most relevant to our story in his phrase "political arithmetic." Petty recognized the importance of a healthy population to the projection of national power and inaugurated the quantitative study of diseases and data relating to health and other problems of the state. In Petty's view, moreover, it was the state's bounden duty to advance medical knowledge as rapidly as possible, and he advocated using hospitals for training physicians and for medical research as effective means to that end. The impact of Petty's work and others' related efforts was only fully realized in the eighteenth century, when Europe's struggle with smallpox reached its climax. In the meantime, smallpox continued to increase in prevalence in Europe.

In 1614, a pandemic of smallpox swept much of Europe and the Near East. Outbreaks were reported in France, Italy, Germany, England, Poland, Flanders, Crete, Egypt, Turkey, and Persia. This upsurge probably was responsible for the first importation of smallpox into the Americas north of Mexico (see chapter 7). Several German-speaking cities were also affected early in the century, including Prague, which lost fifteen hundred citizens in 1606 (Kübler 1901).

Only months before the great pandemic began, a much smaller outbreak in northern Italy had a disproportionately large political impact. There, the duke of Mantua died of smallpox in December 1612, three weeks after burying his son for the same reason. The sudden deaths of the twenty-seven year old duke and his infant son extinguished the direct male line of the Gonzanga family, even though the duke's younger brother renounced his cardinalate and returned from Rome to succeed him. The question of the Mantuan succession raised by the absence of a male heir eventually resulted in the War of the Mantuan Succession, during which France and Austria fought for influence over the heretofore independent duchy (Brinton 1927).

Any hopes Europeans may have had for a respite from smallpox after the epidemics of 1614 were erased by the Thirty Years War (1618–48). Epidemics, including smallpox, erupted in military gatherings and in towns crowded with refugees from the countryside. Helleiner (1967) tells us that troops marching back and forth also helped spread infections. In Ireland, a decade of strife in the 1640s was followed by famine, plague, and smallpox.

By early in the seventeenth century, smallpox was definitely established in the kingdom of Moscow. According to Klein (1974), the Russian word for smallpox—*ospa*, or *vospa*—is first seen in a letter written by a physician in Moscow in 1623. From Moscow, Russians carried the disease east following the conquest of Siberia, with grave consequences for natives of that region. As early as 1630, some areas of Siberia were so devastated by smallpox that it was "impossible to bury the dead" ("Smallpox before Jenner," 1896, 1263). Fifty years later, in one of the earliest regulations against smallpox, the tsar ordered homeowners in Moscow to report any cases of smallpox to the appropriate officials, and he forbade any members of a household where there was a case of smallpox to come near his person. Thus the tsar at least appears to have been aware that smallpox could spread by contagion and took steps to isolate himself from it. Despite the tsar's orders in Moscow, however, a terrible epidemic destroyed entire populations of several Russian towns in 1691.

Inhabitants of the Faroe Islands were infected for the first time in 1650 via a ship from Denmark. Iceland, a favorite site for smallpox importations by Danish ships, had six epidemics between 1616 and 1671 (Kübler 1901; Hirsch 1883).

Meanwhile, in England, parishes in London established an effective reporting system when they began registering church burials by cause of death. These "Bills of Mortality" were published, starting in 1629, providing an almost uninterrupted source of information about epidemics in the metropolis since that date, thus establishing the basis for early statistical proof of smallpox's importance in England. Authorities in Geneva had started keeping records of death from smallpox by age group of the victims beginning in 1580, and as noted above, the tsar initiated a home-based reporting system in Moscow in 1680.

Over a thousand deaths from smallpox were recorded in London in 1634 and in 1649; in 1641, Dixon records, smallpox and plague caused poor attendance in both Houses of Parliament. At mid-century, the disease again attacked European royalty.

Spain, which had had a few comparatively small outbreaks of smallpox in the first half of the century and which suffered a severe epidemic that killed a majority of its victims in nearly all the cities of Andalusia in 1679, lost the heir to its throne, the Spanish Habsburg prince Balthazar Carlos, to the disease in 1646. At the time, the seventeen-year-old prince of the Asturias, immortalized in several exquisite paintings by Velasquez (plate 3), was the only son of Philip IV. The dead prince's fiancee, Austrian Hapsburg princess Maria Anna, married King Philip IV instead and with him produced the last monarch of the Spanish Habsburg line, Carlos II.

Two years after Balthazar Carlos's death, Prince William II of Orange negotiated a peace agreement with Spain, which finally recognized the independence of the United Provinces. William II (plate 4) was stadholder of Holland, and Holland was the most important of the Dutch provinces. Three years after inheriting his stadholdership, William II had arranged a treaty with France, arrested several Dutch leaders, and attacked Amsterdam in maneuvering to assume sovereignty over all of the provinces. But his ambition was halted by smallpox.

According to the Van der Zees' 1973 biography, the twenty-four-year-old prince became feverish on 29 October after returning to the Hague from a long hunt. Smallpox was diagnosed a few days later, after which his pregnant wife, who had not had smallpox, was not permitted to visit him. His mother was able to see her son during his illness since she had already had smallpox. Thus the House of Orange also appears to have had a working knowledge of the concepts of contagion and immunity by this time. When William II died at 9 P.M., on 6 November, 1650, "it was [five] hours before anyone felt brave enough to break the news to [his wife]" (4).[1] Although his son (William III), born eight days after the father's death, eventually ruled England, William II's republican opponents in Holland seized the opportunity of his death to pass the Act of Seclusion, which abolished the stadholdership for over two decades.

Unlucky Maria Anna of Austria, the teenaged archduchess who lost her intended husband to smallpox and was married off to his middle-aged father instead, lost her brother, the heir to the Austrian throne, to the same disease eight years later. The twenty-one-year-old emperor-elect of the Holy Roman Empire, Ferdinand IV died in Vienna on 9 July 1654. At the time of his death, Ferdinand had been crowned king of Bohemia, king of Hungary, and king of the Romans (title of the heir to the throne of the Holy Roman Empire), although his father was still emperor.

Ferdinand's untimely death shifted the line of succession to his fourteen-year-old brother Leopold I, who had been educated for service to the Roman Catholic Church, but who presided instead as Holy Roman Emperor during Vienna's high baroque period in a reign that lasted forty-eight years. It was Leopold I who engaged the services of Austria's greatest warrior, Prince Eugene of Savoy, and with him successfully ended the Turkish threat to Europe at the Siege of Vienna.

For all its unsought beneficence, smallpox exacted a harsh toll from Leopold I. In 1662–63, at a time when his Hungarian subjects were violently restless and when a Turkish army of one hundred thousand men had suddenly invaded Hungary, the emperor was temporarily indisposed by an attack of smallpox. He buried two of his sixteen children because of the disease. In 1691, he wrote to his confessor:

> All my sons and daughters except the King of the Romans are down with the smallpox . . . my youngest daughter born only last year. This angel was well until suddenly the evil began. Barely three days was she sick and this morning early seized with such terrible cramps that her innocent soul winged its way to heaven. (McGuigan 1976, 211)

Smallpox claimed another of his young daughters a few years later. Mercifully, Leopold did not live to see his son Joseph I, the "King of the Romans" mentioned in the letter to his confessor, also die of smallpox.

France, with its relatively large population of about 19 million citizens (compared to about 9 million in Spain, 8 million in Russia, and less than 6 million in England), reported comparatively slight damage from smallpox in the 17th century. The year after it killed the Spanish heir Balthazar Carlos, and three years before it carried away William II of Orange, the disease attacked nine-year-old Louis XIV at Fontainebleau. Louis was comatose for nearly an hour on the eleventh day of his illness, and his toes became infected. Nursed by the regent Anne, he recovered with little scarring despite being bled three times by his doctors. (Cronin 1965). Paris had another severe epidemic in the winter of 1666.

Not all the French victims were as young as Louis XIV. Two of his daughters, Marie Anne and Louise Françoise, caught smallpox in 1686 (when they were twenty and thirteen years old, respectively) and survived, but Marie Anne also infected her husband, the prince of Conti, who died. Ten years later, Madame de Sévigné also died of smallpox, at age seventy.

Compared to France, England suffered severely in the second half of the seventeenth century, though the English may only have kept better records. In London alone (population about five hundred thousand in 1660), over fifty-seven thousand deaths from smallpox—more than five percent of all deaths in the Bills of Mortality—were recorded between 1650 and 1699: an average of over twenty deaths a week for fifty years! Geneva, a town of only about thirteen thousand persons in 1650, recorded slightly less than seven thousand deaths from smallpox between 1580 and 1760. (Creighton 1894, vol. 2). London's Great Plague and Great Fire in 1665–56 were followed by a severe epidemic of smallpox that caused another three thousand, one hundred deaths in 1667–68.

The English royal house of Stuart suffered with its subjects, and was finally extinguished by smallpox (see fig. 2 below). According to Antonia Fraser, when Charles II was invited to restore the English monarchy eleven years after his father's execution, he had already survived a case of smallpox that put him out of action for several weeks in the Hague in the fall of 1648, at a "critical juncture" of the English Civil War. Accompanied by his two brothers, the duke of Gloucester and the duke of York, Charles returned to England from the continent and assumed the crown in May 1660. In September, Henry, duke of Gloucester, fell ill with smallpox at Whitehall Palace. The young duke seemed to handle the infection well, and had been pronounced out of danger by his doctor before he began hemorrhaging and died on the tenth day of his illness. (Sandwith 1910).

Three days after the duke of Gloucester's funeral, Charles and his surviving brother went to the English coast to welcome their sister, Princess Mary of Orange (the widow of William II of Orange), who was arriving from the Hague. She, too, died of smallpox at Whitehall that December (plate 4). Mary's sister, Princess Henrietta, followed her to London, and also developed smallpox, but recovered.

Charles II was succeeded by his brother the duke of York, a Catholic, who became King James II. The crisis caused by James's Catholicism would almost certainly have been avoided had his Protestant brother, the late duke of Gloucester, still been alive as an alternative legitimate male heir to the throne. All of the new king's sons died at an early age, including one who succumbed to smallpox. After three years on the throne, James II fled Protestant England, and was succeeded by his daughter Mary, who had already married her cousin William III of Orange, the posthumous Protestant son of William II. William III and Mary II were declared cosovereigns of England.

Shortly before Christmas 1694, thirty-two year old Queen Mary II (plate 5) was stricken with smallpox at Kensington Palace in London. Macaulay described the sad consequences eloquently in his *History of England* (1914, 5: 2468–70).

> [The King] had but too good reason to be uneasy. His wife had, during two or three days, been poorly, and on the preceding evening grave symptoms had appeared. Sir Thomas Millington, who was physician-in-ordinary to the King, thought that she had the measles; but Radcliffe, who, with coarse manners and little book learning, had raised himself to the first practice in London chiefly by his rare skill in diagnostics, uttered the more alarming words, smallpox. That disease, over which science has since achieved a succession of glorious and beneficient victories, was then the most terrible of all the ministers of death. The havoc of the plague had been far more rapid; but the plague had visited our shores only once or twice within living memory; and the smallpox was always present, filling the churchyard with corpses, tormenting with constant fear all whom it had not yet stricken, leaving on those whose lives it spared the hideous traces of its power, turning the babe into a changeling at which the mother shuddered, and making the eyes and cheeks of the betrothed maiden objects of horror to the lover. Towards the end of the year 1694 this pestilence was more than usually severe. At length the infection spread to the palace, and reached the young and blooming queen. She received the intimation of her danger with true greatness of soul. She gave orders that every lady of her bedchamber, every maid of honour, nay, every menial servant who had not had the smallpox should instantly leave Kensington House. She locked herself up during a short time in her closet, burned some papers, arranged others, and calmly awaited her fate.
>
> During two or three days there were many alterations of hope and fear. The physicians contradicted each other and themselves in a way which sufficiently indicates the state of medical science in that age. The disease was measles, it was scarlet fever, it was spotted fever, it was erysipelas. At one moment some symptoms, which in truth showed that the case was almost hopeless, were hailed as indications of returning health. At length all doubt was over, Radcliffe's opinion proved to be right. It was plain that the Queen was sinking under smallpox of the most malignant type.
>
> All this time William remained night and day near her bedside. The little couch on which he slept when he was in camp was spread for him in the ante-chamber, but he scarcely laid down on it; the sight of his misery, the Dutch envoy wrote, was enough to melt the hardest heart. Nothing seemed to be left of the man whose serene fortitude had been the wonder

of old soldiers on the disastrous day of Landen, and of old sailors through that fearful night among the sheets of ice and banks of sand on the coast of Goree. The very domestics saw the tears running unchecked down that face, of which the stern composure had seldom been disturbed by any triumph or by any defeat. Several of the prelates were in attendance. The King drew Burnet aside, and gave way to an agony of grief. "There is no hope," he cried; "I was the happiest man on earth; and I am the most miserable. She had no fault, none; you knew her well, but you could not know, nobody but myself could know her goodness." Tenison (Archbishop of Canterbury) undertook to tell her that she was dying. He was afraid that such a communication abruptly made might agitate her violently, and began with much management. But she soon caught his meaning, and with that meek womanly courage which so often puts our bravery to shame submitted herself to the will of God. She called for a small cabinet in which her most important papers were locked up, gave orders that, as soon as she was no more, it should be delivered to the King, and then dismissed worldly cares from her mind. She received the Eucharist, and repeated her part of the office with unimpaired memory and intelligence, though in a feeble voice. She observed that Tenison had been long standing at her bedside, and, with that sweet courtesy which was habitual of her, faltered out her commands that he would sit down, and repeated them till he obeyed. After she had received the Sacrament she sank rapidly, and uttered only a few broken words. Twice she tried to take a last farewell of him whom she had loved so truly and entirely; but she was unable to speak. He had a succession of fits so alarming that his Privy councillors, who were assembled in a neighbouring room, were apprehensive for his reason and his life. A few minutes before the Queen expired William was removed almost insensible from the sickroom.

The queen died soon after midnight on Friday morning, 28 December. "And to the waiting Londoners," wrote the Van der Zees, "shivering in a snowbound city, where all the coffee houses and theatres had been shut up, the news was carried by the tolling bells" (1973, 386). William III, whose father had died of smallpox the week before he was born, who had lost his mother to smallpox when he was ten years old, and who had had a severe case of smallpox himself as a child, now prepared to bury his young wife, a victim of the same savage illness.

To refute public charges that the queen's doctors, not her disease, were responsible for her demise, one of her physicians was permitted to publish a clinical account of her final illness. This is especially fortunate for our purposes, since it gives us a detailed view of how some of Europe's best physicians wrestled with the problem of diagnosing and treating a very important patient who had hemorrhagic smallpox at the end of the seventeenth century:

The symptoms of illness on the first day did not prevent the queen from going abroad; but, as she was still out of sorts at bedtime, she took a large dose of Venice treacle, a powerful diaphoretic which her former physician, the famous physiologist Dr. Lower, had recommended her to take as often as she found herself inclined to a fever. Finding no sweat to appear as usual, she took next morning a double quantity of it, but again without inducing the usual effect of prespiration. Up to that time she had not asked advice of the physicians. To this severe dosing with one of the most powerful alexipharmac or heating medicines, the malignant type of the ensuing smallpox was mainly ascribed by Harris, who was a follower to Sydenham and a partizan of the cooling regimen. On the third day from the initial symptoms the eruption appeared, with a very trouble-some cough; the eruption came out in such a manner that the physicians were very doubtful whether it would prove to be smallpox or measles. On the fourth day the smallpox showed itself in the face and the rest of the body "under its proper and distinct form." But on the sixth day, in the morning, the variolous pustules where changed all over her breast into the large red spots "of the measles"; and the erysipelas, or rose, swelled her whole face, the former pustules giving place to it. That evening many livid round petechiae appeared on the forehead above the eyebrows, and on the temples, which Harris says he had fortold in the morning. One physician said these were not petechiae, but sphacelated spots; but next morning a surgeon proved by his lancet that they contained blood. During the night following the sixth day, Dr. Harris sat up with the patient, and observed that she had great difficulty of breathing, followed soon after by a copious spitting of blood. On the seventh day the spitting of blood was succeeded by blood in the urine. On the eighth day the pustules on the limbs, which had kept the normal variolous character longest, lost their fullness, and changed into round spots of deep red or scarlet colour, smooth and level with the skin, like the stigmata of the plague. Harris observed about the region of the heart one large pustule filled with matter, having a broad scarlet circle round it like a burning coal, under which a great deal of extravasated blood was found when the body was examined after death. Towards the end, the queen slumbered sometimes, but said she was not refreshed thereby. At last she lay silent for some hours; and some words that came from her shewed, says

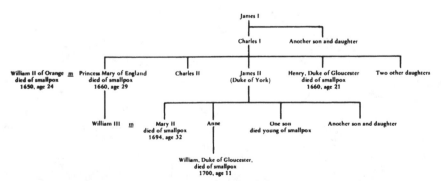

Fig. 2. Effects of smallpox on the House of Stuart, partial family tree

Burnet, that her thoughts had begun to break. She died on the 28th of December, at one in the morning, in the ninth day of her illness. (Creighton 1894, 2: 459)

Mary II died childless.[2] William III ruled alone for eight years and was succeeded by Mary's sister, Queen Anne. Two years before Anne succeeded to the throne, her only child, the eleven-year-old duke of Gloucester, died of smallpox soon after his nurse recovered from the disease. Dixon notes that by ending the Stuart line (See fig. 2), his death precipitated a constitutional crisis that resulted in the Act of Settlement. The act barred another Catholic sovereign and opened the English throne to the House of Hanover.

EIGHTEENTH CENTURY

In the long, global saga of smallpox, eighteenth-century Europe is probably the most dramatic time and place. It was the scene of an epic confrontation between smallpox, which had been gathering force in Europe since the middle of the sixteenth century, and inoculation and vaccination, the first specific countermeasures against it, introduced in the West for the first time. In inoculation, Europeans acquired early in the eighteenth century an entirely new, effective tool for controlling smallpox in a way that had not been possible before against epidemic plague, leprosy, or syphilis. As if it fully appreciated, even anticipated, the limits the eighteenth-century break-throughs would place on its power, the disease embarked on a deadly series of attacks on the royal houses of Europe, the beginnings of which we have already seen. In a regicidal rampage without parallel anywhere else or at any other time, it killed a queen of England, an Austrian emperor, a king of Spain, a tsar of Russia, a queen of Sweden, and a king of France in the eighty years before 1775. This unprecedented surge in monarchal deaths from smallpox is a strong indication that smallpox was significantly more prevalent in eighteenth-century Europe than it had been previously. This is not an artifact of more complete historical records, since earlier royal deaths from smallpox were certainly recorded and were not nearly as frequent as in the eighteenth century. Some of the threatened royal houses exerted a powerful influence, by example, in helping to persuade their subjects to accept inoculation.

Additional evidence of smallpox's increasing impact can be gleaned from the registers of parish burials in London. Edwardes (1902b) notes that the London Bills of Mortality recorded an average of 210 deaths per 100,000 persons from smallpox annually between 1647 and 1700 (60,205 deaths; estimated population of 530,000 in 1685), whereas between 1701 and 1800 they recorded an annual average of 300 deaths from smallpox per 100,000 persons (195,865 deaths; estimated population of 653,900 in

1750). A nineteenth-century British statistician, William Guy (1882), compared the ratios of deaths by smallpox to 1,000 deaths from all causes in the Bills of Mortality for the seventeenth, eighteenth and nineteenth centuries, and reached a similar conclusion (fig. 3). According to Acker-knecht (1965) and Tyson (1901), by 1800 smallpox still caused a third of all blindness and killed an estimated four hundred thousand Europeans each year. But its halcyon days in Europe were over. One shudders to imagine how an increasingly urbanized Europe might have fared if Euro-peans had not discovered inoculation and vaccination when they did.

Smallpox opened the century with an awesome show of force in Iceland. That country had about fifty thousand inhabitants in 1707 when smallpox broke out and infected almost everyone on the island. The outbreak was apparently started by clothing from an Icelandic student who died while fleeing an epidemic in Copenhagen. The student's sister became infected after unpacking his belongings in June, and a meeting of the Icelandic parliament in July amplified the infection:

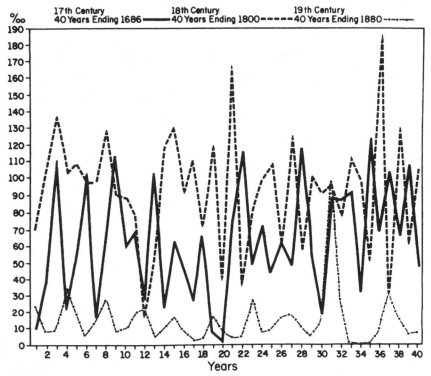

Fig. 3. London smallpox deaths per thousand deaths from all causes, seventeenth to nineteenth centuries. Adapted from Guy (1882).

From the Althing [Parliament] it spread out like a flood through various districts, so that the deaths were over by Christmas in the Southern Quarter and much of the Western Quarter and in many parts of the North. (Roberts 1978, 9–10)

By the time it ended several months later, sixteen to eighteen thousand Icelanders had died of smallpox. The Faroe Islands, Norway, and Sweden all reported smallpox epidemics in the few years before the calamitous epidemic on Iceland. Three years later the disease claimed another three thousand lives in London. Then an otherwise ordinary outbreak in Vienna, where the disease was undoubtedly endemic, spilled over into the royal palace again, with results that were far from ordinary.

According to one biographer of the Habsburgs, Emperor Joseph I seemed "the heaven-sent man to nurture and develop his inheritance at the moment of its first flowering. Fair-haired, blue-eyed, and strikingly handsome under his periwig, generous, kind, physically and morally courageous, an enthusiast for the arts and sciences no less than for war, he was almost too good to be true" (Crankshaw 1971, 246) (plate 6). He spoke seven languages.

Joseph established peace with Hungary in January 1711, the same month his eldest daughter recovered from smallpox. The flurry of baroque building begun in his father's reign continued to transform the Austrian capital. It was for Joseph I that Schönbrunn Palace was begun. Meanwhile Joseph had reorganized and strengthened the state's finances.

On 7 April, the thirty-three-year-old emperor felt ill while dining in the Hofburg. Smallpox was diagnosed, and his physicians, "according to the practice of the times, not only excluded the air from his apartment, but swathed him in twenty yards of English scarlet broadcloth, when the disorder was at its height" (Coxe 1820, 4: 117). On Sunday, 12 April, prayers for the emperor were offered at churches all over Vienna, including the Imperial Chapel and St. Stephens Cathedral, where he had worshipped the previous Sunday (*Wein. Diarium*, 1711, no. 803). But unlike Elizabeth I of England, this promising young sovereign did not recover. He died the following Friday, 17 April 1711, shortly after 10:00 A.M. He had been emperor for six years. After a funeral service in St. Stephens Cathedral, he was buried in the Habsburg crypt beneath the Capuchin church on Monday evening, 20 April.

Fifteen days before Joseph's illness began, the emperor and empress had visited a group of poor mothers and children in a hospital (ibid., no. 797). That act of charity may well have been the source of his infection. Patients with undiagnosed smallpox lying on open hospital wards were a well-known and frequent hazard, as we shall see, wherever smallpox occurred in recent times.

Joseph I's death had important consequences for Austria and

Europe. Austria lost more than a promising emperor. Jeosph's demise also cost the Habsburgs the Spanish succession. The throne of Spain had been disputed since before Carlos II, the last Spanish Habsburg, died in 1700. Because Joseph I died without a son, he was succeeded by his only surviving brother, Charles VI. Charles, who compared poorly with his older brother in almost every respect, hastened back to Vienna from the fighting in Spain, detouring to Frankfurt to be crowned Holy Roman Emperor on the way. But by accepting the Austrian inheritance, Charles was forced to abandon the Spanish throne to the Bourbon claimant, Philip V. Austria's erstwhile allies, who earlier had sought to block the accession of Louis XIV's grandson in Madrid, now changed sides to support Philip V, since they were even more wary of permitting Joseph's brother to reunite the entire Habsburg realm by occupying the thrones of both Madrid and Vienna.

The aging Spanish king Carlos II and his cabinet had at one time favored a third claimant to the Spanish throne, the seven-year-old son of the elector of Bavaria. This prince elector "was waiting in the Netherlands to set sail for Spain when he caught the smallpox and died" in 1699 (McGuigan 1976, 213).

In addition to removing Joseph I from the imperial throne at Vienna and deciding who would win the War of the Spanish Succession, a third important consequence of Joseph's premature death emerged two years later. In April 1713, Charles VI, who had no children at the time, issued the Pragmatic Sanction. This decree secured the dynastic inheritance for his own unborn daughter, in preference to the two daughters of Joseph I or any distant male relative. Since Charles VI also had no surviving son when he died (the old male line of the Habsburgs died with him), he was succeeded by his eldest daughter, Maria Theresa, who thus became the revered Mother-Empress of Austria. In killing Joseph I, smallpox had shifted the Habsburg line of succession for the second time in two generations (fig. 4).

Vienna was not the only European court in mourning because of smallpox in the spring of 1711. Three days before Joseph I died, smallpox ended the life of Louis, the grand dauphin, who was the fifty-year-old heir to the French throne and father of the new king of Spain, Philip V. Louis, too, had seemed to be out of danger earlier that day, but when a delegation of herring-women from Les Halles told him they would have a Te Deum sung in Paris to celebrate his recovery, he replied, "It is not time yet, my poor girls." Soon his "head and face became extremely swollen and the features almost unrecognizable" (Bradby 1906, 308–9). He expired around eleven thirty the same evening, at Meudon:

> If a stranger had come to Meudon that night, he would have witnessed a scene not easily forgotten. The extensive gardens, fragrant with bursting buds and all the promise of spring, were haunted by dim-shapes that

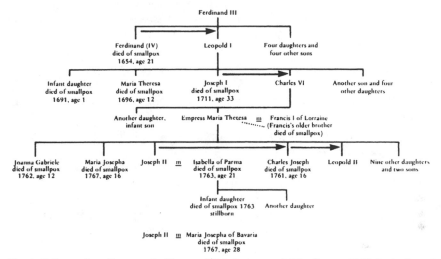

Fig. 4. Effects of smallpox on the House of Habsburg, partial family tree. Shifts in the line of succession to the Austrian throne are marked by arrows.

flitted aimlessly to and fro, from avenue to avenue and from *bosquet* to *bosquet*; but the Chateau itself was plunged in utter silence and darkness, save for one room on the ground floor, where tall candles, placed in a row on either side of the bed, flickered in the draught and shot their uncertain rays into the night through the open windows. Outside this room, half in the light and half in the shadow, a small group of men was kneeling on the terrace, speaking in whispers or muttering prayers, while inside lay the disfigured corpse of the man who, only a few hours before, had been heir to the crown of France, the object of flattery and homage, and the centre of hopes, ambitions, and intrigues. (Ibid., 311)

With the demise of the Sun King's son, the title of dauphin passed to the grandson of a reigning French monarch for the first time. Some time earlier, Louis XIV had looked at his son (the grand dauphin), grandson (the duc de Bourgogne), and great-grandson (the duc de Bretagne) and remarked that never before had the French succession been so secure. The seventy-three-year-old king soon buried all three, each dauphins of France in turn, within eleven months of each other, as they and Marie Adelaide, wife of the popular duc de Bourgogne, succumbed to smallpox (Louis) or measles (the others).[3] Louis was succeeded by his sole surviving great-grandson, the duc d'Anjou, who became Louis XV. The future king's life may have been saved by his governess, who removed him from the contaminated palace.

Statistics from Castiglioni (1941) reveal that eight years after the grand dauphin died of smallpox at Meudon just outside Paris, an epidemic of smallpox killed fourteen thousand Parisians. The duc d'Aumont, the marquis de Lunaty Visconti, the count de Bissy, and the prince of Lorraine were among the victims of another severe epidemic in 1723, which affected nearly every family in Paris, then a city of about five hundred thousand persons (Miller 1957, 180–81). Kübler notes that same year smallpox was raging all over Europe, America, and part of Asia. At long last, however, some relief was on the way.

Up to now, Europeans had relied on isolation and quarantine as their main defense against smallpox. Reports of a more effective way to prevent the dreaded disease began to reach medical circles in London at the turn of the century. In a letter dated 5 January 1700, to Dr. Martin Lister, fellow of the Royal Society, Joseph Lister (a trader for the East India Company) wrote from Amoy, China, to describe the ancient Chinese practice of inoculating persons with infectious material from mild smallpox cases by blowing dust from the powered scabs up their nostrils. This often produced a mild infection in the recipient, who thus became immune at less risk of death than if he had acquired the disease naturally. Another writer reported the Chinese practice to the Royal Society a month later (Miller 1957). At the time of these two letters, which apparently provoked no action, inoculation of smallpox virus into the skin of susceptible persons seems to already have been a popular folk practice among some rural European peasants, who called it "buying the smallpox." Kahn says that Vollgnad and Schultz had reported it in Poland in the 1670s. The Danish anatomist Bartholin described it in 1666 and 1673, it was reported from Scotland in 1715, and Greek peasants were also already familiar with the practice (Dixon 1962; Henschen 1966; Stearns 1950).

Inoculation had been introduced into Constantinople around 1672, apparently having arrived overland from China or Persia via the Circassians.[4] Europeans living in Constantinople learned of inoculation during an outbreak there in 1706. In December 1713, Dr. Emanuele Timoni, an Italian physician, sent an account of inoculation in Constantinople to Dr. Woodward in London, who read it to the Royal Society in May 1714. The following year, a Greek physician, Dr. Jacob Pylarini of Smyrna, published a treatise on the subject at Venice, and this was read to the Royal Society in May 1716. Other reports of the practice were reaching European physicians on the continent around the same time. In Boston, Cotton Mather first learned of it in 1706 while interrogating his African slave.

The failure of European physicians to respond immediately to these reports, in the face of terrible smallpox epidemics, is curious. But it was not altogether irrational. Given a similar level of ignorance about the essential mechanisms and effective treatment of cancer, how many of us would voluntarily submit to being inoculated with malignant cells from someone else's tumor, or would even promote such an idea? Inoculation had to be accepted by physicians and laypeople in order to be practiced, and neither group was prepared to embrace such a risky measure without hesitation, not even in the hope of preventing smallpox.

In her 1957 study, Miller concluded that some of the eighteenth-century physicians were afraid to risk their reputations. Others were blinded by arrogance. Dr. William Wagstaffe, a physician at St. Bartholomew's Hospital in London, fellow of the Royal College of Physicians and Surgeons, fellow of the Royal Society; and one of the main opponents of inoculation, wrote:

> Posterity will scarcely be brought to believe that a method practiced only by a few *Ignorant Women*, amongst an illiterate and unthinking People should on a sudden, and upon a slender Experience, so far obtain in one of the most Learned and Polite Nations in the World as to be received into the *Royal Palace*. (Stearns 1950, 115)

Eventually, however, the receptive intellectual climate, increasing openess to new ideas, and the generally more spirited scientific inquiry that characterized the Enlightenment enabled inoculation to be adopted in Europe, beginning in England.

The new method was finally popularized in England by Lady Mary Wortley Montague, wife of the British ambassador to Turkey (plate 7), with the strong support of a prominent physician, Sir Hans Sloane, and a surgeon, Charles Maitland. An intelligent, strong-willed woman, Lady Mary was an early feminist.[5] At nineteen, she eloped with Edward Wortley Montague, who was elected a member of Parliament three years after their marriage. Lady Montague then "suddenly found herself one of the most popular hostesses in London and a friend of the leading intellectuals of the capitol" (Langer 1976, 112).

Halsband records in his 1956 biography of Lady Montague that the same year her husband was elected to Parliament, an attack of smallpox left her without eyelashes and with a badly pockmarked face. A year and a half earlier, her twenty-year-old brother had died of smallpox. Thus, when Edward Wortley Montague became ambassador to Turkey, his wife had more than a casual interest in the disease, even though she was not a physician. Two weeks after arriving in Constantinople, she wrote her now famous letter dated 1 April 1717, to her friend Sarah Chiswell in London:

> *Apropos* of distempers, I am going to tell you a thing that will make you wish yourself here. The small-pox, so fatal, and so general amongst us, is here entirely harmless, by the invention of *ingrafting*, which is the term they give it. There is a set of old women, who make it their business to perform the operation, every autumn in the month of September, when the great heat is abated.
>
> People send to one another to know if any of their family has a mind to have the small-pox: they make parties for this purpose, and when they

are met (commonly fifteen or sixteen together), the old woman comes with a nut-shell full of the matter of the best sort of small-pox, and asks what vein you please to have opened.

She immediately rips open that you offer her, with a large needle (which gives you no more pain than a common scratch) and puts into the vein, as much matter as can lie upon the head of her needle, and after that binds up the little wound with a hollow bit of shell; and in this manner opens four or five veins.

The Grecians have commonly the superstition of opening one in the middle of the forehead, one in each arm, and one on the breast, to mark the sign of the cross; but this has a very ill effect, all these wounds leaving little scars, and is not done by those that are not superstitious, who choose to have them in the legs, or that part of the arm that is concealed.

The children or young patients play together all the rest of the day, and are in perfect health to the eighth. Then the fever begins to seize them, and they keep their beds two days, very seldom three. They have very rarely above twenty or thirty in their faces, which never mark, and in eight days they are as well as before their illness. Where they are wounded, there remain running sores during the distemper, which I don't doubt is a great relief to it.

Every year thousands undergo this operation: and the French Ambassador says pleasantly that they take the small-pox here by way of diversion, as they take the waters in other countries. There is no example of anyone that had died in it: and you may believe I am well satisfied of the safety of this experiment, since I intend to try it on my dear little son. I am patriot enough to take pains to bring this useful invention into fashion in England, and I should not fail to write to some of our doctors very particularly about it, if I knew any one of them that I thought had virtue enough to destroy such a considerable branch of their revenue, for the good of mankind. But that distemper is too beneficial to them, not to expose to all their resentment, the hardy sight that should undertake to put an end to it. Perhaps, if I live to return, I may, however, have courage to war with them. Upon this occasion, admire the heroism in the heart of your friend. (Dixon 1962, 219–20)

Sarah Chiswell died of smallpox in 1726.

Lady Montague had her five-year-old son inoculated by the embassy surgeon in Constantinople, Charles Maitland, in March 1718. After returning to London, she had Maitland inoculate her four-year-old daughter in April 1721. This was the first professional inoculation in England. Lady Montague then invited several persons to see her inoculated daughter, including Sir Hans Sloane, who had helped care for Lady Montague during her own illness.

Members of the English royal family, particularly Princess Caroline of Anspach, the wife of the Prince of Wales, began to take an interest in the events. They were apparently influenced by Sir Hans Sloane (who was by now president of the Royal Society and the king's physician), by

Caroline's near loss of a daughter from smallpox, and possibly also as a result of Lady Montague's acquaintance with Princess Caroline. However, Genevieve Miller (1957, 1981) concludes that Sir Hans Sloane probably played the most important role of all the nonroyal personalities involved, and that his contributions were later overshadowed by partisan accounts in which Lady Mary's role was exaggerated.

Charles Maitland, who may also have helped enlist the interest of the royal family, was granted royal permission to conduct a trial inoculation of six condemned prisoners at Newgate Prison on 9 August 1721. This event was witnessed by the king's physicians and twenty-five other medical representatives, some of whom were members of the Royal Society or the College of Physicians. According to Moore (1815), the prisoners survived the inoculation, received their freedom, and one was later shown to be immune to smallpox by exposure to two children with the disease. Maitland later inoculated six other persons in London before 17 April 1722, when the Prince of Wales's two daughters were inoculated. King George I no doubt was mindful of the deaths of Queen Mary II and the last Stuart heir to the British throne when he sanctioned his granddaughters' inoculations, which were successful.

These royal inoculations began the firm establishment of inoculation as acceptable medical practice in England. The new practice was not widely accepted immediately, however. Fewer than nine hundred persons were inoculated in England and Scotland in the first eight years after inoculation was introduced (Downie 1951, 251). This was partly because many lay and medical persons were still unconvinced of its efficacy, and partly because of the well-publicized deaths of the son of the earl of Sunderland and of a footman of Lord Bathurst. Both deaths occurred within a month of the royal inoculations and were publically attributed to smallpox inoculation, although probably incorrectly (Moore 1815). It also soon became apparent that persons who had recently been inoculated were a potential danger to the community, since they could spread ordinary virulent smallpox to susceptible persons with whom they were in contact. The inoculees themselves sometimes developed a fatal case of smallpox as a result of their inoculation, although the risk of this happening was much less than the risk of dying from smallpox acquired in the usual way.

Another early medical concern was the prevailing uncertainty about immunity to smallpox and whether taking the obvious risk of being inoculated would lead to permanent protection from the disease. To these medical and social objections, moreover, were added powerful religious concerns, based on strongly held beliefs about whether deliberately inoculating someone with smallpox or allowing oneself to be inoculated, whatever the outcome, constituted interference with God's intentions. Razzell (1977a) maintains that these objections were even stronger in Scotland than in England because of Calvinist beliefs that inoculation implied a distrust in Providence. Proinoculation clergymen based their counterarguments on the contemporary concept that smallpox represented a seed already present in the body; thus inoculation was supported as an acceptable means of expelling that seed artificially rather than as the introduction of a new disease into the body (Miller 1957).

Another powerful force in favor of inoculation was added when Drs. John Arbuthnot, Thomas Nettleton, and especially James Jurin began applying the popular mathematical approach William Petty had championed in the previous century to compare the relative risks posed by natural and inoculated smallpox. In his first paper to the Royal Society of London on this subject in January 1723, Jurin concluded that the risk of dying from smallpox was about two out of seventeen, and that in recent epidemics of smallpox, about one out of every five or six victims died. In comparison, he showed that only one out of every ninety-one persons inoculated in England died of smallpox inoculation (ibid.).

Thus inoculation finally took root as acceptable medical practice in England as a result of several important factors' overcoming substantial skepticism and fear: the well-recognized need for additional protection against smallpox—a need that was reinforced with each epidemic—the appearance in England of knowledge about inoculation then being practiced in Asia, the intellectual climate of the age, the leadership of Sir Hans Sloane and other members of the medical profession represented by the Royal Society, the patronage and example of the royal family, and the spark provided by the indomitable Lady Mary Montague. Just how unusual and necessary the combination of forces that favored inoculation's introduction into England was is illustrated by considering the situation in other continental European countries.

Isolated inoculations were also undertaken in Hungary in 1721, in the electorate of Hanover, where (Klebs 1913, 73) "the inoculation of Prince Frederick (grandson of the English king) acted as a stimulant," and in France two years earlier, without resulting in the practice being adopted then in those countries. In France, which rivaled England fiercely in so many other ways, opposition to inoculation was especially strong and vociferous. According to Miller, the delay in adoption of the practice in France resulted from the "very conservative character of French medical thought," the relatively unimposing personal qualifications of the technique's earliest advocates in France, and the fact that those early advocates were inevitably involved in the consuming political struggle for medical primacy between the royal physicians and the powerful Paris Faculté de Médecine. A "general resistance to new English intellectual ideas" was another major barrier in France once inoculation had begun to be accepted in England, as was the persisting question as to whether a person could suffer from smallpox twice (Miller 1957, 206–7, 269).

The person most responsible for finally overcoming the opposition in France was the well-known mathematician and physical scientist, Charles Marie de la Condamine, member of the Academie Royale des Sciences in Paris. In 1754 La Condamine began a public campaign in favor of inoculation, pointing out that nearly one million deaths from smallpox would have been averted in France if the country had adopted the practice right after it was introduced in England. Smallpox, he said, was "a river that everyone had to cross" one way or another (Edwardes 1902b, 23). In Miller's words, "the personal efforts of La Condamine were a more vigorous reenactment of the role played earlier by Jurin as reporter and analyst, and [La Condamine's] colleagues, Bernoulli and D'Alembert, supplied even more refined mathematical treatment" (1957, 238). Two papers by Daniel Bernoulli and J. L. D'Alembert presenting conflicting statistical analyses of the risks and benefits of inoculation contributed to "the ultimate development of the calculus of probability" (ibid., 225).

After La Condamine, the most important French propagandist on behalf of inoculation was Voltaire, who according to Mason's 1975 biography, saw inoculation practiced while he was in England in the late 1720s and returned to France a passionate believer and vocal advocate of the technique. To La Condamine's quantitative mercantilist arguments on inoculation's value to the French state, Voltaire added his own more qualitative entreaties, imploring his fellow Frenchmen to adopt inoculation "for the sake of staying alive and keeping their women beautiful" (Halsband 1953, 404).

Inoculation finally began in France in April 1755. A year later, the duc d'Orleans, Louis Philippe, invited a well-known inoculator, Dr. Theodore Tronchin, to Paris from Geneva to inoculate his two children. All France awaited the outcome of what some considered to be a reckless step. Thus, when "the recovered children were taken to the opera by their mother," wrote Miller, "they were greeted by spontaneous applause" (1957, 219). Parisian women celebrated the occasion with a new fashion—*Bonnets a l'inoculation*—hats with dotted ribbons signifying the spots of smallpox. By 1769, the practice had been officially accepted in France.

It was the same Genevan physician, Dr. Tronchin, who began the first inoculations on the European continent at Amsterdam during an epidemic of smallpox in that city in 1748. Inoculation began to be adopted in Switzerland in 1749, in Italy, Denmark, and Sweden in 1754–56, and in Russia and Austria in 1768. In *The Adoption of Inoculation for Smallpox in England and France*, Miller examines in detail how this powerful medical innovation was introduced into those two countries. Janssens (1981) recently described some aspects of smallpox's introduction into Holland.

We shall observe how smallpox came to be introduced into some of the other countries mentioned in due course.

Meanwhile, smallpox continued to kill Europeans with a vengeance.[6] London recorded major epidemics in 1719, 1723, 1725, 1736, and 1746, though as in other large cities, the disease was constantly present even in nonepidemic years. Over three thousand Londoners perished in the epidemic of 1723. Twice as many Romans died of the same cause in 1746, and again in 1754. There were large outbreaks in Paris, Leipzig, and Hanover in 1734–35, and in the autumn of 1750, smallpox was epidemic once again in Geneva.

In the large cities, especially, children suffered most of all, as they had since the disease began its ascendency in Europe in the sixteenth century. Most children born in eighteenth-century London reportedly had had smallpox by the time they were seven. Of 6,705 persons who died from smallpox in Berlin between 1758 and 1774, only 45 were more than fifteen years old; and of 25,349 deaths from smallpox recorded in Geneva between 1580 and 1760, 83.1 percent had not reached their fifth birthday. Razzell notes in *The Conquest of Smallpox* that the danger of contracting the disease in British cities was so great that poorer folk hesitated to migrate to the cities, as did students from North America, and Miller observes that persons who had not yet had smallpox found it almost impossible to get a job in London working for a family or in a hospital.

In 1733, a Greenlander newly returned from Denmark was the cause of another outbreak in his homeland. Two or three thousand persons died in that epidemic, which affected three out of every four Greenlanders. In his *History of Greenland*, Crantz said missionaries on the island during the terrible outbreak of 1733–34,

> were almost everywhere shocked with the sight of houses tenanted only by the corpses of their former occupants, and dead bodies lying unburied on the snow. . . . In one island the only living creatures they found were a little girl covered with the smallpox, and her three younger brothers. The father, having buried all the rest of the inhabitants, had laid himself and his youngest child in a grave of stones, bidding the girl to cover him with skins; after which she and her brothers were to live upon a couple of seals and some dried herrings til they could get to the Europeans. (1820, 2: 12–16)

If the royal families of Spain and Russia had immediately followed the courageous examples of their English and Hanoverian counterparts, and accepted inoculation as soon as it was shown to be safe in Europe, the history of those two continental powers would have been different. But in the second quarter of the eighteenth century, most European royal families were as wary of inoculation as were their subjects. As a result, Spain and Russia both lost young monarchs to smallpox more than two years after George I's granddaughters were inoculated.

Even before inoculation was introduced into England, Philip V, the first Spanish Bourbon, had tired of the hard-won throne that smallpox had helped him claim. There was a smallpox epidemic in Asturias that year (1721), but the prince of Asturias, Philip's heir Luis Ferdinand, was not affected. In January 1724, Philip V abdicated,

> Having pondered deeply the past four years and meditated long and thoughtfully on the miseries of this life, through all the illnesses, wars and tribulations which God has seen fit to visit upon Us during the twenty-three years of Our Reign, and not unmindful that Our eldest son, Don Luis, sworn heir to this Our Throne, is now come of age, married and endowed with judgment and talent enough to rule and govern this kingdom wisely and with justice . . . (from the Decree of Abdication, cited in Hargreaves-Mawdsley 1973, 83)

Philip retired to San Ildefonso, in the palace he had built 50 miles (83 kilometers) north of Madrid to remind him of Versailles. Bergamini notes in his 1974 study that he may have resigned the Spanish throne with the intention of claiming the French kingship held by his sickly nephew Louis XV.

Sixteen-year-old Luis Ferdinand accepted the Spanish crown at Escorial on 15 January (plate 8). Spaniards greeted his accession enthusiastically, since unlike his father, the tall blond prince was "by birth, habit and inclination, attached to the customs and manners of Spain"(Coxe 1815, 3: 55). Luis I and his French wife Isabel de Orleans made a triumphal entry into Madrid.

King Luis returned Spanish Habsburg etiquette to the court, but had little chance to do much else (Bergamini 1974). Philip and his Italian-born queen Elizabeth Farnese, who was Luis I's stepmother, continued to issue orders from San Ildefonso. Luis's immature wife so scandalized the Spanish court with her informality and her "strong penchant for water, for food, and for indecency" that the young king had her arrested at one point (ibid., 63). The intrigues and clashes between Luis and his parents plunged Spain into a dangerous crisis, as a result of which "either the son must have descended from the throne, or the father have changed his nominal for a real renunciation of power, if not his retreat for imprisonment" (Coxe, 1815, 3: 78–79). Smallpox resolved the crisis.

Seven months after his accession, Luis visited his parents at San Ildefonso from 7–12 August. Bergamini tells us that three or four days after returning to Madrid, the king of Spain and the Indies fainted at Mass, but was quickly revived. The king didn't leave the palace on the seventeenth and eighteenth, and on the twentieth he wrote his father, telling him, "I just went to bed, I have a cold" (Cardenas 1976, 490).

Smallpox was diagnosed the next day when Luis's doctors noticed a rash as they were applying a tourniquet to bleed him. The king's parents were told he had "benign smallpox" (*viruelas benignas*), a term that may have meant his physicians thought he had chickenpox (*Variola benigna*). Most members of the Spanish court evidently were firm believers in the contagionist theory, since they fled to the safety of another palace, abandoning fifteen-year-old Queen Isabel, who insisted on staying with Luis even though she had not had smallpox.

Communities and convents were asked to pray for the king's recovery, effigies of saints were carried in processions, and the remains of two saints whom the king especially revered were brought to his room in vain. Luis's rash began to fester on 25 August, his seventeenth birthday. By the twenty-ninth he was intermittently delirious and remained so the next day, when his father, through intermediaries, had the king sign a document approving his return to the throne. The archbishop of Madrid administered extreme unction (Danvilla 1902; Coxe 1815, vol. 3).

Luis died between two and three o'clock in the morning Thursday, 31 August 1724, in the eighth month of his reign, at Buen Retiro Palace. Cardenas thinks he may have been infected during excursions into the seedier districts of Madrid.

The king's body was embalmed, dressed in his full dress ceremonial uniform, and exhibited to the public in the Hall of the Kingdoms at Buen Retiro Palace.[7] Thousands of Spaniards viewed the remains of "Luis, el Buen Amado," while "as in the day of his birth, the women cried, and the prudent made intrigues" (Vega 1943, 178). How many caught smallpox from Luis's corpse, we do not know. On Sunday evening, 3 September, a funeral procession of Spanish officials and Luis's wife, which included neither his parents nor his brother, carried Luis Fernando de Borbon to his burial place in the Pantheon of the Kings at Escorial. There his remains were entombed in one of the nearly identical baroque sarcophagi, with the inscription, "Ludovicus I Hispan. Rex."

Luis's widow, whom he otherwise might have divorced, regained the favor of the king, his parents, and the country, by her courageous devotion at his sickbed. She contracted smallpox, but recovered and later retired to Paris. Philip V officially resumed the Spanish throne on 7 September, king of Spain for the second time by the grace of smallpox. He, his wife, and their ministers returned immediately to San Ildefonso, where they remained secluded for forty days, the standard period of "quarantine," to avoid contagion. Maneuvering at court now focused on the untenable positions of those who had supported Luis against his parents during his short reign. In the country at large,

> there was a notable lack of enthusiasm . . . upon the re-accession of the gloomy, middle-aged monarch. The bitterness would undoubtedly have been overpowering if Spain had known that it was destined for a twenty-two year deja vu of meaningless wars over Italian real estate. (Bergamini 1974, 67)

Luis's younger brother Don Ferdinand, now the prince of Asturias, recovered from an attack of smallpox in May 1728, a year when epidemic smallpox broke out in Valencia and spread to other regions. Philip V suffered a complete mental and physical breakdown early the same year, and tried to abdicate again in June, but was blocked by his wife (Coxe 1815, vol. 3; Reira 1977).

Despite the very public tragedy of Luis I, however, inoculation came to be used in Spain only in a small part of Andalusia at first. According to Kübler (1901) not until 1774 was the practice introduced into Madrid, and even then it was not widely disseminated. Thus Spain, which later took up vaccination with alacrity, was even more conservative than France in adopting inoculation. This Spanish conservatism is all the more intriguing since medieval Spanish Moors presumably knew about, and possibly practiced, inoculation.

Two years before Philip V's abdication, Peter the Great of Russia had issued his order requiring notification of any person with smallpox in his new capital on the Baltic. In 1719, Peter's French-born chief architect for St. Petersburg, Alexandre LeBlond, died of smallpox less than three years after arriving in Russia, but not before he completed plans for the gardens of Peter's magnificient palace on the Gulf of Finland, Peterhof (Petrodvoretz), built the main thoroughfare of Nevsky Prospect, and started some other projects (Massie 1980). Having executed his son Alexis for treason a few years earlier, the tsar issued an order in 1722 in which he renounced primogeniture and decreed that henceforth the successor to the Russian throne would be chosen by the reigning tsar. Thus when Peter I died a year after Luis I's demise, he was succeeded by his commoner wife, Catherine I. In 1727, Peter's eleven-and-a-half-year-old grandson, Peter Alexievich, succeeded Catherine I as Peter II (plate 9).

Since Peter II's mother had died at his birth and his father Alexis had been executed, the boy tsar was under the complete influence of one of the families of the Russian nobility, the Menshikovs, who promptly betrothed him to one of their daughters. At the outset of the new regime, Prince Menshikov, in the name of the tsar, forbade anyone living in houses where someone had smallpox from appearing at court or even at the palace. This ruling was reaffirmed several months later after the Menshikovs had fallen from power and been replaced by the Dolgorukys, another leading Russian family (Von Richter 1817).

In January 1728 the court moved from St. Petersburg to Moscow for Peter II's coronation in the Assumption Cathedral at the Kremlin. After the coronation, Peter and the Dolgorukys refused to return to St. Petersburg, reversing his grandfather's plans. As the boy tsar put it, "What am I to do in a place where there's nothing but salt water?" Or, more ominously, "I will not sail the seas as my grandfather did" (Bergamini 1969,

148). The government mint was also returned to Moscow, and according to Bergamini, even the mention of St. Petersburg was forbidden. Russia's new capital and fledgling navy were about to wither away. In keeping with his altered circumstances, Peter II was engaged again in November 1729, this time to Catherine Dolgoruky. They were to be wed at the end of January. Peter, who already understood German, French, and Latin, was maturing fast, and showed signs of restlessness at being manipulated by the Dolgorukys.

Von Richter (1817, vol. 3) records that Prince Sergei Dolgoruky's children came down with smallpox around this time, whereupon the prince allegedly ignored his own strict order and continued to appear at court. Whether this was really the source of Peter II's infection is uncertain. The fourteen-year-old tsar felt feverish on the night of 17 January, and it was assumed at first that he had caught a cold from standing in very cold weather with his head uncovered during a ceremonial review of his troops that day (Arseniev 1839). The definitive diagnosis was made on the twenty-first.

From the twenty-third to the twenty-eighth there was still some hope of recovery, even though the seriousness of his illness was fully appreciated. The tsar's condition then deteriorated suddenly, and he was already unconscious when the last rites of the church were administered to him on the twenty-ninth. He expired around 1:30 A.M. on 30 January, as nobles from all over Russia were gathered in the Kremlin on what was to have been his wedding day.

The Dolgorukys, whose control of an entire country was at stake, were not prepared to watch Peter II die without having chosen a successor. In a desperate attempt to remain in power, they created a most remarkable deathbed drama.

> During the final moments, Prince [Alexis] Dolgoruky in desperation thrust his daughter into the expiring Tsar's bed. Coitus having taken place, the prince was to announce, Catherine was rightful successor to the throne. (Bergamini 1969, 149)

Dolgoruky's scheme didn't succeed. But even in her old age, Cowles reported, Peter's intended bride remembered him as "my lovely eagle" (1971, 64).

Peter II was the last of the old male Romanov line. Bell (1836) argues that had he lived, he likely would have continued to reverse the reforms of his illustrious grandfather. His successor, a half niece of Peter I, transferred the Russian court from Moscow back to St. Petersburg.

Russia was at war with Sweden in 1741, when the fifty-three-year-old queen of Sweden, Ulrica Eleonora, contracted smallpox (plate 10). She had been elected queen with limited powers after her brother died in 1718, but officially transferred what little royal power remained to her husband, Frederick I, two years later. Ironically, according to Miller (1957) Queen Ulrica Eleonora's brother, King Charles XII, had apparently obtained a copy of Dr. Emanuele Timoni's writings on inoculation to prevent smallpox while he was in Turkey in 1713. Yet Sweden, like Spain and Russia, also delayed taking up inoculation. During the war with Russia, Sweden's army was weakened by low morale, hunger, and disease, some of which may also have been smallpox, since widespread outbreaks were reported in Sweden five years earlier (Svanstromi & Palmstierna 1934; Stromberg 1931; Zetterberg et al. 1966).

The official account of Ulrica Eleonora's death tells the course of the queen's illness (Govt. of Sweden 1741). Seventeen days after submitting to her usual quarterly bleeding, Ulrica Eleonora complained of chills, headache, cough, and fever. A day later, 20 November, the queen's back began to ache, but she was able to hear the sermon by the rector of Riddarholmen Church across the street from the palace, before being forced to withdraw into bed again. At the service, she especially ordered to be read "the verse she already since a long time had chosen for this day: Set thine house in order, for thou shalt die (Isaiah 38: 1)."

After the pocks, which first appeared on her face the following evening, increased in number and size, and the queen's face began to swell, Frederick visited her bedside hourly and ordered prayers to be said for her health in all churches. Queen Ulrica herself "knitted her hands together, and . . . called to the Highest to help, to stand by the Nation in the circumstances of the near future, and [bestowed] her blessings on all her true subjects." After briefly seeming to improve (it is interesting how frequently false signs of improvement were reported in royal vicitms), she died a few hours after becoming delirious and slipping into a coma. Of her death at Wrangelska Palace on the morning of 24 November the official account reported, "it happened so quietly that one at first had to shine a candle on the Queen before one could be convinced of this calamity taking place in Sweden."[8]

Since she had no children, Ulrica Eleonora's death raised the question of the Swedish succession. Denmark and Russia vied for the right to nominate a successor, the latter "as a condition for the return of Finland" (Scott 1972, 246–47). The Russians, who feared a union of Denmark and Sweden, prevailed in the matter of the Swedish succession, but they too, continued to suffer from smallpox.

The Russian tsarina Elizabeth had lost her fiancé, Prince Karl Augustus of Holstein-Gottorp, to smallpox not long before they were to be married. Perhaps the memories of that loss and the loss of her beloved nephew, Peter II, caused her to be extra cautious about the disease. Her government again declared smallpox a reportable disease soon after her accession. She forbade those in contact with persons who had smallpox to appear at court until four weeks after the patient in their house recovered; patients themselves had to wait seven weeks. The same year, according to Klein (1974), in preparation for a journey from St. Petersburg to Moscow, she ordered all smallpox patients to be removed from houses along the route to villages further away, and no one was to leave the contaminated houses when she and her entourage were in the vicinity. Thus, the Russian government, which had not yet embraced the practice of inoculation, sought strenuously to protect the tsarina by means of isolation and to protect the Russian public by requiring that cases be reported.

Three years later, the Russian empress's respect for smallpox was tested when another of her nephews, later Peter III, came down with the disease at Khotilovo, midway on a winter journey from Moscow to St. Petersburg. His doctors held out no hope for his life. Peter's fiancée, who had not had smallpox, was advised by her mother to abandon him, which she did. The tsarina had already reached St. Petersburg when she was told of her nephew's illness, and she turned back to care for him.

Peter survived, but in the words of his fiancée, later Catherine the Great, he had become "quite hideous" (Bergamini 1969, 207). Elizabeth arranged the reunion of the couple in a dim room at the palace in an attempt to soften the impact of Peter's appearance. "Unhappy as his childhood had been, Peter's real tragedy probably dated from his smallpox," which eroded his self-confidence by destroying his appearance (ibid.). If Bergamini's assessment is correct, this was one of the most consequential scarrings in history. Gantt (1937) records that Elizabeth's government issued Russia's first quarantine order, for persons with smallpox, a decade later.

At mid-century, inoculation was widely known in Europe, but as we have seen, it had still not been widely adopted on the continent outside Holland and Geneva. Indeed, in the decade and a half before 1740, inoculation appears to have been practiced less frequently in England than it had been shortly after its introduction, because of a lull in smallpox epidemics. Except for moderate epidemics in 1731, 1734, and 1736, London experienced something of a respite from epidemic smallpox between 1726 and 1745, although the disease remained endemic there. But improved inoculation techniques, a better understanding of the disease itself, and continuing murderous epidemics greatly increased the popularity of inoculation throughout Europe in the second half of the eighteenth century.

In England, inoculation's popularity resurged again in the 1740s, assisted by Dr. John Kilpatrick of Charleston, who came to London from South Carolina in 1743 with news of how he had successfully used inoculation to end a severe epidemic in Charleston five years earlier. Kilpatrick advocated inoculating with material taken from the arm of a previously inoculated person rather than from the pustules of a smallpox patient. He was not the first to do this, however: Charles Maitland had used that technique in 1722. In 1746 the London Small-Pox and Inoculation Hospital, the first of its kind in Europe, was instituted to care for inoculated patients during the period of their infectiousness and for poor persons with naturally acquired smallpox. According to Miller 1957, the Small-Pox and Inoculation Hospital and the new Foundling Hospital in London, where inoculation had been made mandatory for all children in 1743, were the only places in England that provided inoculations free at this time. However, religious objections to inoculation had almost disappeared.

Renewed British enthusiasm for inoculation was also stimulated by an unusually severe epidemic. The Bills of Mortality recorded over three thousand five hundred deaths from smallpox in London alone in 1752, more than seventeen percent of all the deaths in London that year. Many English physicians' resistance to inoculation was further dissipated when the College of Physicians in London strongly endorsed the practice in 1755, the same year inoculation began in France (Creighton 1894, vol. 2; Miller 1957).

The 1760s brought three important advances into focus, each of which contributed further to the medical Enlightenment. The first began around 1762, when Robert Sutton perfected, and later with his six sons and other English physicians began to employ widely, modified techniques for inoculation. Zwanenberg and, to some extent Razzell (1977a), give us a clear description of this process.

From the beginning, English inoculators had made deeper incisions for inoculation than was customary in Constantinople. They did so to make sure that their patients got inoculated smallpox and as a consequence of their erroneous belief that the "innate seeds," or "poison," of smallpox had to be allowed to escape from the body as the inoculation healed if the process was to be successful. In addition, the perceived need for weeks of elaborate, supervised medical care and diet before and after the inoculation had quickly become an integral part of the practice in England, with the result that it was an expensive operation. This need for careful preparation derived from the belief that luxurious living and a rich diet predisposed one to severe smallpox. By recommending much smaller incisions, or no incision at all, and careful selection of matter to be inoculated, the Suttons sharply reduced the severity and complications of the practice, including the frequency and density of secondary rashes. This minimized the personal risk previously associated with inoculation in England.

By also recommending that inoculees should be isolated during their convalescence, or that an entire community should be inoculated simultaneously, the Suttons decreased the potential danger convalescent inoculees posed to their communities. However, the reduced risk to communities following those Suttonian precepts may have been offset somewhat by the Suttons' advocacy of the "cold treatment," which required "airing" of inoculated patients, although patients were supposed to air themselves privately at home or on the grounds of special inoculation houses.

The other significant innovation of the "Suttonian method" was their shortening of the period required for preparing patients for routine inoculation. Even before the Suttons, some patients and their inoculators dispensed with preparation altogether when faced with an epidemic. Daniel Sutton began recommending a preparatory period of only eight to ten days, even while his father was still recommending a month of preparation. Eventually the need for any routine preparation was abandoned entirely, thus resuming the simpler practice Lady Mary had witnessed in Constantinople half a century before.

By the early 1760s, the Sutton brothers had inoculated some 30,000 persons using their modified method, of whom 1,200 died. Daniel Sutton alone inoculated nearly 14,000 persons between 1764 and 1766, and eventually claimed to have inoculated 40,000 persons with only 5 deaths. By reducing two of the last major objections to inoculation (personal risk of complications, and length of preparation), the Suttonian method was responsible to a large extent for the widespread popularity of inoculation in Europe until Jennerian vaccination advanced the concept further and made inoculation obsolete. By the end of the eighteenth century, it had become quite common to conduct a general inoculation for all susceptible persons in a community where smallpox broke out.

The second advance of the decade came in 1764 and 1767, when Dr. Angelo Gatti, formerly professor of Medicine at Pisa, published two treatises on inoculation in Brussels. Gatti's two volumes marked "the final demise of belief in the innate seed as the cause of smallpox; he stated clearly his belief that the 'variolous matter' was introduced into the human organism from outside, and subsequently transmitted from human body to human body. Once introduced, it reproduced itself and multiplied indefinitely." (Wilkinson 1979, 11). Gatti built on the works of two English predecessors, Benjamin Marten and Thomas Fuller, who in the 1720s and 1730s had published their conclusions that smallpox was acquired by inhaling contaminated air and was caused by a specific, distinct organism.

It will be recalled that in the early part of the eighteenth century, the European belief that smallpox was due to an inevitable change in innate seeds that were present in every human being at birth competed with the doctrine of an epidemic constitution, which attributed the disease to an unfavorable change in the atmosphere; with the corpuscular theory, which likened the contagion to tiny particles that affected the body in a manner analogous to poison; and with the less popular animalcular theory, according to which smallpox was caused by tiny, living, "animated atoms." In the course of the eighteenth century, concludes Miller, "the most simple change which can be demonstrated is that the material origin of the disease shifted from a location *inside* the body to one without, and linked with this was the increasing conviction that smallpox [was] a *specific* disease attributable to a specific material cause" (1957, 242). Miller considers the European experience with inoculation to be largely responsible for this "significant shift in emphasis." The general acceptance of the contagionist view was aided by the dispute over inoculation in France in the 1760s, when opponents of inoculation used that view as the basis for their arguments for controlling smallpox by isolation and quarantine, instead of by deliberate exposure through inoculation.

The same year that Gatti published his seond text at Brussels, William Heberden read a paper, "On the Chicken-pox," at the Royal College of Physicians in London. Although Fuller and one of his contemporaries had written of chickenpox as a distinct disease some forty years earlier, it was Heberden's paper published in 1768, that described varicella clinically and definitively established it as a separate disease, different from smallpox. This helped reduce the confusion about second attacks of smallpox and about the ability of a successful inoculation to prevent subsequent attacks, which had been another source of opposition to inoculation. One can only guess, for example, how many times inoculators in search of a mild case of smallpox would have mistakenly inoculated their patients with chickenpox virus (Razzell 1977a).

In 1754, the year before the College of Physicians endorsed inoculation in London, the British royal house of Hanover was reminded what smallpox had done to their Stuart predecessors. The Prince of Wales (later George III) fell ill with smallpox, but recovered. As king, he saw his four-year-old son Octavius die a few days after he was inoculated in 1783 (Creighton 1892; Derrick Baxby 1982, personal communication). He was the last immediate member of the British royal family to suffer from the disease.

As in England, the virus also reminded the French royal family of its power over princes and coupled that warning with a ferocious epidemic among residents of the capital. In 1752 the Dauphin Louis, son of Louis XV and father of Louis XVI, fell "dangerously ill" with smallpox. The French king, believing himself immune because he thought he had already had smallpox, solicitiously spent "whole days and nights" in the dauphin's room (Seward 1976, 152). The dauphin survived, and according to Cronin's 1974 study it was said that he fell in love with Marie Joseph, who was already his wife, as a result of her loving care for him during his illness. (Louis XV's favorite daughter, Louise Elizabeth, by then duchess of Parma, died of smallpox in 1759)

Unlike the English, however, neither the French public nor the French royal family were yet ready to be inoculated en masse. Despite the successful inoculation of the duc d'Orleans's two children in 1756, the debate about the practice continued among French physicians. Gatti, arriving in Paris in 1761, said he found "more brochures for and against inoculation than inoculations" (Klebs 1913, 79). When Paris suffered another severe outbreak of smallpox in 1762–63, the French blamed it on inoculation, and their parliament banned the practice in Paris and other towns. Across the English Channel, the response to comparable epidemics in London was renewed enthusiasm for inoculation.

In Sweden, which had lost its queen to smallpox a few years before, and where inoculation began almost simultaneously with the first efforts in France, the crown prince, later Gustav III, was inoculated. After the mid-eighteenth century, Sweden sought to combat smallpox with quarantine, isolation, and disinfection as well as inoculation. In some parts of that country, "smallpox houses" were established in the 1750s to deliberately expose children to smallpox and get that important crisis in their lives over with. Still, Kübler records that over two hundred and ninety thousand persons died of smallpox in Sweden during the last half of the eighteenth century. An unknown number were claimed during another epidemic in Iceland in 1762. A year later, there were outbreaks in Venice, Florence, and London. Vienna had five major epidemics between 1742 and 1759, before the virus attacked that city's royal family again.

Why so many of the Austrian Habsburgs died of smallpox has never been adequately explained. It may have been, as one historian suggests, that the billeting in town of courtiers and servants who worked in the Hofburg and the compact geography of the walled inner city "brought the [Viennese] court far closer to the ordinary life of the town than happened elsewhere as a rule" (McGuigan 1976, 202). The growth and increasing density of European cities almost certainly were major factors contributing to smallpox's increasing incidence among less exalted European urbanites.

Maria Theresa had been queen of Hungary and Bohemia for twenty years when smallpox visited the Habsburgs again in the 1760s. She was empress by marriage, and also in practice, but her husband, Francis Stephen of Lorraine, bore the title of Holy Roman Emperor. That crown could not be given to a woman. Maria Theresa's father had agreed to let her marry Francis Stephen, whom she adored, only after Francis's older brother Clement, to whom Maria Theresa was to be engaged, died of smallpox shortly before he was to leave for Vienna. The two progenitors of the House of Habsburg-Lorraine had sixteen children, of whom ten survived to adulthood. The empress-queen was thus well prepared to heed the ancient admonition to her house: "Let the strong fight wars; thou, happy Austria, marry: What Mars bestows on others, Venus gives to thee." Variola intercepted Venus many times at Maria Theresa's court (plate 11).

In 1761, the empress's favorite son, sixteen-year-old Archduke Charles Joseph, died of smallpox. The next year she buried her twelve-year-old daughter, Joanna Gabriele, for the same reason. The year after that, in November 1763, her son Joseph lost his much loved wife Isabella of Bourbon-Parma to the disease. Isabella was seven months pregnant when she was stricken and gave birth to a premature daughter who also died. Considering Joseph's strained relationship with his mother after he became emperor (Joseph II) when his father died, Isabella's intelligence, beauty, and her ability to get along well with her mother-in-law made her "one of the most fascinating might-have-beens of history" (Crankshaw 1969, 259). Two of the empress's other children, including Maria Antonia also had smallpox during the epidemic of 1763, but they recovered.

Joseph was married again in 1765, this time to the homely Maria Josepha of Bavaria, entirely for political reasons. Two years later, she too developed a smallpox rash and died at Schönbrunn Palace after five days on 28 May 1767. Joseph refused to marry again and had no surviving children. He was succeeded by his younger brother Leopold II, since Charles Joseph, who was two years older than Leopold and would ordinarily have been next in line, had died of smallpox (see fig. 4 above).

Maria Theresa had tried to comfort her frightened daughter-in-law on 23 May, the day Maria Josepha's rash began. Three days later, Boutry's 1903 account tells us, the empress herself developed a rash, which suggests that she and her daughter-in-law were infected about the same time, possibly by the same unknown source. At the news of their beloved empress's serious illness, crowds of Viennese filled the churches, joined religious processions, and crowded about the Hofburg. Her son-in-law Prince Albert of Saxony-Teschen came up to Vienna from Pressburg to convey his wishes for her recovery and got smallpox for his trouble. His mild rash appeared on 19 June. According to Moffat's biography, the empress was never unconscious and eventually recovered, but with some scarring. She attended a special thanksgiving service in St. Stephen's Cathedral, and a medal was struck to commemorate her recovery.

After the empress recovered, the court resumed preparations for the wedding of her daughter, Archduchess Maria Josepha, to the king of Naples. The preparations were nearly complete when the bride-to-be developed smallpox. She died, in Moffat's words, "still clinging to her brother" Joseph, on 15 October. Her sister Joanna Gabriele had also been engaged to the king of Naples, Fernando IV, when she died of smallpox five years earlier. Fernando finally married their younger sister, Maria Carolina.

Among others, Maria Josepha's imminent wedding attracted the Mozart family to Vienna, where it was hoped the eleven-year-old prodigy would perform at the festivities. When the wedding was canceled, and the epidemic raged out of control in the city, Mozart's family fled Vienna, but young Wolfgang was already infected. He became violently ill, with his eyelids swollen shut for nine days. Fortunately he recovered, with only a few pockmarks.

Maria Josepha had been taken by her mother to the imperial burial vault beneath the Capuchin church on 4 October, St. Francis's day, to pay their respects at the two-year-old tomb of the deceased emperor, Francis Stephen of Lorraine. They did not know then that the sarcophagus of Maria Josepha of Bavaria, who had died of smallpox that spring (her unembalmed corpse was placed in the crypt two hours after she died), was still unsealed. When Maria Josepha's smallpox rash appeared two days later, it was concluded that she had been infected while at the royal tomb, and Maria Theresa believed for the rest of her life that she had been responsible for her daughter's fatal infection. In a letter to another daughter on 4 October 1771, the empress wrote, "It is four years today since Josepha went with me to the vault and caught smallpox" (Moffat 1911, 311). The concept of an extended incubation period between acquisition of the infection and onset of the rash was just beginning to be appreciated in European medical circles partly as a result of inoculation (L. Wilkinson, personal communication). Since it takes at least a week, and usually two weeks for the smallpox rash to appear after a person is infected, and since Maria Joseph's rash appeared on 6 October the archduchess had to have been infected several days before she accompanied her mother to the Habsburg vault.

The final royal victims of the outbreak in 1767 were Archduchess Marianna and Archduchess Elizabeth, who McGuigan describes as "the great beauty of the family" and whose rash appeared 21 October. The twenty-four-year-old Elizabeth, who was known to be especially vain, had been infected by her sister, Maria Josepha. When she realized what her diagnosis was, Elizabeth immediately called for a mirror, "taking leave of those features she had so often heard praised, and which she believed would be greatly changed before she should see them again" (Moffat 1911, 312). She did not die of the infection, but the scarring she feared became real. Both archduchesses died years later, ravaged, pockmarked spinsters who spent the latter part of their lives as abbesses in charge of convents, Elizabeth at Innsbruck and Marianna at Prague.[9]

One can only wonder what Maria Theresa's chancellor Prince Kaunitz, who according to Crankshaw had a "pathological fear of smallpox, even the mention of it" must have done with himself at her court in the 1760s (1969, 275).

The empress's Dutch doctor, Leyden-trained Gerard van Swieten, who preferred the red treatment, bleeding, and dark rooms for his smallpox patients, had opposed inoculation. After the terrible ordeal of 1767, the empress and van Swieten wrote to England's King George III and his personal physician and through them secured the services of another Dutch physician, Dr. Jan Ingenhousz. Ingenhousz came to Vienna and successfully inoculated Archdukes Ferdinand and Maximillan, and an archduchess in 1768. On the same occasion, Maria Theresa established a smallpox hospital in Vienna, and inaugurated inoculation in Austria by inviting sixty-five of the first children inoculated there to dinner in the gallery of Schönbrunn Palace, waiting on them herself, assisted by her own children (Coxe 1820).

When Louis XV wrote to express concern that his great-grand-daughter had been inoculated, Emperor Joseph II enclosed with his reply a short note from six-year-old Archduchess Theresa (daughter of Joseph and Isabella) to the king of France:

> Knowing that you love me, dear grandpapa, I assure you that I am astonishingly well. I had only fifty pocks, which give me great pleasure. (Moffat 1911, 313)

The number of "pocks" or pustules was an anxiously awaited sign of the severity of induced infections.

In Austria, therefore, the momentous epidemic in the royal family and the empress's reaction to it finally overcame the resistance to inoculation. Despite the tragedy in Austria, the French royal family still did not feel inspired to adopt inoculation. But Maria Theresa's antithetical contemporary, the Russian empress Catherine the Great, did.

In July 1768, the same year Dr. Ingenhousz introduced inoculation among the Habsburgs in Vienna, an extraordinary courier arrived in London from St. Petersburg. He was the second such courier to arrive that month. Both had the same purpose: to persuade Dr. Thomas Dimsdale, who was a friend and former teacher of Dr. Ingenhousz and probably the most prominent practitioner of the Suttonian method of inoculation besides the Suttons themselves, to journey to Russia to inoculate their empress Catherine II and her son the Grand Duke Paul. Earlier that year, Dimsdale had met the Russian ambassador to London at the home of Dr. John Fothergill, an influential Quaker physician who was later indirectly connected with the introduction of Jenner's vaccine to the United States.

The tsarina had no lack of reasons for wanting to protect herself and her people against smallpox, and it is interesting to consider what caused her to make up her mind in 1768. Clendenning (1973) believed she may have been influenced by the death of her foreign minister's fiancée, Countess Anna Sheremetev, from smallpox soon after her accession in 1762, by a recent victory of proinoculation forces in France against conservatives of the French church and university, and by the essay *Sur l'Insertion de la petite vérole* written in 1731 by Voltaire, whom she admired greatly and with whom she corresponded. But, Bishop (1932) found that the earliest known reference to inoculation in their correspondence is in a letter from Voltaire dated after Catherine had been inoculated. The tsarina no doubt was also influenced by the death of Tsar Peter II from smallpox, and by the "hideous" appearance of her own assassinated husband, Peter III, following his attack of smallpox. In addition, an epidemic attributed to Russian soldiers had killed over twenty thousand of her Siberian subjects in the past year. But the recent tragedy at Maria Theresa's court was probably uppermost in Catherine II's mind when she dispatched her couriers to England.

Dimsdale was an independently wealthy, highly regarded, middle-aged physician who was understandably reluctant to undertake such a risky assignment. After much persuasion, he agreed. He and his son, who was then a medical student in Edinburgh, left London with an escort on 28 July 1768 and arrived in St. Petersburg a month later via Amsterdam, Berlin, Danzig and Riga.

When they arrived in St. Petersburg, Dimsdale and his son were cloistered under guard in a large house. Two days after his arrival, Dimsdale was greeted by the Russian foreign minister, Count Panin, who told him,

> You are now called sir to the most important employment that perhaps any gentleman was ever entrusted with. To your skill and integrity will probably be submitted nothing less than the precious lives of *two* of the greatest personages in the world; with whose safety the tranquility and happiness of this great empire are so intimately connected that, should an accident deprive us of either, the blessings we now enjoy might be exchanged for the utmost state of misery and confusion. (Rappaport 1907, 61–62)

Had Dimsdale not been reluctant to come to St. Petersburg in the first place, the enormity of his mission must surely have weighed on him after Panin's salutation (no doubt the Suttons' recent improvements in inoculation must have seemed inadequate to him now.) Dimsdale and his son were housed, feasted, and entertained luxuriously at the Russian court, but as he wrote, "Many corroding cares disturb me, and embitter all this greatness which I am not able to enjoy" (Fox 1919, 88).

On the fourth day after his arrival, Dimsdale was presented to the empress in a private audience at her summer palace. "She is," he wrote, "of all that I ever saw of her sex the most engaging. She has a way of pleasing, without appearing to have an art" (Bishop 1932, 327). In subsequent interviews, the empress asked several intelligent, penetrating questions about inoculation. But when Dimsdale tried to get her to let her own physicians assist him with her inoculation (and share any blame, should things go wrong), she refused, saying:

> You are come well recommended to me; the conversation I have had with you on this subject has been very satisfactory, and my confidence in you is increased; I have not the least doubt of your abilities and knowledge in this practice; it is impossible that my physicians can have much skill in this operation; they want experience; their interposition may tend to embarrass you without the least probability of giving any useful assistance. My life is my own, and I shall with the utmost cheerfulness and

confidence rely on your care alone. . . . I have also to acquaint you, that it is my determination to be inoculated before the Grand Duke, and as soon as you judge it convenient; at the same time I desire that this may remain a secret business, and I enjoin you to let it be supposed that, for the present, all thoughts of my own inoculation are laid aside. The preparation of this great experiment on the Grand Duke will countenance your visits to the palace, and I desire to see you as often as it may be necessary, that you may become still better acquainted with what relates to my constitution, and also for adjusting the time, and other circumstances, of my own inoculation. (Ibid.)

Dimsdale said he "bowed and promised obedience, but with great anxiety" (Fox 1919, 89). When he suggested hopefully that some trial inoculations might first be conducted on other persons of similar age, sex, and constitution, the empress told him "that if the practice had been novel, or the least doubt of the general success had remained, that precaution might be necessary; but as she was well satisfied in both particulars there would be no occasion for delay" (Bishop 1932, 327).

Dimsdale was summoned to the Winter Palace with a young boy whom he had previously inoculated late Sunday evening, 12 October, six weeks after his arrival. Led up a secret back stairway to the empress's bedroom, he inoculated her once in each arm. The next morning, she left the Winter Palace for Tsarskoe Selo, her summer residence several miles outside the capital, where Dimsdale supervised her convalescence. After a few days, she developed fever, pain, and a moderate number of pustules, but was able to return to St. Petersburg in perfect health near the end of October. A prolonged convalescence or death of the empress at this time would have been very inconvenient, since war broke out unexpectedly between Russia and the Ottoman Empire that month. Dimsdale inoculated the fourteen-year-old grand duke on 2 November, and he also had a favorable outcome.

When the successful inoculations became known, the nobles of St. Petersburg rushed to follow the empress's example. As in Vienna that same year and England nearly a half century before, gold medals were struck to commemorate the royal inoculations. According to Fox (1919), Dimsdale inoculated more than 140 persons in St. Petersburg, and more than 50 others in Moscow, all of whom recovered. By instructing Russian physicians in the technique, he and his son helped establish inoculation hospitals in both cities. Catherine later wrote to Voltaire and boasted that "more people had been inoculated here in one month than in Vienna in a year" (Durant 1967, 454), a statement that seems to confirm the influence of events in Austria on the Russian empress's decision to be inoculated.

The child from whose arm the virus was taken to inoculate the empress was made a noble for his role in the operation. The Russian senate cited the empress for her bravery with an inscription that read "She saved others to the danger of herself." Her public bravado and real courage notwithstanding, Catherine had quietly taken care to ensure Dimsdale's personal safety if she or the heir to the throne had died as a result of the inoculations. The empress, "in order to render his escape from Russia easy, secretly ordered relays of horses to be ready for his flight all along the line, from the capital to the frontier of her dominions" (Molloy 1906, 2: 354).

Dimsdale did not have to flee Russia. Instead, the empress gave him permission to add the wing of the Black Eagle of Russia to his coat of arms. She also awarded him a fee of ten thousand pounds, plus two thousand pounds for travel expenses, a pension of five hundred pounds per year, diamond-studded miniature portraits of herself and the grand duke, made him a councillor of state, and proclaimed him an hereditary baron of the Russian Empire. According to Clendenning's account, a noble whose children had been inoculated presented him with a bag of gold coins so heavy, Dimsdale said, that he limped while carrying it out of the room. These overwhelming manifestations of gratitude may also be taken as striking illustrations of how deeply Dimsdale's benefactors feared smallpox. Dimsdale's patent of nobility stated in part:

> We Catherine the Second by the Grace of God Empress and Autocratrix of all the Russias . . . make known [that] in justice to the rare merit of Thomas Dimsdale English Gentleman and Doctor of Physic whose virtue and laudable concern for the good of mankind . . . induced him . . . to apply all his . . . faculties towards improving the inoculation of the smallpox, as the only rational preservation of the human species against that mortal disease, and [who] has raised this practice to such a degree of perfection, as that all the apprehensions of danger from the smallpox in the natural way may be . . . dispelled; who, regardless of his private Interest, and intent only upon accelerating human Happiness, did not hesitate to lay open to the World his Discoveries; who . . . refused not on our invitation to leave his Family and to visit our Court, purely to render Us all the services in his Power, . . . and who at last did with remarkable Care Skill and Success actually inoculate as well Us Ourselves and Our beloved Son the Czarowitz and Grand Duke, as also many inhabitants of Our Capitol, and who thus removing the anxious Fears of our Faithful Subjects destroyed at the same time that baleful Hydra Prejudice, and the dreadful apprehensions of this (hitherto) fatal disease. We have been pleased to testify to the said Thomas Dimsdale our grace and favour, by such . . . marks of distinction as shall not only tend to his . . . Honour for ever, but may also excite his Posterity and other Learned Men, . . . to pursue such studies and Investigations of Nature as may prove equally beneficial to the human Species. (Fox 1919, 92)

Baron Dimsdale returned to Russia thirteen years later when he was invited to inoculate the grand duke's two sons, Princes Alexander and Constantine.

Klebs (1914) tells us that an attempt to introduce inoculation in St. Petersburg in the 1750s, without royal sponsorship and example, was unsuccessful, although Tooke records that some Siberian tribes had apparently already known about inoculation before Dimsdale entered Russia. They used a fish bone dipped in pus from a smallpox patient to inoculate themselves.

When Dimsdale taught Russian physicians to inoculate, smallpox epidemics were recurring at regular intervals among the various populations in the Russian Empire. Despite inoculation's introduction among the noble families of Moscow and St. Petersburg, at the end of the eighteenth century smallpox was still killing an estimated two million Russians annually (Bishop 1932).

The toll of deaths from smallpox was even greater in the Polish provinces of the Russian Empire. Referring to the latter, Tooke observed: "We may confidently state the mortality at six or seven out of ten, and such as escape this fate are almost always cruelly disfigured. Hence it is also that no country in Europe so swarms with blind people as Poland" (1800, 2: 70–71). Here, too, as in England, Austria, Russia, and apparently Sweden, inoculation's debut as an acceptable medical practice was associated with the royal court.[10] Two years before the Russian empress was inoculated, the first surgeon to the king of Poland paid a visit to Daniel Sutton in England. When smallpox inoculation was first reported from Poland a year after Catherine's ordeal, the Polish king's court physician and the rector of the Cracow Academy were its chief promoters. In neighboring Prussia, Frederick the Great summoned an English inoculator to Berlin in 1775 to instruct Prussian physicians in an attempt to popularize the practice (Zwanenberg 1978; Chizynski & Rozewska-Chizynska 1972; Klebs 1913).

Smallpox, of course, wasn't the only infectious disease with which Catherine had to contend. An epidemic of plague in Moscow in 1771 "brought such scenes of terror, superstitious savagery, and violence that much of the population seemed to have gone beserk" (Coughlan 1974, 269). The Russian empress sent her companion Gregory Orlov to the city, and he successfully restored order. To commemorate his return, Catherine built a triumphal arch on St. Petersburg's Nevsky Prospect and had it inscribed "To Him Who Saved Moscow from the Plague." The next year, when she had taken a new lover, the Empress and Autocratrix of all the Russias used the legitimate excuse of a smallpox quarantine to keep Orlov out of St. Petersburg (ibid., 270).

The French, meanwhile, still banned inoculation in their cities. Klebs estimated that up until this time, two hundred thousand inoculations had been performed in England, compared to about fifteen thousand in more populous France. Voltaire, writing the Russian empress in February 1769, was almost beside himself:

Oh, Madam, what a lesson Your Majesty is giving to us pretty Frenchmen, to our ridiculous Sorbonne and to the argumentative charlatans in
our medical schools! You have been inoculated with less fuss than a nun
taking an enema. The Crown Prince has followed your example. Count
Orlov goes hunting in the snow after his inoculation against the Smallpox. . . . We French can hardly be inoculated at all, except by decree of
the Parliament. I do not know what has become of our nation, which used
at one time to set great examples in everything. (Clendenning 1973, 123)

The French re-called inoculation from the countryside when their
new king, Louis XVI, was inoculated in June 1774. His frivolous young
queen's milliner even designed a fanciful hairstyle, *pouf a l'inoculation,* to
celebrate the operation's success. This turnabout in the French attitude
toward inoculation resulted from the totally unexpected death of Louis
XV from smallpox.

The aging king spent a pleasant spring evening dining with his
thirty-one-year-old mistress, Madame du Barry, and her husband at
Trianon the day before he became ill. Louis was sixty-four, and had been
king of France for fifty-nine years, and he was still reputed to be "the
handsomest man at court" (Seward 1976, 169) (plate 12). The next day,
27 April, he awoke with a slight headache, pains in his back, and shivering. By evening, the aches and pains were worse, and he was feverish. His
doctors brought him back to the main palace at Versailles in his dressing
gown on 28 April. As the king's symptoms intensified, the six physicians,
five surgeons, and three apothecarys in attendance decided to bleed him.
Since a third bleeding was almost always followed by the last sacrament,
Louis's doctors bled him only twice, to minimize his alarm and that of the
court. They took care, however, "to make the second bleeding so heavy
that it would take the place of a third," withdrawing "four large basin-
fuls," according to one witness (D'Angerville 1924, 349). No specific
diagnosis had been made, but it was obvious that the king of France was
very ill.

In the meantime, Madame du Barry had remained at Louis's bedside,
angry that he had been moved from Trianon to Versailles in the first
place. His physicians were at pains not to manifest unwarranted concern
for the king's condition, however, since if he were extremely ill, as to
require three bleedings for example, he would have to receive the last
sacrament. And in order for him to receive the last sacrament, Madame
du Barry would have to be sent away. This last act could mean trouble for
those who were indirectly responsible for it, if the king recovered and du
Barry regained her influential position. The court was divided into those
who intrigued for or against her removal.

Louis was afraid for his health almost to the point of cowardice. Each
of the fourteen medical people attending him were repeatedly called to
the edge of the state bed, one after the other, to examine some part of His

Most Catholic Majesty's person. The grand master of the wardrobe, who was present, wrote that, "during all these inspections great care was taken to keep the light, which bothered him and of which he had already complained, out of the King's eyes, the rays being allowed only to shine on the part it was desired to illuminate" (ibid., 351).

Finally, on the fourth day of his illness, an accidental illumination of the king's face revealed an unmistakable rash. He had smallpox, the possibility of which had not been seriously considered before the rash was discovered. According to the 1971 article "L'inoculation et Louis XV," Louis and his doctors believed he had had smallpox thirty years before and therefore was immune. Relieved, however, at having a specific diagnosis at last, even if it was smallpox, Louis's doctors "left the King's room to make the announcement to the royal family, saying that at last they knew what the matter really was, that there was no room for doubt, that the King was prepared for it and that all would go well" (D'Angerville 1924, 354). One of the doctors broke the news to Madame du Barry. Louis's grandson and heir, who had not had smallpox, was barred from the king's apartments. The king's three daughters, who also had not had smallpox, refused to leave their father's bedside.

Whether or not the king should be told he had smallpox was discussed at some length, the grand master of the wardrobe and others fearing that the mere knowledge that he had such a dread disease would kill him. Finally the king was told, whereupon he calmly ordered Madame du Barry, in whose presence—according to a French historian quoted by Major (1936)—he had often "forgot . . . the burdens of the kingdom," to leave the court. "Go to Rueil . . . and there await my orders, but be always assured of my affection" (Cabanes 1897, 56–57).

He received the last sacrament on 7 May and became delirious the following day. By 9 May "he was motionless, his mouth open, his face neither deformed nor showing any sign of agitation, but towards the end swollen and copper-coloured" (Cronin 1974, 51). According to Cabanes, "The body of the King was falling to pieces, in a state of living putrescence, and the smell was horribly fetid" (1897, 56–57). On Tuesday, 19 May 1774, Louis XV died, shortly after 3:00 A.M.[11] When a candle in his bedroom window was extinguished as a prearranged signal of his death, the new king and his wife, who had been keeping a vigil from their apartments across the courtyard, immediately left Versailles for the safety of another palace. The entire court went with them, except for the few whose duties required them to remain with the corpse.

The elaborate formalities and ceremonies usually followed on the death of a French king were prudently ignored. The Faculty of Medicine at Paris wrote regarding their right to be represented at all royal autopsies, and the king's chamberlain requested the chief surgeon to proceed with an autopsy. But the surgeon informed the lord chamberlain, "your duties oblige you to hold the head of the defunct. I declare to you, if the body is opened, neither you nor I nor anyone present at the autopsy will be alive a week later" (Major 1936, 123–24). No autopsy was performed, nor was the body embalmed. Instead, Louis's deteriorating corpse was placed in double lead coffins, covered with lime, vinegar, spices and wine, and hastily escorted to the royal crypt at Saint-Denis. The funeral ceremonies and lying-in-state of Louis XIV had lasted seven weeks. His great-grandson's body was lowered into the crypt of the Bourbons in less than two days. Seward (1976) reports that it was alleged that one of the workers who helped put Louis's coffin into the crypt died of uncontrollable vomiting brought on by the stench.

From this account, it is evident that the idea of smallpox's contagiousness was well appreciated at the French court by the 1770s. At the same time the diagnosis and treatment of smallpox, despite Sydenham's improvements, were much less advanced in France and elsewhere in Europe. Louis's diagnosis and treatment were scarcely any better than that afforded to Mary II of England at the end of the seventeenth century.

In Paris, news of the dissolute king's illness and death caused no outpouring of sadness. On the contrary. D'Angerville (1924) tells us that in contrast to the occasion of the king's serious illness three decades before, after which his relieved countrymen began calling him "Louis, the Well-Beloved," by May 1774, some Frenchmen were calling his successor "Louis, the Longed-For." (It was, of course, "Louis the Longed-For" who the French sent to the guillotine only fifteen years later.) In France it was widely rumored that the king had caught smallpox from a teenaged girl who had been coerced into sharing his bed a few weeks earlier. Others said the king was infected during a chance encounter with the funeral procession of a peasant victim of smallpox. Smallpox was not epidemic in Paris that year, but it was epidemic in the town of Versailles. The countess of Provence had contracted the disease shortly after her marriage, and the Spanish ambassador to Louis's court had recently died of it. (Inoculation was finally taken up in Madrid the same year.)

In all, fifty persons at court had smallpox soon after the king's illness, including two of his faithful daughters. Ten of them died. At Choisy, twenty-year-old Louis XVI spent the first nine days of his reign in quarantine, "unable even to see his ministers" (Cronin, 1974, 57–58). Louis and his brothers were inoculated in June and had to be isolated again for that reason.

What effect, if any, Louis XV's death from smallpox in 1774 may have had on the French Revolution fifteen years later, or on France's role in the American Revolution, we shall never know. Had he lived longer, wrote the historian Desmond Seward (1976), Louis XV might have saved the French monarchy; as it was, his unpopular reign probably contributed to its demise. But as fateful as Louis XV's death may have been, France soon paid another steep political price for neglecting inoculation.

Four years after he came to the throne, Louis XVI's government was at war with England, having entered the American War of Independence on the colonials' side in an effort to limit English power and protect France's interests in the New World. Spain, Europe's other major naval power, joined her French ally by declaring war on England in June 1779. By August that year, France had assembled forty thousand men to invade England at a time when much of Britain's military might was on the other side of the Atlantic, fighting the Americans. Jenkins described France and Spain's intentions in his *History of the French Navy* (1973, 158):

> The plan for the invasion of England was comparatively simple. Two armies, each of twenty thousand, were to be assembled with their transports, one at St. Malo, the other at Le Havre. D'Orvilliers was to take the main French fleet from Brest, join the Spanish fleet, and the combined force of over sixty of the line, which would give them odds of three to two over any force the English could put to sea, was to take command of the Channel. The troop transports were then to unite north of Cherbourg and be escorted to land the soldiers on the Isle of Wight and round Portsmouth, destroying the English naval base in the Channel preparatory to a march on London.

According to Thursfield (1940) the French and Spanish fleets united, and the combined armada of sixty-six ships and fourteen frigates appeared off the coast of Plymouth, "with the wind in their favor." Napoleon later considered that command of the English Channel for two days would be ample time for a successful invasion of England. The "Other Armada" of 1779 dominated the Channel for more than three days. Admiral Hardy and his thirty-eight British ships were nowhere in sight. To the English on shore, wrote the British parlimentarian and historian George Otto Trevelyan, "nothing was certain except that the most powerful armada that ever walked the waters had inserted itself between the British fleet and the British arsenals and dockyards" (1912, 1: 193). As the *Cambridge Modern History* stated, "Never perhaps has England been in more serious danger of invasion than in July 1779" (Ward et al. 1909, 376). Ill-defended Plymouth awaited its fate.

Thursfield summarized Trevelyan's account of what happened:

> And yet the French did not attack. It was for them the golden opportunity, but they lay there for three days and made no effort. The reason was that they had smallpox on board, and far from being in a condition to fight, they were so weakened that it would have been impossible to maneuver their ships. On August 16, their sick were "at least equal" to the number of sound men. Their line-of-battle ships had many of them from 50 to 60 percent of their crews [out of combat] and the dead were flung overboard in such numbers that it is recorded that "the inhabitants

of Plymouth ate no fish for a month." On August 18, a wind increasing to
a gale blew from the east and the weakened French and Spanish fleets
were blown a hundred miles into the Atlantic. . . . So ended a threat of
invasion, which came nearer to success than either that or the Armada or
that of Napoleon. (1940, 318)

Variola ruled the waves. Far from securing the invasion of England,
the "Other Armada" captured one British ship. Mortified, the French and
Spanish allies blamed each other for the disaster. Both were at fault.

The Spanish fleet under Admiral Don Luis de Cordoba had arrived at
the rendezvous from Cadiz on 23 July, more than six weeks late. Admiral
d'Orvilliers's ships had set out from Brest on 4 June with smallpox and
"putrid fever" (typhus) on board. Soon, "first one [French] ship and then
the other began to signal that she had a number of cases of serious illness
aboard. In the first half of July putrid fever and smallpox began to gather
momentum" (Patterson 1960, 162). The French were also running short
of supplies, so that by the time the apparently powerful combined force
appeared off Plymouth on 16 August, "it was already almost at the end of
its tether and practically powerless. Sickness was continuing to spread in
French and Spanish vessels alike" (ibid., 205). In addition to smallpox and
typhus, scurvy apparently claimed some of the victims. More than eight
thousand sailors, mostly Frenchmen, died at sea (Jenkins 1973; Patterson
1960; Del Perugia 1939; Coulter & Coulter 1961, vol. 3; Tormo 1949).

Smallpox saved the British, but it did not spare them.[12] Nearly twenty-
five hundred deaths from the disease were recorded in London in 1779,
and it claimed another thirty-five hundred Londoners two years later.
During the last two decades of the eighteenth century, smallpox killed
over thirty-six thousand persons in London, and an equal number in
Glasgow. This constituted almost one out of every ten deaths in London,
and nearly a fifth of all the deaths in Glasgow in that period. In Glasgow
even more than elsewhere, the overwhelming majority of the victims were
still young children, since nearly all surviving adults were immune. In
English towns, nine of every ten persons who died of smallpox were
under five years old.

Smallpox was always present in Britain's densely populated large
cities, even between epidemics. In London's population of about 750,000
for example, 1,039 deaths from the disease were recorded in 1773, a non
epidemic year. In the more sparsely populated countryside, it commonly
appeared only in epidemics in intervals of several years. Thus, for young
adults from rural areas who had previously escaped infection, smallpox
was one of the most serious risks they faced in the big cities.

On the continent also, smallpox was still terribly destructive. Its
continuing toll is only weakly reflected two centuries later by the bare
numbers of victims that remain for our consideration. Copenhagen,
which increased from 60,000 inhabitants in 1750 to 84,000 at the end of

the century, lost 12,309 persons from smallpox in the same period. In Sweden, major epidemics in 1779 and 1784 killed over 27,000 persons in those two years alone. Rosen von Rosenstein, a Swedish physician, reported that smallpox killed ten percent of all Swedish infants each year. In Russia, Sir Alexander Crichton, the tsar's British physician, reported that one-seventh of all Russian infants died of the disease annually. In France also, La Condamine had said that one of every ten persons born in that country died of smallpox. Berlin recorded six smallpox epidemics, which carried off about a thousand inhabitants each, between 1766 and 1795. The epidemic in 1795 was thought to have been started by freshly inoculated persons, and epidemics in Weimar (1788) and Hamburg (1794) were attributed to the same cause. In Vienna, over sixteen thousand persons were infected during an outbreak in 1790, of whom about fifteen hundred died. Iceland had another epidemic in 1786.

The year of Jenner's discovery, 1796, smallpox killed over three thousand five hundred persons in an epidemic in London. Throughout Great Britain and Ireland, the disease claimed an estimated thirty-five thousand more lives that year, and in the German-speaking states, over sixty-five thousand deaths were attributed to it. Europe (excluding Russia) was losing over four hundred thousand citizens each year to death by smallpox, which was also responsible for more than a third of all the blindness in Europe. As recently as the middle of the eighteenth century, a French physician estimated that about one fourth of all mankind was being killed, blinded, or disfigured for life by smallpox.

The tragic, agonizing experience of one otherwise typical young Englishwoman who died within a month of Jenner's discovery illustrates how smallpox often ruined the lives of countless anonymous ordinary individuals, even when it didn't kill them. Miss Anna Rhodes's memorial monument is preserved in London's Victoria and Albert Museum (on loan from the Diocese of London):

> Erected by a Sister in Memory of her beloved ANNA CECILIA, Daughter of Christopher Rhodes esq; of *Chatham* in the County of *Kent.* She departed this life, June 2d 1796, aged 32. Her Remains were deposited in the 42d Vault of this Chapel. Distinguished by a fine Understanding, and a most amiable Disposition of Heart, She was the Delight of her Parents, and the Admiration of all who knew her. At the Age of 17, the Small-pox stripped off all the Bloom of youthful Beauty, and being followed by a dreadful Nervous-disorder, withered those fair Prospects of earthly Happiness which were expected from her uncommon Affection, Sensibility and Tenderness. After enduring this afflictive Dispensation many Years, when it was difficult to say which exceeded, her Sufferings or her Submission; her Friends' Concern for her Sorrows, or their Admiration of her Patience; She was released by Death, and received into that World where there shall be no more Pain, but GOD himself shall wipe away Tears from every Eye.

Whether Miss Rhodes's condition was caused by psychological damage from severe scarring of her face or was a result of direct neurological damage from the virus, is unknown.

Shortly before the eighteenth century ended, smallpox claimed one more Spanish prince. The seventy-two-year-old reigning monarch, Carlos III, had five sons, one of whom was Fernando IV, the king of Naples and Sicily who earlier had lost two Viennese fiancées to the disease. Coxe (1815) records that Fernando's talented brother, Don Gabriel, became infected while ministering to his Portuguese wife and their newborn infant, both of whom died of smallpox about three weeks before he succumbed on 23 November 1788. This was apparently the last such tragedy from smallpox among European royalty. Edward Jenner discovered vaccination less than a decade later.

Despite the disease's continuing ravages, by the end of the eighteenth century, inoculation had reduced smallpox's impact in European communities where it was widely practiced. This more general improvement in the public's health must be distinguished from the personal health of individuals who were successfully inoculated, personal benefits having been manifest as soon as inoculation began in Europe in 1721. Peter Razzell, a sociologist with a special interest in historical demography, presents evidence of inoculation's favorable impact in rural districts of England in his 1977 study *The Conquest of Smallpox*. Indeed, in an earlier article in the *Economic History Review* Razzell attributes the increase in life expectancy at birth in eighteenth-century England to the introduction of inoculation against smallpox. As he also noted, recent medical studies suggest that natural smallpox infections sometimes damaged the testes, thereby reducing the fertility of surviving male victims. Thus inoculation's effect on population growth in Europe may have included a significant reduction in the prevalence of under fertility in adult males (Phadke et. al. 1973).

Inoculation's beneficial impact on public health in the latter part of the century resulted partly from the increased practice of "general inoculations" of entire villages and towns simultaneously when smallpox threatened, a practice that the Suttonian method facilitated. After the Suttons perfected their cheaper, safer method in the 1760s, many more poor people were inoculated without charge. The substantial costs of caring for ill paupers during smallpox epidemics led some parishes to pay willingly for inoculations for the poor. In some instances, burial costs were deemed so great that many parishes compelled everyone within their jurisdiction to be inoculated.

In contrast to the comparatively widespread, systematic practice of inoculation in the countryside, inoculation in large towns and cities was more haphazard and in Razzell's words, "greatly neglected." As a result, in London at least, the risk of dying from smallpox increased during most of the eighteenth century, with only a negligible decline towards the end. According to Guy (1882) in the London Bills of Mortality, the proportion of deaths from smallpox to 1000 deaths from all causes in successive twenty-five year periods of the eighteenth century was 73.2, 75.4, 96.6, and 91.7 (see fig. 5 below). This increase appears to have been a continuation of the momentum of increasing smallpox among Europeans since the sixteenth century. Whether sporadic inoculations in London contributed to the increase, and if so how much, is not clear.

England's John Haygarth published a plan in 1793 that built on a scheme he had proposed to John Fothergill fifteen years earlier. In his *Sketch of a Plan to Exterminate the Casual Small-Pox From Great Britain,* Haygarth proposed systematic inoculation throughout the country, isolation of patients, decontamination of potentially contaminated fomites, supervised inspectors responsible for specific districts, rewards for observance of rules for isolation by poor persons, fines for transgression of those rules, inspection of vessels at ports, and prayers every Sunday.

By the end of the eighteenth century, inoculation had had a definite, if limited impact on the incidence of smallpox in Europe. However, as Miller (1957) points out, more important was that as the "chief *medical* contribution of the Enlightenment," it helped advance Europeans' understanding of the disease significantly. Thus, the experience with inoculation as an effective specific tool against smallpox, in Europe and North America especially, enabled inhabitants of those two continents to exploit Jenner's vaccine almost as soon as it was discovered. In that sociological, nonbiological sense, Jennerian vaccination was not an abrupt break with the past, but the direct descendant and heir of inoculation.

Edward Jenner, 1749–1823

Edward Jenner was born 17 May 1749 at Berkeley, Gloucestershire, England (plate 13). Orphaned at age five, he was raised by his oldest brother. After preliminary schooling he studied surgery and pharmacy as an apprentice to Daniel Ludlow of Sodbury, beginning in 1762. It was during this period at Sodbury that he said he first heard a country girl remark that she could not be infected with smallpox because she had already had the cowpox. This knowledge had been extant in England for over a century, and not only among "country girls." Around the middle of the seventeenth century, the duchess of Cleveland, one of King Charles II's favorites, is said to have remarked that she did not fear losing her beauty, and thus her position at court, through disfigurement from smallpox since she had had cowpox (Major 1936).

In 1770, Jenner went to London, where he studied at St. George's Hospital under John Hunter for two years. Jenner and Hunter shared a mutual interest in natural history, which was part of the basis for their long friendship. According to Dixon (1962), Jenner turned down an appointment as naturalist on Captain Cook's voyage in 1772 in order to begin practicing medicine on his own at Berkeley in 1773.

Over the next two decades, Jenner practiced medicine, continued to indulge his interest in natural history, and kept in close touch with his friend and teacher, John Hunter. During one exchange over a question of natural history soon after Jenner returned to Berkeley, Hunter admonished his former pupil to experiment instead of speculating (Baron 1827).

Although Jenner's studies on cowpox overshadowed all his previous work, he made several important discoveries during this early period of his life, described by LeFanu in his 1951 study. He was the first to associate angina pectoris with changes in coronary arteries seen at autopsy (the true significance of this finding was first realized by Jenner's colleague, C. H. Parry) and he devised a method for purifying tartar emetic by recrystallization. He also was the first to describe the unusual behavior and adaptation of the cuckoo, which lays its eggs in the nest of a hedge sparrow or other bird and whose young use transient depressions in their backs to eject the nest's rightful tenants, hatched or unhatched. Hunter submitted Jenner's paper on the cuckoo to the Royal Society, and Jenner was elected a fellow of the society the next year, largely on the strength of that paper and its illustrious sponsor.

Jenner married in 1788, the same year his paper was submitted to the Royal Society. Dixon records that he also took a drawing of a cowpox-infected milker's hand to London that year, and showed it to several medical men. Cowpox, a relatively mild disease of cattle, usually caused a few blisters on the udders of infected animals. Susceptible persons sometimes acquired the infection on their hand after milking infected cows. Such infections in people could be painful and caused scarring. Cowpox was also known to occur on the European continent.

The year after Jenner's marriage there was an outbreak of "swinepox" among pigs in Gloucestershire, and he took the opportunity to inoculate his infant son and two of his neighbor's servants with material taken from a pustule on the son's nurse, who had caught the infection. Early in 1790 Jenner inoculated the nurse and his son with smallpox virus, which elicited no reaction. He did not pursue the experiments with swinepox any further, so far as is known, perhaps because the epidemic in animals had ceased. But a year later, he began collecting cases of "cowpoxed milkers who were said to have resisted smallpox inoculations" (Kahn 1963, 604). As an inoculator himself, Jenner had several opportunities to observe such people in his medical practice. He himself was already immune to smallpox, having had a severe reaction when he was inoculated as an eight year old. He received his M.D. from St. Andrews University in Scotland in 1792, a year before John Hunter died of angina pectoris.

On 14 May 1796, Jenner inoculated James Phipps with cowpox lymph taken from a sore on the hand of Sara Nelmes, a milkmaid who had recently been infected. A week later the child developed a mild reaction to the inoculated cowpox, similar to that expected after a favorable smallpox inoculation. On 1 July, Jenner inoculated the boy with pus taken from a patient who had smallpox, which produced no significant reaction. The previous inoculation with the benign cowpox virus had made Phipps immune to smallpox. Jenner described his own reaction in a letter to a friend dated 19 July 1796:

> I was astonished at the close resemblance of the Pustules in some of their stages to the variolous Pustules. But now listen to the most delightful part of my story. The Boy has since been inoculated for the Smallpox which as I ventured to predict produced no effect. I shall now pursue my Experiments with redoubled ardor. (LeFanu 1951, plate 29)

Jenner informally submitted a brief paper describing this single experiment and the traditional beliefs about cowpox protecting against smallpox to the Royal Society in 1797. Because his evidence was so slim and his conclusion so audacious, the paper was quietly returned "with a note that if he valued his reputation already established by his paper on the cuckoo, he had better not promulgate such ideas as the use of cowpox for the prevention of smallpox" (Kahn 1963, 604).

When a fresh outbreak of cowpox next made that virus available to him again early in 1798, Jenner boldly inoculated five more children and challenged three of them with smallpox inoculation later. He then published an account of his experiments himself, along with accounts of unsuccessful attempts to inoculate others who had already had cowpox naturally. He announced his findings to the world in London in June 1798 in a pamphlet entitled *An Inquiry into the Causes and Effects of Variolae Vaccinae, a Disease, Discovered in some of the Western Counties of England, particularly Gloucestershire, and known by the Name of Cow Pox.* Jenner coined the term *variolae vaccinae*, smallpox of the cow, to describe the infection he said he had been thinking about for over twenty-five years.

It was, wrote Edward Edwardes in his *Concise History of Small-Pox and Vaccination in Europe*, "as if an Angel's trumpet had sounded over the earth" (42). In London, Dr. George Pearson performed several vaccinations himself, conducted a nationwide survey of English physicians for more evidence of resistance to smallpox or inoculation after cowpox infection, and published his results, which supported Jenner's main thesis, the same year. Dr. William Woodville, who was in charge of London's Small-Pox and Inoculation Hospital, took advantage of a local dairy's outbreak of cowpox to vaccinate several hundred persons in early 1799. Unfortunately Woodville vaccinated with cowpox and inoculated with smallpox in his smallpox hospital, and many of his "vaccinees" developed generalized rashes due to smallpox.

Knowledge that an attack of cowpox made one resistant to smallpox or to smallpox inoculation was widespread in cattle-raising districts of England for some time before Jenner's experiments, as we have seen. After Jenner's first paper on cowpox was published (he published three more before 1802), others began to claim that they had "vaccinated" with cowpox material before him. Some of these claims were valid. A Dr. Fewster read a paper entitled "Cowpox and Its Ability to Prevent Smallpox" to the London Medical Society in 1765, but then let the matter drop. Jobst Bose in Göttingen, Germany (1769), Plett, a Danish teacher in Holstein (1791), and Jensen, a farmer in Holstein (1791), had each inoculated with cowpox. Perhaps the best claim was that of Benjamin Jesty, a cattle breeder in Dorset, England, who had inoculated his wife and two sons with cowpox in 1774 to protect them during an outbreak of smallpox. There were also unsubstantiated reports of ancient cowpox inoculations in India, and of much more recent cowpoxing in Baluchistan and Mexico, none of which can be verified (Kahn 1963; Dixon 1962; Edwardes 1902b; *History of Inoculation*, 1913).

However, Jenner's unique contribution was not that he inoculated a few persons with cowpox, but that he then proved that they were immune to smallpox. Moreover, he demonstrated that the protective cowpox matter could be effectively inoculated from person-to-person, not just directly from cattle. Strictly speaking, Jenner did not "discover" vaccination, observed Edwardes, he "introduced" it.

Only a few years after his discovery, Jenner predicted that "the annihilation of smallpox—the most dreadful scourge of the human race—will be the final result of this practice" (LeFanu 1951, 58). Dumont, a Frenchman, asserted that since smallpox was to blame for thirty-five out of every one hundred blind Europeans before Jenner introduced vaccination, "were this [prevention of blindness] its only result this alone would suffice to render Jenner's name immortal" (Seely 1871, 234).

Jenner received many honors, including two parliamentary grants of ten thousand pounds and twenty thousand pounds. He maintained a worldwide correspondence after 1798, was the first president of the Royal Jennerian Society (1803) and the first director of England's National Vaccine Establishment (1808), both of which he helped found to provide vaccine supplies for practitioners. His deputy and successor in the latter post was James Moore, author of *A History of the Smallpox*. Jenner was never knighted nor made a member of the Royal Society of Medicine. According to a fascinating recent biography by Paul Saunders (1982), Jenner conducted much of his work on behalf of vaccination from Cheltenham, a fashionable spa at the foot of the Cotswolds, although Berkeley remained his primary residence. He retired in 1815, the year his wife died of tuberculosis. He died at home in Berkeley of a stroke on 23 January 1823 and was buried in the local church. The home he built for James Phipps a few yards away is now the Jenner Museum.

NINETEENTH CENTURY

Despite the considerable improvements in smallpox inoculation technique introduced in the second half of the eighteenth century, the advantages of vaccinating with cowpox were recognized almost immediately. Both techniques conferred immunity to smallpox, but cowpox vaccination was much safer for the individual vaccinees, and unlike inoculation, it entailed no risk of spreading smallpox to other persons in the community. These important distinctions were mentioned by Mr. Henry Cline, who performed the first vaccination in London in July 1798, in a letter to Jenner dated 2 August 1798:

> I think the substituting of cow-pox poison for the smallpox promises to be one of the greatest improvements that has ever been made in medicine: for it is not only so safe in itself, but also does not endanger others by contagion, in which way the small-pox has done infinite mischief. The more I think on the subject the more I am impressed with its importance. (Baron 1827, 1: 152)

Vaccination was also simpler and cheaper, since vaccinees did not have to be isolated for two or more weeks, as persons inoculated with smallpox did.

The result was that Jennerian vaccination was adopted much more rapidly in Europe than inoculation had been and quickly spread around the world, supplanting inoculation. Thus by 1801, more than one hundred thousand persons had been vaccinated in England, whereas only 897 persons were inoculated in Great Britain, the American colonies, and Hanover combined during the first seven years after inoculation was introduced into Europe and North America. In the decade before 1814, about two million vaccinations were performed in Russia. In France about 1.7 million persons were vaccinated in the four-year period 1808–11 (Edwards 1902b; Razzell 1977a).

Within three years after it was published in London, Jenner's *Inquiry* had been translated into German, French, Spanish, Dutch, Italian, and Latin. Kahn (1973) records that George Pearson sent vaccine to over a hundred physicians in Europe in 1799, the year vaccination began in Hanover and in Vienna. According to Bowers (1981), Jean de Carro, a Swiss graduate of the University of Edinburgh medical school, performed the first successful vaccinations in Vienna in late August with vaccine provided by a former classmate, Alexander Marcet. De Carro in turn provided vaccine that was used to begin the practice in Constantinople late in 1800. After receiving a fresh supply early in 1801 from Dr.

Luigi Sacco of Milan—Italy's foremost vaccinator, who in the autumn of 1800 had discovered natural cowpox infections in a herd of Swiss cattle at a fair in northern Italy—de Carro sent vaccine to Baghdad in 1802, whence it was forwarded by ship to India the same year. Jenner himself had made special efforts to get vaccine to India and North America, and William Woodville personally assisted at vaccination's inauguration in Paris in 1800. Vaccination also began in North America in 1800, and in Berlin and Moscow in 1801. For several years, Hale-White notes in his study of nineteenth-century doctors, Berlin held an annual festival on 14 May to commemorate Jenner's discovery.

Royal patronage and example were not as critical to the introduction of vaccination in Europe as they had been nearly a century before in the struggle to establish inoculation, but the pattern still held in several countries. According to Edwardes, King Frederick William of Prussia was "the first sovereign to adopt vaccination in his own family" (1902b, 49). In Russia, it was the empress dowager who arranged for vaccine to be imported from Breslau, Prussia and ordered that the first child vaccinated, an orphan, should be named "Vaccinoff," educated at public expense, and given a pension for life. She also sent Jenner a diamond ring. Baron (1827) records that the king of Denmark promoted vaccination in his country by appointing a committee to collect information about the new method and develop regulations to govern its dissemination. In Poland, Countess Zamoiska, sister of the late king, obtained vaccine from de Carro in Vienna and initiated vaccination in her nation, beginning with her own grandchild. It was the king of Spain, however, who underwrote the most dramatic efforts by far to promote vaccination. He sent vaccine from Spain to his dominions in North and South America and Asia by a living chain of orphan boys, who were vaccinated in succession during the voyages (discussed further in chapter 6).

The diffusion of cowpox vaccine and of would-be vaccinators in the early nineteenth century was impeded temporarily by the Napoleonic Wars, which at the same time were an incentive for vaccinating the armies concerned. The duke of York ordered the British army to be vaccinated in 1802. Napoleon issued similar orders for his troops three years later, a year after another imperial decree, commemorated by a medal, ordained the vaccination of French civilians. Napoleon's slight delay was not because he didn't appreciate fully the military value of Jenner's discovery. On several occasions, Napoleon liberated captured Englishmen in response to petitions from Jenner. Once, when he was inclined to refuse a pardon, Napoleon was shown an appeal from Jenner, whereupon he declared, "Ah, Jenner, I cannot refuse Jenner anything!" (Ah, Jenner, je ne puis rien refuser a Jenner!) (Major 1936, 130–31). The emperor of Austria and the king of Spain also freed prisoners of war following appeals by the English discoverer of vaccination. Some English travelers used a simple certificate signed by Jenner, who personally vouched for the bearer, instead of a passport.

Despite its manifest popularity and rapid spread, vaccination was not embraced without opposition, even in England. As had been the case when inoculation was introduced, scientific, religious, and social objections were evident from the very beginning of the vaccination era. Because it greatly simplified the way artificial immunity to smallpox was induced, and thereby made their practice obsolete, vaccination was not welcomed by numerous inoculators, who reacted to the threatened loss of fees for their services. Kahn (1963) mentions a British surgeon named John Birch who opposed vaccination because it would eliminate a disease that he regarded as a merciful means of reducing the country's poor population. (Malthus's "Essay on the Principles of Population" was published the same year as Jenner's *Inquiry*.) As we shall see, more serious social opposition emerged in the last half of the nineteenth century when efforts to make vaccination compulsory collided with growing sentiments of personal freedom of choice, especially in Great Britain.

Some religious leaders also opposed vaccination at first. The 1913 *History of Inoculation* quotes one who declared that "smallpox is a visitation from God, but the cowpox is produced by presumptuous man; the former was what heaven ordained, the latter is perhaps a daring violation of our holy religion" (87). More typical, however, were the actions of priests in Naples and Palermo who Bowers described leading processions of people to be vaccinated, despite their own view that vaccination was "discovered by one heretic and practiced by another" (1981, 19). In Bohemia, village priests recited the names of smallpox victims from their pulpits quarterly, and reminded parents of their responsibility "before God for neglecting the vaccination of their children" (Raska 1976, 228). Some pastors in Germany, Switzerland, and England not only were advocates, but actually vaccinated people themselves. According to Baron (1827), Reverend Finch of St. Helen's, Lancashire, reportedly vaccinated more than 3,000 persons. In Geneva, one minister permitted a physician to hand out literature promoting vaccination to parents when they brought their children to be baptised. During an epidemic in Rome in 1814, the pope endorsed vaccination as "a precious discovery which ought to be a new motive for human gratitude to Omnipotence" (Saunders 1982, 329).

The most difficult opposition provaccinators faced grew out of the scientific skepticism and doubt resulting from the still inadequate understanding of the causative organisms of the disease and their effects on humans. Recall Cline's reference to the cowpox "poison." The logic of smallpox inoculation had by now been generally accepted, if not wholly understood. But for all its advantages, cowpox vaccination was in one respect more objectionable than inoculation, because vaccination required infecting humans with a disease of animals. Some laymen could not believe that having one disease could protect a person against a different disease, and the fact that cowpox came from animals enhanced their skepticism. Dixon notes that others were understandably put on guard by rumors that cowpox was a venereal disease of cattle. Cartoonists unabashedly depicted people who grew horns, tails, or acquired other bovine characteristics after being vaccinated. One woman complained that after her daughter was vaccinated, she "coughed like a cow, and had grown hairy over her body" (*History of Inoculation*, 1913, 87).

Serious questions about the efficacy of vaccination arose from the uncertainty, which persists to this day, about exactly what Jenner's vaccine was and where it came from. The nature and relationship, if any, of the "grease" disease in horses, swinepox, and cowpox of that period are still unknown (Baxby 1981, 1977; Downie 1951; Razzell 1977b). Apart from Jenner's much-criticized early assertion that his vaccine originated in the "grease" disease of horses—a disease, he believed, that first had to pass through cows before being vaccinated into humans—there was the problem that "grease" was a name used for several different infections of horses, only one of which could confer immunity to smallpox. Moreover, cows also suffered from other infections that might appear to be cowpox, but that provided no protection against smallpox. Even when vaccinations were performed with vaccine taken from the pustule or scab of a previously successfully vaccinated person, the vaccine lesion of the donor could not be approached indiscriminately, because of possible secondary infection and contamination or inactivation of the virus. Then as now, ineffective, bacterially contaminated vaccine often left a scar similar to that caused by cowpox or vaccinia virus, and this caused much controversy between Jenner and his critics. Almost at the outset Jenner formulated his "golden rule," which was that vaccine should be taken from vaccine pustules only around the fifth to eighth day, before the "effloresence" appeared, to be sure of getting active cowpox virus (LeFanu 1951).

In addition to the confusion about vaccination's efficacy, controversy about the duration of the immunity it provided was another fertile source of opposition. Whereas smallpox and smallpox inoculation usually provided immunity for life against the naturally acquired smallpox, Dixon tells us that as early as 1804 there was increasing evidence that some successfully vaccinated persons could still contract the disease several years after their vaccination, although it was usually much milder ("varioloid") in such cases. Jenner's unshakeable belief that cowpox vaccination conferred lifelong immunity to smallpox led him to contend, mistakenly, that any apparent failure of immunity must be due to faulty technique or vaccine. Jenner's obvious fallibility on this issue was exploited by antivaccinationists until revaccination was introduced in 1829.

A final drawback of Jennerian vaccination that concerned its backers and was also seized upon by early opponents was its safety. Arm-to-arm vaccination sometimes transmitted other diseases such as erysipelas or syphilis. The danger of vaccinal syphilis was apparent in Italy as early as 1814 and in Germany, France, Russia, and other countries somewhat later. In one episode at Rivalta, Italy, for example, sixty-three children were vaccinated with material taken from the vaccinal pustule of an apparently healthy infant who had an inapparent syphilis infection. Forty-four of the vaccinated infants developed overt syphilis, several died of it, and some infected their mothers and nurses (Nott 1867). In theory, the risk of unwittingly transmitting other dangerous infections by arm-to-arm vaccination must have existed also for arm-to-arm inoculations, but if it was recognized then as a problem at all, it apparently was not thought to be so serious.

As we shall see, effective solutions were found during the nineteenth and twentieth centuries to almost all of the objections raised by the early opponents of vaccination. But in the early nineteenth century, vaccination reduced the prevalence of smallpox in Europe so quickly and drastically that the antivaccinationists' objections, all of which were relatively minor when compared to the alternative of uncontrolled smallpox, loomed larger as the perceived threat of smallpox receded. (We should also note here that even the extremely rare, but serious, residual complications of vaccination were the reason routine Jennerian vaccination ultimately became unacceptable late in the twentieth century, after smallpox had been eradicated from various regions.)

As more and more people were vaccinated, smallpox mortality declined and remained at relatively low levels for the first few decades of the nineteenth century. Such epidemics as occurred were less severe and less frequent than in the previous century. In London, for example, the average ratio of deaths from smallpox to one thousand deaths from all causes, which stood at 73.2 in the first quarter of the eighteenth century before inoculation had any significant impact, rose to 91.7 in the last quarter of that century when inoculation was at its height, declined to 51.7 in 1801–25, and to 14.3 by 1851–75. Similarly, comparable ratios in Geneva fell abruptly to their lowest level ever in the first decade of the nineteenth century under the impact of vaccination (fig. 5). Baron (1838) reports that in Sweden, extensive vaccination reduced the number of reported deaths from smallpox from some twelve thousand persons in 1800 to eleven in 1822, and in Denmark, the disease was eradicated altogether between 1811 and 1818, not a single case of smallpox being reported in those years.

In the activist mood made possible by vaccination, some Europeans adopted new legal measures to press the struggle against smallpox. According to Raska's 1976 article, in 1803 the governor of Bohemia

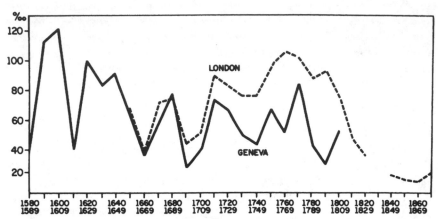

Fig. 5. Deaths from smallpox in London and Geneva per thousand deaths from all causes, 1580–1869. Adapted from Perrenoud (1980) and Guy (1882).

ordered that thenceforth, funerals of smallpox victims were to be conducted without the attendance of family, friends, or even a priest. Over thirteen thousand Bohemians died of smallpox that year. Russia was the first country to outlaw inoculation with smallpox virus in 1805, Prussia followed in 1835, and England in 1842. During a parliamentary debate in England in 1806, the banning of smallpox inoculation was denounced by one member on the grounds that "the liberty of doing wrong was still left among the privileges of freeborn Englishmen," a sentiment that proved to be a portent of things to come (Dixon 1962, 271).

As the effectiveness and comparative safety of vaccination became generally appreciated, governments began to require their citizens to be vaccinated. Vaccination was made compulsory in Bavaria (1807), Denmark (1810), Norway (1811), Russia (1812), Sweden (1816), and Hanover (1821). District vaccination committees were organized in Russia in 1811, but their activities were disrupted during Napoleon's invasion. After 1815 all newborn Russians were supposed to be registered with the local vaccination committee, but Kraechenko (1970) reports there was not yet adequate capacity to vaccinate all who registered. Vaccination was made mandatory in England in 1853 and in France not until 1902. The 1853 act in England proved to be a time-bomb, the effects of which were felt somewhat later.

Smallpox did not yield completely to these early efforts. The disease infected an estimated eight million Russians between 1804 and 1810, killing 827,000 of them ("Smallpox before Jenner," 1896, 1263). Severe epidemics occurred in European Russia in 1814, 1834, and 1846. In Ireland, a famine in 1816 led to large-scale movements of farm families in 1817–18, which in turn increased the spread of smallpox. Iceland had only one large epidemic after vaccination was introduced, in 1819, but Greenland suffered epidemics in 1800, 1809, and 1851. Epidemics began again with renewed vigor in European cities as the century progressed. In London, epidemics of smallpox and typhus broke out simultaneously in 1817–19, and again twenty years later. Smallpox erupted in Edinburgh (1817), Marseilles and Rotterdam (1818), Milan (1822), Berlin (1823), Hamburg (1824), Copenhagen (1824–27), and Paris (1825). Twice, in 1824–29 and in 1837–40, smallpox pandemics affected nearly all of Europe. These two waves were not up to seventeenth- or eighteenth-century standards, but they were serious enough.

The pandemic of 1824–29 extended as far as Constantinople. According to Walsh (1836), after Abdul Hamed, eldest son of Sultan Mahmud the Reformer, died of smallpox in April 1825, the sultan had his other children vaccinated. Other Turks then followed his example. What the sultan didn't know was that his elite military force, the Janissaries, was planning to depose him and put Abdul Hamed on the throne when smallpox intervened. A year later, he destroyed the Janissaries and "at last accomplished a task which had baffled many of his predecessors" (Spry 1895, 170–85).

The second European pandemic in 1837–40 was more severe than the first. London recorded more smallpox deaths in 1837 (2,100) than in any of the past thirty years. In the two and a half years before December 1839, England reported over thirty thousand deaths from smallpox. While worse mortality had been frequent in the eighteenth century, it was less tolerable near the middle of the nineteenth century, when vaccination had been available for more than a generation. The great British epidemiologist William Farr was outraged. In a bitter note to the British journal *Lancet* in 1840, he compared the outbreak to allowing children to be thrown daily, for months on end, from London Bridge. In England, the pandemic of 1837–40 resulted in passage of that country's first Vaccination Act in 1840. The act provided for the first free medical service by empowering local parish leaders to "contract with registered medical practitioners to perform vaccinations" (Dixon 1962, 278).

Farr was correct in suggesting an element of neglect in the epidemics that affected Europe toward the middle of the nineteenth century. As the fear of smallpox declined after Jenner's discovery, fewer persons took the trouble to be vaccinated or to have their children vaccinated. In addition, many persons who had been vaccinated one or two decades before caught smallpox as their immunity waned. Thus Edwardes (1902b) notes that several epidemics around this time were characterized by higher rates of illness in adults than in children, since many children were more recently vaccinated. In earlier times, endemic smallpox ensured that most adults living in cities were permanently immune and children had suffered most during epidemics. In addition, persons in the lower classes, who had least

access to vaccination, were now even more disproportionately represented among those dying of smallpox.

Since smallpox virus was known to provide permanent immunity in
most cases, the increasingly obvious inferiority of a single vaccination led
some British practitioners to revive smallpox inoculation briefly in the
1820s. A safer solution to the problem, namely revaccination, was first
introduced at Wurtemberg in 1829. German states took the lead, and
some of them began to require revaccination of all military recruits as
early as 1833. It was made compulsory for the Prussian army in 1834.
Among the latter, smallpox deaths, which had averaged eighty-eight per
year in 1831–34, dropped to five, nine, three, and seven in the next four
years, and averaged less than two per year over the next thirty years.
English military authorities did not begin to require revaccination until
1858. Although it unfortunately was neither appreciated nor adopted as
readily as Jenner's original discovery had been, the concept of revaccination against smallpox was a very important improvement in Jennerian
vaccination (Creighton 1894; Ackerknect 1965; Edwardes 1902b).

Soon after the answer to the problem of waning immunity began to be
recognized, the solution to another major objection to Jennerian vaccination was also discovered. Up to this time, it will be recalled, most vaccinations were performed with vaccine taken from the pustule or scab of a
previously vaccinated person. Some persons were still inoculated directly
from naturally occurring cowpox, but that disease did not exist everywhere, nor was it always present in districts where it was known. This
usually meant that the vaccine had to be propagated continuously, from
person to person. This was troublesome enough in larger towns, but
impossible in sparsely settled areas. Vaccines passed from arm to arm
were sometimes inoculated back into cattle in attempts to make sure they
retained their cowpox qualities. Moreover, apart from the logistical inconvenience of this method, there was the substantial risk of transmitting
other dangerous infectious diseases we saw above.

In 1843, Negri of Naples solved the problem of arm-to-arm propagation of cowpox when he began deliberately passing cowpox from cow to
cow. He scarified the animals' sides before inoculating them, which also
provided a much larger source of vaccine virus than was previously
possible. Nott tells us in his 1867 article that inoculated cows were led door
to door, and children were vaccinated with virus direct from the cow at
their doorstep. Propagating the vaccine in cows provided a reliable,
regular source of an assuredly effective vaccine that was also safer. This
method spread throughout Europe, arriving in France in 1864, Germany
in 1865, and England in 1881. Negri's superior method restored the cow
as the source of most vaccine.

Thus, by the mid-nineteenth century, practical solutions had been
found to two major problems that had troubled earlier vaccinationists,

but revaccination and Negri's method were not yet universally accepted in Europe, even within the medical profession. Similarly, while some European states had enacted compulsory vaccination laws, others had not. First inoculation and then vaccination had reduced the disease's inevitability for individuals and the severity of outbreaks. But, though robbed of much of its historical terror, smallpox persisted. Neither the immunolog ical process provoked by vaccination nor the germ itself were yet satisfactorily understood.

There were generally fewer smallpox outbreaks in Europe in the 1850s and 1860s; Russia counted about a hundred thousand deaths from smallpox in 1856 ("Smallpox before Jenner," 1896, 1263). Two years later, Berlin suffered its largest outbreak in over twenty-five years, when 4,534 people were infected, of whom 406 died ('Bericht über die Pockenepidemie," 124). In Switzerland, there were epidemics in 1849–50, 1853, and 1864–68. But this was merely the lull before Europe's worst pandemic of smallpox in the nineteenth century, the outbreak of 1870–75. That pandemic, which temporarily halted the downward trend of smallpox in Europe, was a direct consequence of the Franco-Prussian War.[13]

France and Prussia declared war in late July 1870. Napoleon III surrendered to the Prussians at Sedan on 2 September. However fighting continued elsewhere in France as French republicans proclaimed a new government in Paris. The Germans besieged the French capital on 19 September. France finally surrendered on 28 January 1871.

When the war began, vaccination was still entirely voluntary for civilians in France and northern Germany, but southern German states required infants to be vaccinated. Revaccination of civilians was not compulsory in either country. Nevertheless, the German Empire was almost free from smallpox when the war began.

In France, where a third of the country's population of about 35 million had never been vaccinated, smallpox had been smoldering in several towns in the southeast, northeast, northwest, and in Paris, since the last quarter of 1869. It was also epidemic in Holland and Belgium. As war became imminent, the conscription and movement of troops and the emigration of thousands of Parisians intensified the epidemic in France. Whereas France had recorded 593 deaths from smallpox as recently as 1866 and 4,164 deaths in 1869, when the outbreak was getting started, the epidemic of 1870–71 killed an estimated 60,000 to 90,000 French citizens. Paris alone reported 10,539 deaths in 1870, and 2,771 more the following year.

In Germany, poorly protected civil populations suffered so much from smallpox that if Bismark attributed the epidemic to the war, he may have wondered who really won. The Prussians began shipping captured French soldiers to camps in Prussia soon after the fighting began. In all, some 373,000 French prisoners of war were incarcerated all over Germany. Many of them carried smallpox with them, and beginning in September–October 1870, the disease spread to German civilian populations in Leipzig, Danzig, Dresden, Essen, Dusseldorf, Berlin, and numerous other cities. Among the French prisoners of war in Germany, 14,178 had smallpox, of whom 1,963 died. According to Rolleston (1933), exposure of German civilians was facilitated by the petty trade in personal effects, including clothes of dead Frenchmen, that developed between civilians and prisoners. In Hamburg, 83 persons died of smallpox in 1870, and 3,647 in 1871. Berlin lost over five thousand of its citizens in 1871. Prussia as a whole recorded 4,200 deaths from the virus in 1870; 59,839 in 1871; and 65,109 in 1872. Overall, at least 162,000 deaths from smallpox were reported in all the German states (population about 45 million) for 1871–72. Because of differences in vaccination requirements for civilians, the epidemic was more severe in northern Germany than in the south.

The French at least had only themselves to blame for their epidemic, since "among the hundreds of German prisoners in Paris, only one was sent to the Bicetre Hospital as a case of smallpox, and his attack was so mild that the diagnosis was doubtful" (Rolleston 1933, 11).

The two armies experienced dramatically different mortality from smallpox during the war. Unlike the German civilian population, the German army was routinely revaccinated every seven years. Of the 800,000-man army, 8,463 caught smallpox and only 459 (5.4 percent) died, suggesting a mitigating effect of waning vaccinal immunity on the fatality rate. The French army, which included more than a million men, of whom over 700,000 were taken prisoner, reportedly had approximately 125,000 men infected by smallpox during the epidemic. Of these, some 23,470 died—a fatality rate of about 18.7 percent. Thus the French army lost almost as many men to death from smallpox as the total number of German soldiers killed in the war (28,208). The French were ill-prepared for the war, but the impact of smallpox on their army must have made matters worse. Hirsch (1883) records that in one *Gardes mobiles* unit of 1,158 men, for example, over half the men contracted smallpox during the war.

Although most of the fighting had been limited to the two principal belligerents, the smallpox epidemic the war brought about was not. It spread all over Europe, were it was especially severe in Belgium, Holland, and Austria, and metastasized to North and South America, the West Indies, and Africa. Refugees from the Fall of Sedan carried smallpox to Belgium, which reported 4,163 deaths from smallpox in 1870; 21,315 in 1871; and 8,074 in 1872. Other refugees carried smallpox to England the same autumn, where 2,580 deaths due to smallpox were reported in 1870; 23,126 in 1871; and 19,094 in 1872.[14] From England the epidemic spread to Scotland and Ireland. Holland had 706 deaths in 1870; 12,476 in 1871; and 2,297 the following year. In Sweden the epidemic peaked later, with about 1,100 deaths in 1873, over 4,000 the next year, and 2,019 in 1875. Stockholm, which was more lax then the rest of Sweden in enforcing that country's vaccination laws, buried 1,206 victims of small-pox in 1874 alone. French troops pushed into western Switzerland by German soldiers caused more epidemics in that country. Zurich, Basel, Bern, and Geneva suffered heavily. Austria reported more than 141,000 deaths from smallpox in the years 1872–74, with Vienna and Prague most severely affected. Italian volunteers who fought for the French on the Côte de'Or carried smallpox back to Italy. European Russia had epidemic years in 1872 and 1875.

Low, who reviewed the incidence of smallpox all over the world in the late nineteenth century, estimated that in all, at least a half million Euro-peans died of smallpox in the pandemic triggered by the Franco-Prussian War. (1918, 4). Although this wave of epidemics was not as severe as those Europe had suffered repeatedly in the eighteenth century, it was by far the worst such catastrophe in the nineteenth, and it violently shocked Europeans out of their complacency about controlling smallpox.

The pandemic of 1870–75 discriminated sharply between civilian populations of states with compulsory vaccination laws for civilians, such as England, Scotland, Sweden, and Bavaria, and states without such laws, such as Prussia, Austria, and Belgium. The latter had smallpox mortality rates about three times as high as the former, and young children under ten years comprised most of the deaths in states where vaccination was not compulsory (Edwardes 1902b). In addition, the value of revaccination was illustrated by the Prussian army's epidemiologic experience during the war.

This costly lesson in public health policy resulted in direct legal actions in England and Germany, but not in Austria (fig. 6), or in France. In England, Parliament passed the Vaccination Act of 1871, which pro-vided for local inspectors to enforce previous Vaccination Acts by pros-ecuting offenders. The Vaccination Acts of 1840, 1853, and 1867 had made the practice universally available free of charge, obligatory in in-fancy, and compulsory under penalties. Germany enacted the Vaccina-tion Law of 1874, which required all German children to be vaccinated before their second birthday, and revaccinated at about age twelve. Another positive consequence of the epidemic caused by the Franco-Prussian War was that Weigert seized the opportunity presented by the outbreak in Breslau during 1871–72 to undertake an unprecedented study of the pathology of smallpox, examining two hundred victims (Bloomfield 1958).

With good enforcement, the new legislation virtually eliminated smallpox as a major public health problem in Germany after 1874 (see fig. 6) Enforcement of the 1871 act was more gradual in England, where

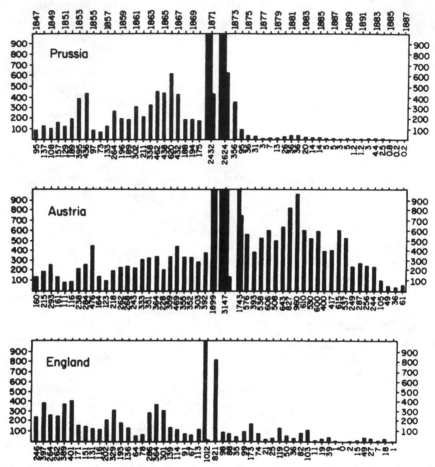

Fig. 6. Deaths per million from smallpox in nineteenth-century Prussia, Austria, and England. Adapted from Edwardes (1902b).

efforts to implement that public health legislation provoked a widespread public reaction rooted partly in English objections to being compelled to do anything by the state and partly in the confusion that still prevailed about how smallpox spread, and about the efficacy of vaccination.

In the 1870s British medical and public opinion, like that of other European states, was still polarized between anticontagionists, who attributed epidemics such as smallpox to atmospheric conditions or unsanitary surroundings, and adherents of the germ theory, who believed such epidemics were caused by spread of specific infectious agents, or "viruses." Thus, the London physician quoted above who wondered whether the excessive discharges of gun powder in Paris during the siege of 1870–71 had cleansed that city's atmosphere, thereby eliminating epidemic smallpox in Paris, was probably not jesting entirely, if at all. Even Dr. William Guy, who in 1882 presented a detailed paper to the Statistical Society of London demonstrating conclusively the dramatic decline in smallpox in the nineteenth century (which was not accompanied by a similar decline in other diseases such as measles or whooping cough), and who concluded that vaccination, and not general sanitary improvements, was responsible for smallpox's unique decline, felt compelled to invoke the "atmospheric condition" to explain the unusual epidemic of 1871.

> That atmospheric condition, whatever it may be, to which our epidemics are due, was so favourable to attacks of smallpox that the barrier of vaccination, though effective in ordinary years, proved insufficient in this. (1882, 424)

Many anticontagionists felt the specificity inherent in the contagionist theory and vaccination threatened efforts to attack what they considered to be the root causes of all diseases, namely "foul air, overcrowding, and filthy streets" (McLeod 1967, 109). Commercial interests also favored the anticontagionist view, since they preferred measures that did not require quarantining goods and people.

In addition, while the failure of a single Jennerian vaccination to provide lifelong protection against smallpox was obvious to many antivaccinationists, it was still the subject of debate in British medical circles. Moreover, erysipelas, syphilis, and other secondary infections were complications objectionable to much of the British public, which despite their legislature's reaction to the epidemic of 1871, remained relatively unimpressed by the vastly reduced threat of smallpox. It will be recalled that Negri's improved technique of producing vaccine in cows was not adopted in England until about 1881, and even then it was protested by some medical officers, "who were mainly old-guard adherents of the arm-to-arm technique" (MacLeod 1967, 193).

Against this background of medical uncertainty and controversy, rising individualism, and a diminished public perception of the threat posed by smallpox, aggressive efforts to enforce the Vaccination Acts in England by prosecuting negligent parents led to a violent upsurge in resistance to vaccination. Brown and McLean (1962) note that numerous British parents whose children died as a result of illegal inoculation were tried and convicted for manslaughter, adding more fuel to the public debate. The resultant opposition by prosecuted parents, wrote R. M. MacLeod, "merged with the rising tide of working-class opinion and with the efforts of radical reformers who saw in the vaccination question the embodiment of impersonal and uncompromising governmental intervention in the daily life of the individual" (1967, 108).[15]

One of the most notorious hotbeds of opposition to the vaccination laws in England was the town of Leicester, site of a massive demonstration against the Vaccination Acts in 1885. During the demonstration, a copy of the Acts was publically burned before a crowd of more than twenty thousand persons from all over England. More significant was Leicester's espousal of what came to be known as the "Leicester Experiment." Instead of compulsory vaccination, the Leicester Board of Guardians, which was responsible for carrying out the Vaccination Acts, had emphasized isolation of smallpox patients, disinfection of their quarters, quarantine of contacts, and mandatory notification of cases, since the 1870s. According to a 1980 article by S. M. F. Fraser, this appears to have been the first time that quarantine was used to control infection in contacts. Fraser argues that the method "was established in Leicester before the antivaccinationists became a major influence there" (332). At the time, the town's reliance on measures other than vaccination was radical. Opponents likened Leicester to "a town where the brick-built homes are gradually being replaced by wooden ones" (Tomkins 1886, 827–28). But by and large, the stringent containment measures worked, minimizing transmission of smallpox in Leicester during the last quarter of the nineteenth century. They were particularly effective after 1901, when the local medical officer of Health was able to modify the original method by adding selective vaccination. The "Leicester Experiment," as modified by Dr. C. K. Millard in 1901, foreshadowed the strategy of "selective epidemiologic control" that was used to successfully eradicate smallpox between 1968 and 1977.

In most other English cities, unfortunately, resistance to compulsory vaccination was not accompanied by equally vigorous efforts to control smallpox by other means. At the centennary of Jenner's experiment with cowpox, Gloucester, whose cathedral contained a memorial statue of the doctor from nearby Berkeley, was in the grips of a severe smallpox epidemic (1895–96). There were almost two thousand cases in the town of about forty thousand persons, of whom 434 died in thirteen months ("The Story of Gloucester," 221–23). This epidemic, wrote one observer, "proved one of the most disastrous, for the size of the town, in modern times. Whilst it lasted, Gloucester was a plague-stricken city, hotels were deserted, and trade seriously injured" (Millard 1916–17, 119). Major (1936) reported that even the small village of Berkeley had over seven hundred cases of smallpox that epidemic year. In Sheffield, funerals of smallpox victims were cited as an important source of infection in addition to attendance at "public houses and theatres" by workers ill with smallpox who were being paid to stay home (Hobson 1963).

During the controversy over compulsory vaccination in England, Louis Pasteur, who with Robert Koch did more than anyone else to produce evidence in support of the germ theory, attended an international medical congress in London in 1881 and chose on that occasion to openly acknowledge his indebtedness to England's native son, Edward Jenner:

> I cannot complete this address, however, without testifying the great pleasure I feel that it is as a member of an international medical congress meeting in England that I finally communicate to you the vaccination of a disease [chicken cholera] probably more terrible for domestic animals than smallpox for man. I have given to the term vaccination an extension which science, I hope, will consecrate as a homage to the merit of and to the immense services rendered by one of the greatest of Englishmen, your Jenner. I am indeed happy to be able to praise this immortal name in the noble and hospitable city of London. (Mellanby 1949, 924)

The sustained agitation by antivaccinationists and the British medical profession's failure to provide effective leadership on behalf of the method resulted in the collapse of compulsory vaccination in England. Under the new Vaccination Acts of 1898 and 1907, parents needed only to state their "conscientious objections" as a legally valid reason for not having their children vaccinated. Embarrassed Britons working in India wrote letters to medical journals at home inviting the conscientious objectors to come see what smallpox was doing there.

By the early 1880s smallpox had returned elsewhere in Europe, to normal prewar levels or less, except in Italy, Spain and Austria.[16] Spain reported nearly 5,500 deaths from smallpox in 1879. In Austria, smallpox deaths continued to occur at higher rates than before the war until 1890 (see fig. 6 above). Health authorities were aware of a thousand cases of smallpox in Milan on 9 July 1888. European Russia had fresh epidemics in 1878 and 1881–82. Only 155 deaths from smallpox were reported in all of Germany in 1886, and those occurred mainly in areas bordering Russia, Austria, and Switzerland. That same year, there were 202 deaths from smallpox in Paris alone, 204 in Vienna, 256 in Moscow, 275 each in Genoa and London, 470 in Rome, 1,558 in Budapest, and 2,501 in Marseilles. In Stockholm, no one died of smallpox that year, and by 1896, all of Sweden was enjoying its first smallpox-free year.

Even as the disastrous controversy in England set back the cause of vaccinationists in that country, overall efforts to control smallpox were advanced at the end of the nineteenth century by another Englishman's discovery, which paved the way to better vaccines. For several decades, various European vaccine establishments had added glycerine to cowpox lymph as a diluent and later as a preservative. In 1891 Monckton Copeman demonstrated the selective germicidal effect of glycerin on bacteria in calf lymph vaccine. Glycerin helped reduce bacterial contamination of vaccines, thereby increasing their effectiveness and reliability, and reducing the incidence of undesirable secondary infections. This established the basis for improved, more stable vaccines produced in calves and helped complete the shift away from arm-to-arm vaccination. Claims for priority of discovery by Italian, German, and French workers attested to the importance of this development. "Filterable viruses" were demonstrated for the first time a year later.

TWENTIETH CENTURY

At the turn of the twentieth century, Russia, Spain, Italy, Portugal, and France were reporting the greatest number of deaths from smallpox in Europe. Germany and the Scandanavian countries had exceptionally low amounts of smallpox, since their populations were well vaccinated. Austria, like Germany, was also experiencing relatively little smallpox following a rapid decline in the disease during the 1890s. The approximate numbers of deaths from smallpox reported by various countries during the first decade of this century are listed below (figures from Low 1918; 1910 population given in parentheses):

European Russia, including Poland (134 m)	400,000
Spain (20 m)	37,000
Italy (35 m)	18,000
Portugal (5.9 m)	14,000
France (39 m)	11,000
Great Britain and Ireland (45 m)	5,000
Belgium (7.5 m)	4,000
Germany (65 m)	386
Austria (28 m)	312
Sweden (5.5 m)	35
Norway (2.3 m)	35
Denmark (2.8 m) (urban)	13

As might be expected, Russian travelers often carried smallpox to other parts of Europe. Ships from Russian ports were a recognized hazard in Scandinavia. Most of the few cases still being reported in Germany were from areas near the borders and often occurred in foreigners, especially Russians and Italians. In 1910 almost thirty percent of all cases of smallpox reported from Germany were Russians. Despite its strong antivaccinationist movement, Britain, shielded perhaps partly by the English Channel, reported its last large outbreak of *V. major* in 1902. France apparently had its final large outbreak of *V. major* in 1907, although I have not been able to obtain statistics for France from 1914 to 1919. There were especially large urban epidemics during this period in Madrid (1,284 deaths from smallpox in 1900), Marseille (1,895 deaths in 1907), London (1,314 deaths in 1902), Glasgow (1,389 deaths in 1901), Warsaw (797 deaths in 1904), Paris (487 deaths in 1901), and Moscow (485 deaths in 1908).

The disruption and mass movements of World War I caused a resurgence of smallpox in Russia and several neighboring countries. The disease was particularly rampant in Russian Poland during the war. Heavy fighting in Galicia and Bukovina early in the war was accompanied by a flare up of smallpox cases (42,000 in 1915 and 1916) in those provinces of the Austrian Empire. In 1915, a moderate-sized outbreak in Vienna was aggravated by the absence of over half of the city's vaccinators, who were doing military service elsewhere. A year later, Austria vaccinated three-quarters of its population in an attempt to check virulent smallpox epidemics attributed to spread of the disease from Russia.

Invalids of the war, traveling from Russia to Germany in 1917, caused an epidemic while passing through Sweden. Soldiers returning from the Eastern Front were the alleged cause of another outbreak at Vienna in the final year of the war. Switzerland, which had learned its lesson during the Franco-Prussian War of 1870–71, sealed its borders during World War I. Although the borders were closed for political, not sanitary reasons, the effect was to also protect Switzerland from imported smallpox. Only nine cases were reported from 1915 to 1918; none were reported in 1917. In the previous four years, the Swiss had reported an average of more than twenty cases per year.

Italy emerged from the war in the throes of another severe epidemic which claimed over thirty-six thousand lives. An epidemic in Portugal caused over fourteen thousand more deaths in the same period (1918–20). Even well-vaccinated Germany was affected: an epidemic there killed about fifteen hundred people in 1917–20. As bad as the situation had been in Russia before the war, it was even worse afterward. Enormous epidemics of typhus, cholera, and smallpox occurred toward the end of the war and after the Bolshevik revolution. One hundred and eighty-six thousand cases of smallpox were reported in 1919. The new government enacted a mandatory vaccination law on 10 April the same year, in a decree signed by Lenin. Five years later, the Soviet vaccination law was modified to require vaccination in infancy, and revaccination of teenagers.

Austria became smallpox-free in 1924, at about the same time a new, mild type of smallpox, *V. minor*, began to be noticed in England and Switzerland, for the first time in Europe. According to Dixon, this new strain had already spread throughout North America just before the turn of the century, and may have been introduced into England from Salt Lake City, Utah, during a Mormon conference held at Nottingham in 1901. Switzerland had an outbreak of 5,052 cases of smallpox, of whom only 10 died, in 1921–24. In England and Wales, 81,453 cases and 209 deaths were attributed to *V. minor* in the period 1920–34. Following this outbreak, Great Britain became free of smallpox for the first time in 1935.

New epidemics in 1931–33 led to intensified vaccination efforts in the Soviet Union, which eliminated endemic smallpox in 1936. That same year, *V. minor* predominated in Spain, while *V. major* was the most common type in neighboring Portugal. The Spanish Civil War allowed a brief resurgence of fatal smallpox in that country, and over two thousand Spaniards died of the disease in 1939–40. But by the end of World War II, Spain and Portugal were the only European countries that still had endemic smallpox. When those two countries were freed of it by the early 1950s, for the first time the disease ceased to be a matter of concern to most Europeans. Persons unknowingly infected while traveling or living in areas of Africa or Asia where the disease was still endemic became the main threat to a smallpox-free Europe.

Between 1950 and 1971, smallpox was introduced into Europe forty-nine times, giving rise to 958 indigenous cases in seventeen countries. Most of the imported cases of smallpox came from Asia, and most of the consequent cases were infected in hospitals, where unrecognized cases were admitted before the correct diagnosis was made. In an extraordinary outbreak at Meschede, West Germany, in 1970, a patient with undiagnosed smallpox infected 17 other persons in the hospital without having had direct contact with any of them. Gelfand and Posch report in their 1971 article that smoke tests later implicated the pattern of air currents leading away from the patient's room as the unusual mode of infection.

Two years after the outbreak at Meschede, Europe was shocked again when a large outbreak of smallpox suddenly erupted in Yugoslavia, where the disease had been carried by a pilgrim returning from Mecca. Investigators traced this surprise attack to a silent chain of infection that reached from Afghanistan across Iran and Syria to Iraq, where the homeward-bound Yugoslav pilgrim was apparently infected while visiting religious sites in Baghdad. He had a mild case, did not seek medical attention, and "at no time was he confined to bed" (WHO 1972, 161–62). The resulting epidemic in March and April was the largest outbreak of smallpox in Europe since World War II, and the first outbreak in Yugoslavia in forty-two years. One hundred and seventy-four Yugoslavs contracted smallpox, of whom thirty-five died. There was also one related case in the Federal Republic of Germany. This was the last time smallpox was imported into Europe, but not its last appearance there. That unwelcome distinction was reserved for Jenner's homeland, where a new problem, peculiar to the twentieth century, materialized.

On 11 March 1973, exactly a year after the outbreak in Yugoslavia, an unsuspecting technician at a research institute in London became ill eleven days after having watched another worker harvest smallpox virus from some eggs in which the virus was being grown for research purposes. She was hospitalized, but had a highly modified, sparse rash, and smallpox was not suspected until the twelfth day of her illness (22 March). By then, she had been on a general hospital ward for a week and had infected a young couple who visited a relative in an adjacent bed. Both visitors died of smallpox, the first such deaths in England and Wales in eleven years. A nurse who cared for one of the two fatal cases herself became the last victim in this outbreak, but she survived (WHO 1973).

Five years after the laboratory-associated outbreak in London, the virus mysteriously escaped from a similar research facility in Birmingham, England, and infected a forty-year-old medical photographer who worked on the floor above the smallpox laboratory (WHO 1978; McGinty 1979). The photographer, Mrs. Janet Parker, became ill on 11 August 1978, almost ten months after the world's last case of endemic smallpox was quarantined in Somalia, East Africa. She was hospitalized thirteen days later, when smallpox was diagnosed, but died one month after her illness began. Nearly three hundred persons with whom she had been associated were quarantined. Of these, only her mother, who had been revaccinated soon after Mrs. Parker's disease was diagnosed, developed the infection, which was manifested by only a few pustules.

As Mrs. Parker lay isolated in a smallpox hospital, her disease was partly to blame for the deaths of two other persons who were not infected. Mrs. Parker's father died of a heart attack soon after visiting at her bedside, and the forty-nine-year-old director of the smallpox laboratory where her infection had presumably originated, Professor Henry Bedson—a world-reknowned authority on the disease—committed suicide while quarantined at home, eight days after Janet Parker's astonishing diagnosis was made.

Twelve years before Mrs. Parker was infected, another medical photographer who worked in the very same rooms as she did contracted *V. minor* and initiated a large outbreak in Birmingham. At the time it could not be proven that his illness originated in the laboratory since he might have been infected by a person from an endemic area with unrecognized smallpox (McGinty 1979). When Mrs. Parker was infected in 1978, there were no such endemic areas remaining. The report of the official inquiry into the outbreak in 1978, Europe's last, concluded cautiously:

> We do not know how the virus reached Mrs. Parker, but we believe one of two routes to have been the most probable. The first involved airborne spread, the virus travelling in a service duct to a room immediately above the pox virus laboratory suite. This room contained a telephone that was frequently used by Mrs. Parker. The second was by direct or indirect contact transfer from a visitor from the Department of Medical Microbiology to Mrs. Parker in her darkroom. (U. K., Dept. Hlth. 1980, 61)

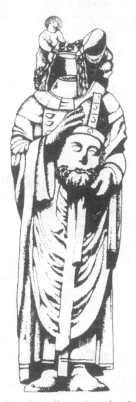

Fig. 7. St. Nicaise, patron saint of smallpox. Drawing by Chris L. Smith.

St. Nicaise: Patron Saint of Smallpox

St. Nicaise (Nicasius) was bishop of Rheims and had already constructed a church on the site of the present Cathedral of Rheims when the Huns pillaged eastern France in the middle of the fifth century A.D. This invasion by the Huns was disrupted by outbreaks of a pestilential disease, but before retreating, they killed the bishop and his sister on the steps of his church in 451 or 452. According to tradition, Nicaise

> went forth attended by his clergy to meet the enemy, singing hymns: one of the barbarian soldiers, however, struck off the upper half of his head, but the saint, nevertheless, continued to sing his stave until, after a few steps, he fell dead. (Shrewsbury 1956, 214)

In another version, the martyred bishop supposedly "returned to the cathedral after his assassination, carrying his skull in his hand, and . . . only fell dead when he reached the altar" (ibid.).

Since Nicaise had recovered from an attack of smallpox only the year before (which suggests that smallpox may have been the pestilence affecting the Huns) and had attributed his recovery to self-anointment with holy oil, he became the patron saint of smallpox victims after his canonization. Some sources report that Nicaise was martyred by the Vandals in 407, but his later martyrdom by the Huns is more probable, according to *Butler's Lives of the Saints* (Thurston & Attwater 1956).

An English manuscript in the Royal Library at Stockholm, dating from about the eleventh century, attests to the long-standing association of the French saint with smallpox. According to Shrewsbury (1956, 215), the reference reads in part:

> Saint Nicaise had apokke small.
> and mekyl grewans he had wythall;
> He preyed to God yt hum dere bowte,
> Yat quo so indyrly hym be sowte,
> Yat he hym from ye pockys schuld were
> Zif he on hym hys name wrete bere.

Another inscription in Latin, dating from about the tenth century, in the Harleian collection of the British Museum includes a prayer "for the consecration of an amulet against the smallpox" (ibid.):

> In the name of our Lord Jesus Christ, may the Lord protect these persons, and may the wish of these virgins ward off the smallpox. St. Nicaise had the smallpox, and he asked the Lord (to preserve) whoever carried his name inscribed: O St. Nicaise! thou illustrious bishop and martyr, pray for me a sinner, and defend me by thy intercession from this disease. Amen.

These two manuscripts notwithstanding, St. Nicaise was apparently only rarely recognized in modern times as the patron saint of smallpox victims, where he was known at all. Shrewsbury notes that the bishop's obscurity may have resulted from medieval Europe's obsession with epidemic plague for three hundred years before the mid-seventeenth century; from the fact that most surviving adults were immune to smallpox, whereas plague threatened adults and children whether they had had plague before or not; and from the fact that the Reformation had diminished Europeans' faith in saints, especially in Protestant countries, just as smallpox was becoming widespread in Europe.

A flagstone near the pulpit of the present Rheims cathedral marks the site of St. Nicaise's martyrdom, and one of the altars is dedicated to him. On the exterior of the cathedral, the bishop is dramatically depicted in a larger-than-life statue above the north entrance, holding his head, still wearing its bishop's miter, in his hand (plate 14). Inside, another headless statue of the saint faces the nave from above the main entrance. There, with the cathedral's great rose window at his back, the patron saint of smallpox must have "witnessed" Louis XV's coronation.

St. Nicaise was the principal, but not the only object of prayers by variolous Christians and their relatives. Successful intercessions on behalf of smallpox victims were also attributed to other saints, including St. Sebastian, St. Roche, and St. Barbara. Bleichsteiner (1954) described a cult in which St. Barbara was worshipped as a kind of smallpox goddess in Soviet Georgia and similar incarnations of smallpox gods or demons in Armenia and nearby areas. Most interesting is the strong association of St. Barbara and these other deities with the color red. As with the smallpox goddess in India, Georgian smallpox victims feared that modern medical treatment would anger the smallpox spirit, and some groups refused vaccination for that reason. Others regarded the patients themselves as "blessed" embodiments of the smallpox deity. Bleichsteiner reported that the cult of St. Barbara was also manifest in Nenning, Luxemburg, where smallpox was once known as "Barbara-pox."

Three

Heavenly Flowers

CHINA AND THE ISLAND NATIONS along the coast of the East Asian mainland—Japan, the Philippines, Indonesia, Malaysia, Papua New Guinea, Australia, and New Zealand—comprise a diverse group of countries we shall arbitrarily consider together. The islands were only partly isolated from the comings and goings on the mainland. Commercial and cultural ties linked countries of this region long ago, providing opportunities for dissemination of smallpox and other diseases. Indian middlemen sold spices and gold from Java, Bali, and Sumatra to Roman merchants before A.D. 300. Later, India's sea route to China included calls at local ports in some of the islands. By the seventh century A.D., Arab traders had settlements on Java, from which they traded with China as well as with their own countries in the Near East. According to Parker (1907), Chinese pilgrims also visited Java during this latter period and reported an unusual disease that they attributed to contact with "poisonous women."

In addition to being the largest, most influential country in the region, China has the longest historical record, followed by Japan. China and Japan had especially strong cultural and religious ties. Elsewhere, historical records of the period before Europeans "discovered" the islanders in the sixteenth century are generally scanty. Not surprisingly, the earliest evidence of smallpox in this region is from China.

As we saw in chapter 1, smallpox appears to have been introduced into China from Central Asia by the Huns around 250 B.C. Because of the size and density of its population, the disease probably was already endemic in northern China by the beginning of the Christian era. Nevertheless, during the reign of Emperor Kwang Wu Ti of the Han dynasty, smallpox apparently was introduced into China again, this time from the south, and was regarded as a new disease. The second importation occurred after one of the emperor's most reknowned generals, Ma-Yuan, was sent with a 40,000-man army to suppress an uprising of native Wuling tribes in present-day Hunan Province in A.D. 48 or 49. Ma-Yuan and his deputy disagreed over the route they should take after entering hostile territory, and the general led his army into a district where an epidemic was in progress. The result was that more than half of the Chinese expeditionary force, including General Ma-Yuan, succumbed to the dis-

ease. The remnants of Ma-Yuan's army returned home with their prisoners, bringing "captive's pox," or "barbarian pox," into China. No detailed
clinical description of this disease survives, but it probably was smallpox.
A Chinese treatise written by Ko Hung in the fourth century A.D. specifically suggests that the Huns were the source of this imported epidemic
(MacGowan 1884; Tao 1936; MacGowan 1897).

China's increasing commercial contact with other countries could
have been responsible for smallpox's appearance in Hunan Province at
this time. Around the time of Ma-Yuan's disastrous experience, there
began to be increased direct and indirect traffic between China and other
peoples of Central and Southeast Asia, Arabia, Persia, and India; by land
and sea, via the "Silk Road" and the "Burma Road." The Burma Road
between China and Southeast Asia passed directly through Hunan Province.

Only a generation after Ma-Yuan's expedition, in A.D. 90, another
Chinese general "penetrated so far west as to discover the 'Western Sea'
[apparently the Caspian Sea] and adjoining countries, and it was in the
ranks of [Pan-chao's] army that some Chinese scholars suppose small-pox
to have been brought to China" (Dudgeon 1871, 115). By this time,
however, an even more likely route for importing smallpox had been
opened: Messengers sent by the Chinese emperor returned from India to
introduce Buddhism into China in A.D. 65.

Only in the fourth century A.D. do we find the first unmistakable
description of smallpox in China. Huard and Wong (1968) attribute that
description to the alchemist-pathologist Ko Hung (281–340). Ko Hung's
text, the *Chou-hou pei-tsi fang* (Prescriptions for emergencies), couldn't
give a clearer diagnosis:

> Recently there have been persons suffering from epidemic sores which
> attack the head, face and trunk. In a short time these sores spread all over
> the body. They have the appearance of hot boils containing some white
> matter. While some of these pustules are drying up a fresh crop appears.
> If not treated early the patients usually die. Those who recover are
> disfigured with purplish scars which do not fade until after a year. This is
> due to poisonous air. The people say that it was introduced in the reign of
> Chien Wu when that king was fighting with the Huns at Nang Yang. The
> name of "Hun pox" has been given to it. (Wong & Wu 1936, 82)

He goes on to say that this fourth century epidemic was seasonal and
progressed from west to east, along with the Hun prisoners.

Two well-known scholars of Chinese medicine, Needham and Gwei-
Djen (1962, 464), traced a "very clear description of a smallpox
epidemic," which they date at about 497, to a sixth-century enlargement
of Ko Hung's treatise. One edition of this text apparently also refers to an
epidemic that "broke out in the east, gradually coming down westward,

till it spread all over the country" in 653 (Tao, 1936, 187). By 561, China was divided between rival dynasties, a Tartar-governed North and Chinese-governed South, and a Northern ambassador dispatched to the Southern court was described as having "just passed through the feverish disease, and his face was covered with scars" (Parker 1907, 88). Thus smallpox appears to have been well known in China by the sixth century, a period when Japan was coming more and more under China's cultural influence both directly and indirectly, via Korea.

After two unsuccessful attempts earlier in the same century, Buddhism was introduced into Japan in 552 by envoys of the king of Kudara (Paichke, in southwestern Korea), who brought a gold-plated image of Buddha and sacred books to the Japanese emperor, Kimmei. The Korean ruler was seeking the emperor's help against the threatened encroachment of two other kingdoms in the north and east of the Korean peninsula. Irwin (1910) records that soon after the emperor decided to allow the new religion to be worshipped in Japan, a pestilence ravaged the country, and conservative Japanese officials blamed the epidemics on worship of the new faith. Buddha's golden image was thrown into a canal, and the new temple was burned.

A quarter century later, the king of Kudara sent another statue of Buddha to Japan, with some two hundred volumes of sacred books, Buddhist priests, nuns, and a temple architect. These were followed in 584 by yet two more images of Buddha, brought from Korea by returning Japanese officials. The current emperor of Japan, Bidatsu, ordered his subjects to worship the Buddha diligently. Once again a severe pestilence followed introduction of the Buddhist images. According to the chronicles of Japan,

> Again the land was filled with those who were attacked with sores and died thereof. The persons thus afflicted with sores said:—"Our bodies are as if they were burnt, as if they were beaten, as if they were broken," and so lamenting, they died. (Aston 1896, 104)

Some Japanese began to believe their indigenous Shinto gods were punishing the nation for having embraced Buddhism. The images of Buddha were again thrown into a canal, the temple was burned, and Buddhist nuns were stripped and flogged. But as the epidemic showed no sign of responding to these penitential countermeasures, other Japanese began to wonder whether the pestilence was punishment for destroying the images of Buddha. National consternation peaked when at last, "the Emperor and the Ohomuraji" (the head of all clan leaders) were "suddenly afflicted with sores" (ibid.). In a desperate attempt to halt the epidemic, Bidatsu reversed his recent decision and ordered the Buddhist temples to be rebuilt—but forbad proselytizing. Soon after issuing that directive in the autumn of 585, the forty-eight-year-old emperor died in his fourteenth regnal year, apparently the first royal victim of smallpox in Japan (Davis 1916; Ponsonby-Fane 1959; Aston 1896).

Emperor Bidatsu had not designated an heir among his seventeen children, so he was succeeded by his sixty-nine-year-old brother, Emperor Yomei. Two years later, this emperor also died suddenly of the disease, which was still epidemic. Shortly before dying, he became the first Japanese emperor to personally embrace Buddhism (Ponsonby-Fane 1959).

According to Sansom's *History of Japan*, in the "fierce succession quarrels" that followed Yomei's death, disputes about the adoption of Buddhism were an additional cause of strife. Yomei was succeeded by Sujun, a son of the former emperor Kimmei. But Sujun was assassinated after five years, whereupon Bidatsu's widow, Suiko, assumed the throne as Japan's first reigning empress. She was the sovereign for thirty-five years (593–628). According to one traditional account, it was Yomei's son Crown Prince Shotoku who vowed to erect a temple dedicated to the "Buddha of Medicine" when his father was striken in 585. Finished in 607, the Horyuji became the national center and shrine of Japanese culture, the "very source of Japanese civilization and art" (Harrison 1978, 638). Thus smallpox apparently exerted a profound influence on Japan's political and religious life from the very beginning of its sojourn in that country.[1]

Evidence that the pestilence of 585–87 was smallpox rests largely on the description of the outbreak given in the Japanese chronicles cited above. The disease could have been brought to Japan directly from China, or it may have been introduced in one of the entourages that accompanied the Buddhist images from Korea. It may also have entered Japan as a consequence of secular traffic from Korea, especially in the first instance, since until 562, the Japanese maintained a small enclave on the southeast tip of Korea, directly across from Kyushu. Henschen, in his *History and Geography of Diseases*, reports that smallpox was introduced into Korea in 583. Thus, if the outbreak in Japan in 552 was also smallpox, and if the disease became established in Japan thereafter, then it is conceivable that smallpox was introduced into Korea from Japan, rather than from China. It would seem more probable, however, that smallpox was introduced into Korea from China in 583, caused typically large initial epidemics in Korea, and was carried from Korea to Japan a year later with Buddhism. It apparently was not endemic in Japan before the introduction around 585, even though it may have been imported earlier in that century.

Until early in the eighth century, the Japanese lived in scattered settlements. In 710, Nara was established as Japan's first true city, giving the emperor a capital worthy of the name for the first time. This concentration of city dwellers also provided smallpox with heretofore unknown opportunities.

Both Schmid (1896) and Murdoch (1910) record that only twenty-five years after Nara was founded, a Japanese fisherman shipwrecked on the coast of Korea was rescued and returned to the Japanese island of Kyushu, where he soon developed smallpox. The fisherman's infection began a series of outbreaks that raged for over two years. From Kyushu, the epidemic spread to the main island, Honshu, reaching Nara around 735. Hundreds of Nara's five hundred thousand inhabitants died, including many nobles at court and four brothers of the powerful Fujiwara family. Each of the brothers had headed a branch of the family, which virtually ruled Japan, before all four "died in a single year from smallpox at comparatively young ages" (Reischauer 1937, 185). Had the Fujiwara family not suffered this blow, it might have successfully resisted the rise of a Buddhist monk, named Dokyo, who became chancellor of the realm under Empress Shotoku and who Sansom says nearly succeeded in being named the empress's successor before she died in 770.

The epidemic of 735 continued to spread beyond Nara, and in the words of the Japanese chronicles, "smallpox was very mortal in all parts of the Empire" (Kaempfer 1906, 1:296). The ferocity of this epidemic caused an increase in religious fervor, facilitating once again the spread of Buddhism in Japan. Shinto priests again tried to blame the epidemic on the foreign religion, but Emperor Shomu, who was Buddhist himself, ordered a monastery and seven-storied pagoda to be erected in each of the country's seventy-one provinces, hoping thereby to gain relief from the epidemic.

As the epidemic still raged, Shomu feared that his attempts to placate the new god were inadequate, and decided to build a colossal statue of Buddha, "in the hope that so great a proof of devotion would put an end to the troubles" (Davis 1916, 82). The Japanese people were ordered to contribute to the construction of the statue, and the year before it was completed, the emperor himself carried earth in his hands to help build the platform around its base. Some 437 tons of bronze and nearly 300 pounds of gold were required for the casting. Technical problems and a revolt in Kyushu delayed the project, but the *Nara Daibutsu* was finally completed in 748 after seven unsuccessful attempts. The inaugural ceremony was attended by "the Emperor Shomu and all the princes, princesses, nobles, dignitaries and civil and military functionaries" (Sansom 1974, 1: 90). Fifty-three feet high, this Great Buddha can support three men in its palm. It is one of the largest and best-known images of Buddha in the world, as well as the world's largest bronze casting (plate 15).

The epidemic of 735–37 is sometimes referred to as the first epidemic of smallpox in Japan, but as we have seen, it appears to have been at least the second, and perhaps the third time the disease was introduced into that country. There were two other epidemics of smallpox in eighth-century Japan (in 763 and 790), and in the ninth century epidemics were recorded in 814, 853, and 899.

Epidemic smallpox hammered Japan six times in the tenth century, in 915, 925, 947, 974, 993 and 998. Why this apparent surge in the frequency of epidemics occurred in the tenth century is not clear. It may have been related to increased travel between Japan and China after conditions of the sea voyages improved around the middle of the previous century. A Great Purification Ceremony was performed in futile attempts to halt the outbreak of 915. Buddhist prayers were read, an amnesty was proclaimed, the Japanese people were freed from all unpaid tribute in kind and from half of that year's annual forced labor, and their taxes were commuted. The epidemic infected Emperor Daigo, which may explain the vigorous "containment measures," but he survived. In the outbreak of 947, the retired emperor, Suzaku, and the reigning emperor, Murakami, were both infected. Taking no chances, the government ordered provincial officials to make offerings to Shinto shrines and to have Buddhist prayers read for the emperors' recovery. They survived. Another great amnesty was proclaimed in response to the next epidemic (Reischauer 1937).

The epidemics made a deep impression on tenth-century Japan. They may have been the reason an astonishingly persistent prescription for smallpox victims, the "red treatment," apparently made its historical debut at this time in the Land of the Rising Sun. Eleven years before the century's fifth epidemic erupted, a Japanese medical book, *I Shinho*, was published, which according to Castiglioni (1941) and Cartwright (1972) contains the earliest known reference to the hanging of red cloth in the sickroom of patients ill with smallpox, and the first mention of special isolation hospitals for smallpox victims. As we shall see the red treatment persisted in various forms down to twentieth-century Europe and the United States. Engelbert Kaempfer, a European physician who visited Japan at the end of the seventeenth century, reported that Japanese physicians "think it very material in the cure of the smallpox, to wrap up the patient in red cloth. When one of the Emperor's children falls sick of this Distemper, not only the room and bed are furnished with red, but all persons that come near the patient, must be clad in gowns of the same colour" (1906, 1: 296).

The *I Shinho*'s reference to special isolation hospitals for smallpox victims is even more significant than its mention of the red treatment. We do not know what the Japanese really thought of that infection at the time, but some of them had clearly concluded that isolation of patients was useful.

The *I Shinho* was published the same century that the Arab physician Rhazes published his *Treatise on the Smallpox and Measles* and that Chien Chungyang published the first known medical description of smallpox in China. Needham (1954) cites evidence that Rhazes was visited by a Chinese medical scholar in Baghdad, but whether Rhazes' houseguest arrived before the physician finished his own treatise is not clear. MacGowan (1884) argues that Chien Chungyang is said to have used the modern Chinese character for smallpox—a combination of the characters for "lentil-bean" and "sickness"—for the first time in his text. Dudgeon (1871) reported descriptions of the disease in at least two books—*Chieu pien so yen* and *Tow chen cheng tsung*—from about the time of the Northern Sung dynasty (960–1127). One of them may have been the work of Chien Yi (1023–1104), a pediatrician, who differentiated smallpox, chickenpox, measles, and scarlet fever over six hundred years before that distinction was made in the West (Huard & Wong 1968).

ELEVENTH–FIFTEENTH CENTURIES

By most accounts the practice of inoculation (variolation) to prevent smallpox appeared in China for the first time during the Northern Sung dynasty. Interestingly, it is frequently described by Chinese sources as being practiced first in southwestern China, toward the border with India, where inoculation had been known since before the Christian era. According to Chinese tradition, the delicate practice of "planting the flowers"—the Chinese sometimes called the smallpox pustules "Heavenly Flowers"—was developed after a famous premier, Wang Tan, had lost all of his children to the disease. When, in his old age, Wang Tan fathered another son and sought to protect the child from the disease, a Buddhist nun near Tibet prescribed blowing the scabs from a mild case of smallpox into the boy's right nostril (plate 16).[2] She also advised that scabs used for this purpose should be about fifteen to twenty days old during hot weather and forty to fifty days old in winter. The nun then returned to her Sacred Mountain and told her followers that she was an incarnation of the goddess of mercy come to save children from dying of smallpox (MacGowan 1884). The legend says that after that pronouncement all the women worshipped her as the goddess of smallpox, to whom many shrines were devoted (fig. 8).

According to Wong and Wu (1936), historians of Chinese medicine, the Chinese method of inoculation was discovered by a philosopher who lived in the O Mei Mountains at Szechuen, on the border with India. Hes and Rutkovska (1973) attribute the origin of the "nostril insufflation method" to Yo-mei-shan, who is said to have inoculated the emperor Chen Tsung himself (1023–63) in the same era. Ball (1904), on the other hand, cites evidence that inoculation was discovered in China as early as the end of the second century A.D., for the purpose of protecting a grandson of Prince Tchiu-Siang. I am aware of no other evidence to support the latter account. The most plausible explanation of inoculation's commencement in China seems to be that stated by D. J. MacGowan (1884), who on the basis of his inquiries into late nineteenth-century China, suggested that a Buddhist nun popularized the practice in the eleventh century and that she may have been taught inoculation by a Tibetan monk who had learned it in India. It appears not to have been widely practiced in China until sometime later, as we shall see.

North of densely settled China (population about 100 million toward the end of the thirteenth century), smallpox was probably not yet endemic among the scattered, fractious nomadic tribes at the beginning of the thirteenth century, when they converged under the leadership of a "Universal Ruler," Ghenghis Khan. By founding the Mongol Empire, Genghis Khan united much of the Asian mainland during the thirteenth and fourteenth centuries, from Baghdad to Korea. After capturing Peking in 1215, the Mongols ruled the Northern (Chin) and Southern (Sung) regions of China for about a century (1271–1368) under a single new dynasty, the Yuan. "While the Mongol supremacy lasted," we are told, "it was easier to travel by land from Europe to China than it had ever been before, or than it was ever to be again until the nineteenth century" (Strayer et.al. 1961, 458). In addition to Marco Polo, the Mongol court in Peking was visited by French and papal ambassadors, employed "dozens of Europeans," and attracted Chinese and Mongol visitors from all over the empire. Smallpox, which up to then was reportedly unknown in Peking, is said to have been introduced into that city from the south during the Yuan dynasty.

Toward the end of the dynasty, from 1344 to 1362, unspecified pestilences ravaged nearly all of China. Apart from the publication of another treatise in 1323, however, there seems to be little specific reference to smallpox in China during this period. During the succeeding Ming dynasty, Chinese sources began to mention smallpox more frequently and stated regularly that the disease was infrequent among the Mongols, compared to the Chinese. Thus, "Chinese contacts constituted the gravest danger for the Mongols," whether such contact occurred at horsefairs along the border or in border raids (Serruys 1980, 41–43).

Epidemics of unknown causes hampered Mongol attempts to extend their empire. MacGowan (1897) records that during the Yuan dynasty, an army of Mongols and Chinese developed an illness that became widespread and killed great numbers of them while they marched across Annam to Cambodia. The weakened imperial army started to retreat but the Cambodians attacked and killed two Chinese generals in their triumph. The Mongol dynasty did not try to invade Cambodia again. In the Mongols' last attempt to invade Japan, one of the two fleets dispatched by Kublai Khan lost three thousand of its seventy thousand men from an unknown illness (Brinkley & Kikuchi 1915). The remainder of the combined force was defeated by the Japanese and by a timely storm.

Smallpox continued to infect the Japanese and their emperors, who had no knowledge at all of inoculation. Thirteen-year-old Emperor Goichijo was very ill with smallpox during a large epidemic in 1020, but recovered after he proclaimed an amnesty. Five years later, another smallpox epidemic raged throughout the empire from May to October. Other epidemics followed in 1036, 1072, 1085, and 1093.

Toward the end of the eleventh century, smallpox dealt the Japanese royal family another blow. Emperor Shirakawa (r. 1072–1086) had been especially anxious to have a son born of his union with Kenko, who was a daughter of the Fujiwaras. The emperor's special prayers were answered when Kenko gave birth to a boy, Prince Atsubume. Shirakawa's hopes turned to grief when Prince Atsubume and another royal prince, Atsukata, both died of smallpox in 1077. When Shirakawa abdicated in 1086, another of his sons, Horikawa, whose mother was not a Fujiwara, became the new titular emperor as Shirakawa began the system of "cloister government" and continued to function as the governing sovereign until he died in 1129. This shift of authority from maternal, Fujiwara relatives of titular sovereigns, whom a Fujiwara could control while serving as regent, to the paternal relative, the former emperor, was possible in part because of the coincidental failure of Fujiwara empresses to bear surviving sons during this period (Sansom 1974).

Japan suffered four more major epidemics of smallpox in the twelfth century (1113, 1143, 1175, and 1192). The third outbreak claimed lives throughout the empire, and also infected fourteen-year-old Emperor Takakura, but he survived. In addition to attacking the reigning emperor of Japan, the epidemic of 1175 ushered in a decade of turmoil and suffering from epidemics, bad weather, earthquakes, famine, and fire, for which the Japanese people, as usual, blamed their leaders. This set the stage for the dramatic downfall of one influential warrior clan, the Taira, and the rise of their rival, the Minamoto, during a protracted conflict known as the Gempei War (1180–85). The historian George Sansom believes that one of the major factors contributing to the Taira's defeat in this struggle was the "absence of determined leadership" after the sixty-three-year-old head of that clan, Taira Kiyomori, died suddenly in 1181 at Kyoto. Kiyomori may have died of smallpox. According to Sansom:

> It was in the early spring of 1181 that he took to his bed. The most reliable diary of the time reports on March 13, 1181, that the Zemmon (Kiyomori) is suffering from a high fever, and all contemporary accounts agree in describing him as suffering torments, crimson in the face, and "burning like fire." . . . We find it recorded on March 21 that he had died on that day. (Ibid., 287)

Kiyomori's victorious counterpart, Minamoto Yoritomo, consolidated his rise to power by becoming in 1192 the first permanent, hereditary shogun.

Among several famous members of the Minamoto clan whose exploits have been preserved in Japanese legends and romances, one other is of special interest to us. Chinzei Hachiro Tametomo (1139–70), Yoritomo's uncle, was reknowned as "the most skillful archer in the whole of the realm at that time" (Ozaki 1909, 3). Before his own clan came to power, Tametomo's enemies exiled him to the island of Oshima, southwest of present-day Tokyo. Many stories are told of this exceptionally large, strong man's prowess, including one apocryphal tale in which he prevented a smallpox demon from landing on the island. Tametomo was thus credited with the island's freedom from that disease, and the grateful residents raised a shrine in his honor that still exists today. His image, printed in red ink, was one of the most popular pictures Japanese families used to hang on the walls of their homes to protect or help cure family members from smallpox (plate 17), another manifestation of belief in the red treatment.

Japan recorded seven widely separated epidemics of smallpox in the thirteenth, fourteenth, and fifteenth centuries (in 1209, 1277, 1311, 1361, 1424, 1452, and 1454), suggesting that the disease had by then become endemic, subject only to occasional flare-ups when enough susceptible persons accumulated in the population. Sansom tells us that starting around 1225, a "series of calamities" affected the whole country over the next several years, including famine, smallpox, and assorted natural disasters. In 1329, a large outbreak of another unspecified pestilence in Kyoto gave Emperor Go Daigo an excuse for frequent pilgrimages, which he used to remain on the throne beyond his alloted ten years. Forty-five years later, when the Japanese Empire was wracked by constant warfare between Northern and Southern emperors, one of the rival emperors established a benevolent hospital for treatment of smallpox victims.[3]

Sixteenth Century

Only in the sixteenth century do we find the first accounts of smallpox among the inhabitants of other islands off the coast of East Asia. When, where, and how smallpox first reached these peoples is not known. It could have been introduced by any number of sources along a variety of routes. Indian merchants could have carried it from Rome before the fourth century A.D. Arab traders had dealings with the islands by the seventh century, as did the Chinese. During the early Ming dynasty (1368–1644), Chinese emperors actively supported intensive explorations in countries bordering the Indian Ocean and beyond. Borneo, Java, and Sumatra each sent envoys of their own to the Ming court, thus providing potential opportunities for introduction of smallpox when such ambassadors returned or sent messages home. Bantug (1953) cited the lack of an Arabic name for smallpox in local languages as evidence that the Arabs, at least, were probably not responsible for introducing the disease.

Wherever it came from, smallpox was present before Portuguese and other European seafarers began to explore the East Indies early in the sixteenth century. As Phelan (1967a) notes, sixteenth-century inhabitants of the Philippines were spared the nearly complete devastation suffered by their Aztec contemporaries only because the Filipinos already had some immunity to smallpox before the Spanish arrived. Nonetheless, later accounts by Europeans are nearly unanimous in observing how powerful the impact of smallpox was among local populations. Some of these reports also indicate that the disease had been present long enough to influence native mythology. One observer, writing about his experiences in the Sulo Islands between Borneo and the Philippines early in the nineteenth century, noted:

> The smallpox commits as many ravages here as in any part of the world for the extent of its population. It is held in the greatest fear and dread . . . if it rages extensively all business is at a stand and the people fly to the other islands. One half of the whole that get the infection die with it. (Moor 1837, 52)

Another traveler, who visited Java around the same time, observed that "the most fatal disorder among them is the smallpox . . . one tenth of all the children born die . . . of this disorder" (Crawford 1820, 1: 33). Skeat and Blogden reported from the Malay peninsula early in the twentieth century that "all of them are, however, in mortal terror of one disease in particular, viz., smallpox, from which many of their tribes have greatly suffered from time to time" (1906, 1: 100).

Some islanders' respect for smallpox was so profound that the wrath of the disease was accounted for in legends of the world's creation. Among one tribe in Borneo, Kinaringan, the Creator, is believed to have received earth to add to the empty waters and sky from an evil spirit named Bisagit. In return, Bisagit demanded that "when Kinaringan had peopled his world with men and women he should allow Bisagit to take a toll of half of them every forty years, by afflicting them with the scourge of smallpox" (Rutter 1929, 228). The legend alludes to the pattern of sporadic, highly destructive epidemics affecting children and adults, which probably was typical of most of the islanders' experience with smallpox. Except for densely populated islands like Java, the disease probably died out after each epidemic, and appeared again only after being reintroduced by seafarers. After a generation or so, much of the population would be susceptible, and able to sustain another epidemic.

The earliest documented epidemic I have found in the islands occurred in 1591, when Father Chirino, a Jesuit, described an outbreak of
smallpox in Manila and the surrounding countryside: "One-third of the
population was in bed and there was not left any person who was not
attacked by it and many died, especially among adults and the aged"
(Bantug 1953, 104). D'Ardois (1961) records that one of the early outbreaks of this period occurred after a Spanish ship, the *Nao de la China*,
carried smallpox to the Philippines from Mexico.

As Europeans were exploring the off-shore islands and providing
evidence of smallpox there for the first time, inoculation was becoming
more widely known and used in China. Inoculation had been a popular
folk practice in some areas, but in the sixteenth century it was incorporated into Chinese scientific medicine. According to Sery (1973) and Das
(1902), in addition to the more convenient *Han Miao*, blowing powdered
crusts up the nose via a long silver tube (plate 16), the Chinese employed
several other methods, including *Shui Miao*, the method of choice, which
involved plugging the nose for six hours with cotton pledgets soaked in
powdered scabs mixed with camphor, herbs, or musk. By the method of
Tou I a susceptible child was made to wear the undergarment of a child
who had smallpox, whereas the *Tou Chiang* technique required smearing
a piece of cotton with fluid from a smallpox blister and inserting that into
the nose (Wong & Wu 1936). Why these methods of introducing the virus
by what appears to have been the natural route of infection, namely the
nose, did not regularly give rise to ordinary, virulent infections, remains a
mystery. One possible explanation, suggested to the author by Dr. D. A.
Henderson, is that the virus inhaled naturally was in sufficiently small
particles to be deposited deep within the lung, whereas particles inoculated by nasal insufflation may have been much larger and were likely to
implant in the nose or throat where a local lesion might be produced. Yet
another method was to rub smallpox pus or crusts mixed with water into
an abraded area of skin. Material for inoculation was sometimes kept in a
sealed vase.

In all, some fifty texts on the treatment of smallpox are known to have
been published in China during the Ming dynasty (Hes & Rutkouska
1973). By the late nineteenth century, inoculation had been carefully
codified: Ten Chinese rules prescribed, among other things, that spring
and autumn were the most favorable seasons for inoculation, that one
should avoid very hot or very cold months for inoculation, that children
should be inoculated at one year of age, and that "inoculation is to be
performed when there is no disease present in the system; good lymph
must be selected, a proper time chosen, and good management adopted,
and then all will go well" (Ball 1904, 754). Thus the Chinese apparently
developed relatively effective empirical techniques for inoculation and
for storing virus for inoculation over short periods. But we know little

about how they or the Japanese thought smallpox spread or produced disease during these early centuries.

Although inoculation was practiced since very early times in India and perhaps in Persia and became widespread in China around the sixteenth century, it apparently was not known to most of the East Asian islanders until much later. Astonishingly, according to Miyajima (1922–23) even the Japanese were ignorant of inoculation until it was introduced from China in the mid-eighteenth century, about the same time it was becoming popular in England and France.

Although inoculation was not known to the islanders until very late, smallpox's contagiousness apparently was recognized, and infected persons and villages were often abandoned forthwith because of it. However, such actions may sometimes have reflected only superstitious fear of a hideous disease. Special isolation hospitals for smallpox victims were recommended in Japan, it will be recalled, as early as the tenth century, well before the London Small-Pox and Inoculation Hospital was established in 1746. Occasionally friends or relatives who had already had smallpox remained behind to help care for victims. Because the risk of infection from corpses of smallpox victims was also appreciated (or feared), tribes in Borneo would throw a rope around a smallpox corpse and use that to drag it to a shallow grave, in order to avoid touching the body directly. Evans's 1953 study of Bornean tribes records that some were afraid to eat corn during an epidemic because of the resemblance to pustules. Both Skeat and Blogden (1906) and Hose (1926) note other more practical tribesmen on Borneo and the Malay peninsula used a unique type of *cordon sanitaire* in an attempt to protect themselves: they hung a rattan rope or felled trees across rivers and streams leading to and from an infected area to prevent spread of the disease, which the Sea Dyaks called "Jungle Flowers," or "Jungle Fruits." Among the Sea Dyaks of Borneo, Dyak medicine men were supposed to be able to cure most diseases, but they acknowledged that smallpox and cholera were beyond their powers. E. H. Gomes, who lived among them at the turn of the twentieth century, wrote that "no witch-doctor will approach any case of these, however well he may be paid" (1911, 19).

SEVENTEENTH AND EIGHTEENTH CENTURIES

With no knowledge of inoculation, but with a more densely settled population, Japan suffered heavily from smallpox in the seventeenth century. The previous century had brought a partial respite from the disease, with only two epidemics recorded, in 1522 and 1550. In 1609, smallpox was again recorded in the royal family, although the details of the case are not clear (Irwin 1910, 1205). According to Williams (1963) four years later the disease struck the port city of Langasaque (Nagasaki), killing over two thousand six hundred persons. One wonders whether it was also smallpox that helped expose a serious conspiracy against the government in 1651, when one of the main conspirators became ill suddenly, and "began to shout secrets in his delirium" (Sansom 1974, 3: 56). A more visible blow, however, came a few years later, when smallpox returned to the royal palace and killed another emperor.

Son of a Fujiwara mother, Emperor Gokomyo was raised from birth by one of his father's other consorts and succeeded to the throne when he was eleven (plate 18). He immersed himself in the diligent study of all subjects useful to the art of governing and preferred Confucianism over Buddhism for that reason (Ponsonby-Fane 1959). "From his earliest youth [Gokomyo] showed sagacity, magnanimity, and benevolence. . . . There can be no doubt that this sovereign conceived the ambition of recovering the administrative authority [from the shogun]" (Brinkley & Kikuchi 1915, 591). Gokomyo spent much time engaged in sword exercises, which made him suspect in the eyes of the powerful shogun, Ietsuna, who was the real administrative authority of the empire. One official warned the young emperor that the study of martial arts did not become the imperial court and would probably provoke a reaction from the shogun. When the emperor ignored this advice, the official threatened to commit suicide "unless the fencing lessons were discontinued." In response to this threat the young emperor calmly replied, "I have never seen a military man kill himself, and the spectacle will be interesting. You had better have a platform erected in the palace grounds so that your exploit may be clearly witnessed" (ibid.). The incident was reported to the shogun, who "concluded that some decisive measure must be taken."

Before the shogun could act, however, and before the emperor could realize his own ambitions, Gokomyo died of smallpox in 1654. He was twenty-two years old. By Brinkley and Kikuchi's account, Gokomyo's sole accomplishments were "the restoration and improvement of certain court ceremonials, the enactment of a few sumptary laws, and the abandonment of cremation in the case of Imperial personages" (ibid.). He also had begun to improve official discipline. Since Gokomyo left no son when he died, he was succeeded by his half-brother.

Ietsuna's predecessor in the shogunate, Iemitsu, himself suffered an attack of smallpox sometime between 1623 and 1651. On that occasion, a new Japanese treatment of bathing smallpox victims in hot water, to which sake, rice water, red beans, and salt were added, was employed for the first time on such an important person, "after a heated discussion among the close attendants and the Shogunal physicians" (Maekawa 1976a). Whether the rationale for this treatment reflected a shared belief in the principles on which Rhazes' heat treatment was based, I do not know. Iemitsu recovered, and the treatment was used subsequently for other shoguns and their children who caught smallpox.

Ietsuna died in 1680, having held the office of shogun for thirty years. He was succeeded by his son Tsunayoshi, who at thirty-four years of age became the fourth shogun of the Tokugawa line. Such was Tsunayoshi's power that Englebert Kaempfer, on his visit to Japan in 1690–92, mistook him for the emperor. Born in the Year of the Dog, this eccentric shogun was convinced that he must show particular mercy to dogs in order to secure the male heir he wanted so badly. Because of this unusual mania, Tsunayoshi is known in Japanese history as the "Dog-Shogun." Tsunayoshi prohibited the slaughter, abuse, and "insulting" of dogs and ordered that stray dogs were to be fed. Each street was required to care for a certain number of them, and those dogs that died were to be buried decently at the tops of hills and mountains. Citizens who violated these orders received severe penalties. Killing a dog became a capital offense.

When Tsunayoshi caught smallpox in 1709, he presumably was treated with the same special bath inaugurated by the third Tokugawa shogun a few decades before, but in Tsunayoshi's case the treatment didn't help. Neither was his devotion to the empire's canine population rewarded, since he died without a son and was succeeded by his nephew.

In 1709, the year the "Dog-Shogun" died of smallpox, the all-powerful virus completed its sweep of the Japanese leadership by killing yet another emperor in the same epidemic. Former emperor Higashiyama was thirty-five years old when he died and had reigned since 1687. Six months before his death, he abdicated in favor of his eleven-year-old son, Nakanomikado, but he had continued to exercise such imperial authority as there was. Higashiyama is credited with having revived certain religious rites at court, including a thanksgiving service for farm crops and a ceremonial rite for investiture of the crown prince.

By the time Shogun Tsunayoshi and Emperor Higashiyama died of smallpox in 1709, Japan's population of about 25 million was at peace, with a rising standard of living and birth rate, and had been almost completely isolated from the rest of the world for seventy years (Sansom 1974). Under the "Exclusion Policy" the Tokugawa shogunate enforced between 1639 and 1853, only Chinese, Portuguese, and Dutch ships were permitted to call at Japan, and those only at the southern part of Nagasaki. Despite this relative isolation, Matsuki (1971) notes that the northern island of Hokkaido recorded an average of one epidemic of smallpox every fourteen to fifteen years in the two centuries following 1624. Ironically, it was during the two centuries of the Exclusion Policy that smallpox inoculation finally reached Japan, though it might have arrived in Japan earlier, but for the country's policy of national isolation.

Sometime between 1654 and 1709, years both marked by the death of a Japanese sovereign from smallpox, a Chinese medical instructor taught a student in Nagasaki what he knew of the pathology and therapy of the disease. The pupil, Seichoku Ikeda, later founded a special school devoted exclusively to the treatment of patients with smallpox. Whether this school included inoculation is not clear, although Furukawa (1971) and Miyajima (1922–23) state that inoculation was first introduced into Japan at Nagasaki in 1744, from China, and that the European method of inoculation was first introduced in about 1790. The European method was probably introduced by the Dutch since Holland was the first country in continental Europe to adopt the practice and Holland and Portugal were the only European countries in contact with Japan. We are also told that around this time, "most of the scientific knowledge [Japan had] so far obtained from the Dutch had been applied to medicine" (Sansom 1974, 3: 191). Why the Chinese method of inoculation became known in Japan so late, despite considerable Chinese influence on other aspects of Japanese culture, is a question more easily asked than answered. It would seem, however, to support evidence that inoculation had not been widely practiced in China for more than a few hundred years.

At the end of the seventeenth century, Kaempfer (1906) noted that the Japanese distinguished three types of poxlike illnesses: *Fooso*, or true smallpox (Variola); *Fasika*, or measles; and *Kare*, or watery pustules (probably chickenpox). He also observed that the Great Pox (syphilis) was recognized in Japan, where it was known as "the Portuguese disease." In 1796, Japan's first Medical Academy in Yedo (later Tokyo) inaugurated a chair devoted to the study of smallpox.

On the Asian mainland, smallpox was also playing an influential role in Chinese affairs, despite the mainlanders' sophisticated knowledge of inoculation. The Manchus, who were another of several tribes in the area north of the Great Wall, were no strangers to smallpox. Years before they overthrew the Ming dynasty and succeeded to the throne of the Celestial Empire in 1644, the Manchu khan and other princes who had not had smallpox were so afraid of catching the infection that they refused to extend condolences in person to the family of a young Manchu prince who died of the disease. Finally, the khan, who had already started calling himself "Emperor (of China)," "met the father of the deceased at a distance of ten *li* [three miles] outside of the smallpox avoiding area" (Parker 1907, 89).

During a council of war held in 1633 at a time when the Manchu khan was uncertain of what his policy should be, his general, Yangguri, "made proposals which determined the future course of China" (Hummel 1944, 2: 898). Yangguri advised that attempts to conquer Korea or the Chahar Mongols or to enter China via Shan-haikwan be postponed in favor of direct raids through weak spots in the Great Wall. According to Hummel (1944) and Serruys (1980), one specific feature of his plan was that only officers who had had smallpox should be sent on these expeditions—a necessary precaution, since their route would take them through territory where smallpox was known to occur. The area the Manchus feared was probably one of the several settlements of Chinese immigrants that sprang up "north of the Great Wall line, outside of Chinese jurisdiction, but regularly going back to their native villages," after the mid-sixteenth century (ibid., 46). A year after Yangguri proposed his plan, it was learned that Linden Khan of the Chahar Mongols had died of smallpox.

As we saw earlier, during the sixteenth century the Mongols were said by Chinese sources to have been in "gravest danger" of contracting smallpox when they came into contact with Chinese. Writing in 1594, a Chinese official on the Chinese-Mongolian border reported that when Mongols got smallpox, "they provide [the sick] with a Chinese to take care of him. . . . [In this respect] they regard China as a house on fire, and they refuse to stay there long for fear of contracting smallpox" (ibid.). When the Manchus, who like the Mongols were a widely scattered people and had therefore remained relatively free of smallpox, established the Ching dynasty, they took care to exempt both Manchus and Mongols who had not had smallpox from what would have been hazardous mandatory appearances at the imperial court in Peking. Serruys cites an imperial document, the *Ta-Ch'ing hui-tien shih-li* (1764), with reference to Manchu officials:

> When the time comes round for Solons and Dahurs to come to court, the military governors and other officials are used to send them to the capital whether or not they have had smallpox before. Last year, seven men contracted the disease; and again, two years ago, six or seven men did so. (Their visits) are not important as far as military matters are concerned, and it is not right to harm so many people needlessly. So we order to inform the military governor of Hei-lung-chiang immediately: from hereon he must not allow to send to the capital those who have never contracted smallpox. (Ibid., 55)

Twenty years later, another edict decreed:

> From hereon, Mongols from the Inner Administration [i.e., Inner Mongolia] and from the Qalqas who are to inherit a rank, and have reached (legal) age, if they have once contracted smallpox, shall come to the capital to be installed, presented at court, and receive their succession. Those who have not yet contracted smallpox, shall proceed to Je-ho [Jehol, north of the Great Wall] to be installed, appear at court, and receive their succession. (Ibid., 49)

Parker (1907) supplies further evidence of the military significance of smallpox in the seventeenth-century struggle for control of China. The same year the Ching (Manchu) dynasty came to power, a Manchu prince was censured for excusing himself from a military campaign on the grounds that he had not had smallpox. The very next year, in a primitive attempt to isolate municipal smallpox victims, an imperial edict commanded all persons suffering from smallpox to remove themselves to a distance of 40 *li* (about 12 miles, or 7 kilometers) from Peking.

The Ching court's fears were well founded, but their precautions were inadequate. Perhaps because they were Manchus and unfamiliar with endemic smallpox, they did not yet know about or trust inoculation. Whatever the reason, around 2 February 1661, Emperor Fu-lin, the first Manchu ruler of China, felt ill on his return to the Forbidden City after visiting a temple, probably the Temple of Heaven just south of the Forbidden City. Hummel (1943) believes he may already have had tuberculosis, since he was noted to be very thin and spat blood. Five days after his acute illness began, orders were issued in the emperor's name forbidding his subjects to stir fried beans. In 1980, I was informed in a letter from Dr. Chen Zheng-ren, director of the National Vaccine and Serum Institute in Peking, that according to Chinese custom, "this kind of saying indicated that he was suffering from smallpox." The next day the twenty-three or twenty-four-year-old Son of Heaven "ascended the dragon." According to Dr. Chen, who examined several Chinese sources,

> all [the emperor's] clothes and things were burnt outside of his living house on the 14th. People saw his mother dressed in black clothes crying in the corridor. His body was moved to Ching-Shan (northern side of the Palace). All officers were lined up from the Palace to Ching-Shan. There were 20 to 30 boys, in black clothes, walking in front of the coffin and followed by the coffin of his wife who died for him. His mother again in black clothes walking behind. Finally, . . . 27 days after his death, all officers went to Ching-Shan and burnt all of their robes and that ended the funeral.

Fu-lin's reign title was Shuh-Chih, Emperor of China, Manchuria, Mongolia, and Korea. One of his uncles, who was regent during the Shuh-Chih emperor's minority, had also died of smallpox around 1650. After Fu-lin's death, the Manchu court decreed that Mongol princes who had not had smallpox should not come to Peking for imperial audiences (Wang 1972).

Having killed the Chinese emperor, smallpox dictated the selection of his successor in an unusually direct way. Despite the emperor's youth, he had eight sons when he died. Of these, the third son, eight-year-old Hsüan-yeh, was chosen to become the new Son of Heaven expressly because he had already had smallpox and so was less likely to die young (Hummel 1943). The long-standing Manchu dread of smallpox, so vividly confirmed by Fu-lin's death, and their realization that as non-Chinese their claims to the throne were enhanced by ruling from smallpox-ridden Peking, apparently outweighed any perceived advantages of selecting one of the older, susceptible sons. (Chen says that Hsüan-yeh was temporarily removed from the palace during his illness five or six years earlier—

which may have spared his father from infection then.) Thus, Hsüan-yeh became Emperor K'ang Hsi. A nineteenth-century portrait shows numerous pock marks on his face (plate 19), which according to Chen's sources were also remarked upon by missionaries from Belgium and France who visited him in his middle age.

Smallpox and the Manchus chose well. K'ang Hsi reigned as emperor of China for sixty-one years and became "one of the most famous inhabitants of the dragon throne" (Hummel 1943, 1: 328). The historian J. MacGowan asserted, "there are few Emperors in the long history of China that will bear any comparison with K'ang Hsi. He was a man of great natural abilities, a wise ruler and a distinguished scholar" (1897, 539). In the opinion of another historian,

> The K'ang-hsi emperor . . . reigned over China longer than any emperor before him and was probably the most admirable ruler of the entire later imperial age. Conscientious, inquisitive, and indefatigable, he had awesome physical and mental powers. He was thoroughly Chinese by culture, wrote literary prose and poetry of good quality, and encouraged literature, art, fine printing, and porcelain manufacture. . . . A careful, frugal, and efficient administrator, the K'ang-hsi emperor made strenuous efforts to ensure honesty in government and to foster Chinese-Manchu harmony. He made six grand tours of inspection around the country to see for himself what conditions were like. . . . No less than in the domestic realm, the K'ang-hsi emperor was a determined and masterly leader in military affairs. (Hucker 1975, 297)

Jonathan Spence published a collection of excerpts from the writings of this remarkable emperor. In them, K'ang Hsi tells us that he had his regular troops "inoculated against smallpox as I did my own children" (1975, 18). The following excerpt reveals the wit and wisdom of this great emperor:

> On appointing Ch'en in 1711, I told him: "When you get to Kwangsi you must ensure harmony between civil and military, and keep troops and commoners at peace. The governor is responsible for the troops, and must drill them constantly. You've been in the Hanlin Academy for many years, so I am going to make a special experiment of appointing you to a senior provincial post, and see how you are able to manage things." At first his memorials were too long and in the wrong format, and he passed on a report that magical *chih* fungus had been found on a mountain top under a fragrant cloud, sure proof of the Emperor's virtue and promise of long life to come; and even though he knew I did not value such auspicious omens, he was duty-bound to send it in to the palace, so I could examine it or use it for medicine. I replied that the *Histories* are full of these strange omens, but they are of no help in governing the country, and that the best omens were good harvests and contented people. Later his memorials were shorter, there was no more *chih* fungus, and he became a sensible governor. (Ibid., 52)

In spite of the early Ching edict requiring all victims of smallpox to leave Peking, the Chinese capital continued to be notoriously dangerous for nonimmune visitors. When K'ang Hsi died in 1722, Mongols who had not had smallpox were exempted from coming to Peking for his funeral. In 1698, the Panchen Lama of Tibet had also excused himself from visiting Peking because he had not yet had smallpox. (Not that he was completely safe at home. Wessels [1924] quotes Jesuit documents from this period that show there were large epidemics of smallpox with enormous mortality rates in Lhasa about once every ten years.) Two years after the Chinese emperor's seventh son died of smallpox in 1747, the son of a Tibetan king, several chiefs, and a group of lama priests declined to go to Peking for the same reason as had the Panchen Lama (Parker 1907).

Long after K'ang Hsi's grandson, Chien Lung (r. 1735–95), himself a "scholar and poet," had succeeded to the Dragon Throne, he extended several invitations to the third Panchen Lama, Lobsang Palden Yeshe, to visit Peking. Ordinarily the Dalai ("all-embracing" or "ocean-wide") Lama at Lhasa exceeded the Panchen ("wise and great") Lama in prestige as well as rank, since the Dalai Lama was the spiritual and civil ruler of Tibet under nominal Chinese leadership, whereas the Panchen Lama had spiritual influence but no real authority as head of the monastery at Tashilhunpo, west of Lhasa. In the late 1770s, the Panchen Lama who repeatedly excused himself from accepting the Chinese emperor's invitations had eclipsed his Dalai Lama in prestige. He was described by a visiting Scot as a man of "remarkable character, learning and ability," with an "affable and friendly nature" Richardson 1962, 65). Emperor Chien Lung persisted with his invitation, since he hoped to exploit the Tibetan leader's spiritual prestige to help improve the empire's authority in Mongolia, where the Panchen Lama was also venerated. After the risks, including the risk of smallpox, were debated again, the Panchen Lama left Tibet in June 1779, and arrived in China by way of Mongolia a year later.

On his arrival in China, he was met by the emperor at the imperial palace at Jehol, north of the Great Wall, as a mark of courtesy. When the Panchen Lama arrived in Peking about a month later, he was housed in the Yellow Temple (*Huang si*), which Emperor Shuh-Chih had built in the previous century for the visit of the fifth Dalai Lama.[4] There in the Yellow Temple, within a few weeks of his arrival, the forty-two-year-old Panchen Lama died of smallpox in November or December 1780, "in spite of all available medical assistance, and though the Imperial Princes and the Emperor himself frequently visited his bedside" (Ludwig 1904, 17). The grief-stricken emperor, who had come to like and respect the genial Tibetan, had a white marble obelisk (Dagoba) erected in the Yellow Temple's courtyard, where the Panchen Lama's "garments, shoes, and prayers" remained after his cremated body was returned to Tashilhunpo in a gold coffin (ibid.,19–21; Destenay 1980).

Thirteen years after the Panchen Lama died in Peking, Lord Macartney, who led the first British embassy to the emperor of China, reported that the confluent form of smallpox was very common in China, sweeping away thousands at a time (Cranmer-Byng 1963).

Apparently, the Chinese did not deliberately keep knowledge of inoculation from barbarians beyond the Celestial Empire. According to the 1913 *History of Inoculation and Vaccination*, during the same generation that inoculation was introduced into Japan from China, K'ang Hsi's successor, Emperor Yung Ching, sent Chinese physicians to "Tartary" (Siberia) to help relieve a smallpox epidemic in 1724—an early example of international assistance in fighting an epidemic. Needham and Gwei Djen (1962) record that thirty-five years earlier, the Russians had sent a special mission to China to study the use of inoculation against smallpox. Although an English physician in the Russian Service, Thomas Harwin, also participated in that mission, which occurred nearly five years before Queen Mary II died of smallpox, and over forty years before Tsar Peter II died of it, the first account of Chinese inoculation against smallpox did not appear in Western Europe until 1700.

One western Mongolian tribe, the Kalmucks (Khoits), were still being battered by periodic epidemics during the mid-eighteenth century, much as the Manchus had been before the Ching era. In 1739, the Chinese emperor warned a Kalmuck mission to his court to avoid a certain southerly route if they had not already had smallpox. Six years later, there was a large outbreak in one of the Kalmuck regions. A Kalmuck prince named Batur Ubasi and a young Turbet Mongol prince both died of the disease during this period.[5] Eventually, the emperor decreed that young Mongol princes who were engaged to marry Manchu princesses must be sent to Peking for inoculation and education (Parker 1907).

In the late eighteenth century, the Chinese emperor ordered a large stone tablet to be erected at the other end of his empire at the entrance of the chief shrine on a road leading into Lhasa. Positioned so that all pilgrims would see it, the tablet described the procedures to be followed when smallpox broke out (plate 20). (Apparently, no such tablets were erected on the roads leading into Peking.) Also under orders from the Chinese emperor, the Dalai Lama built special hospitals for smallpox patients in Lhasa, where they were provided with food and cared for by special officers (Das 1902). Moore (1815) quotes Saunders, surgeon to an embassy in Tibet, as saying smallpox victims' houses and sometimes entire villages were burned down in attempts to halt the disease. Probably unbeknownst to the Tibetans, villagers on the island of Sumatra were using the same drastic methods.

On 2 November 1749, a dispatcher in Madras provided one of the earliest specific references to the disease in the Asian islands south of Japan when he mentioned "difficulties in disposing of the ships . . . in Sumatra owing to an epidemic of smallpox" (Dodwell 1920, 83). Garrison

(1914) says there was an exceptionally destructive epidemic in the "East Indies" in 1770–71; and in 1783, Marsden estimated that about one third of the Sumatran population had died in a terrible epidemic over the past three years:

> It is reagarded as a plague, and drives from the country thousands whom the infection spares. Their method of stopping its progress (for they do not attempt a cure) is by converting into an hospital or receptacle for the rest, that village where lie the greatest number of sick, whither they send all who are attacked by the disorder, from the country round. The most effectual methods are pursued to prevent any person's escape from this village, which is burnt to the ground as soon as the infection has spent itself, or devoured all the victims offered to it. (Marsden 1966, 191)

Others also attested to smallpox's role in seriously depopulating the coastal districts of West Sumatra in the eighteenth century.

NINETEENTH CENTURY

Early in the nineteenth century, an attempt by the British East India Company to force the population of Sumatra to cultivate pepper caused many natives along the west coast of the island to move about, which contributed to intermittent epidemics. By 1818, one witness estimated that about two-thirds of the four thousand would-be pepper planters along the coast had emigrated or died of smallpox (Bastin 1957).

Toward mid-century, another Briton, Sir James Brooke, established a small "personal empire" at Sarawak, on the adjacent island of Borneo, in an effort to extend British rule in that area. Visiting the state of Luwu on Celebes in April 1840, this first "White Rajah of Sarawak" observed that smallpox had followed a recent civil war, killing more people than had died in the fighting (Mundy 1848). A few years later, Sir James himself almost died of a severe attack of smallpox. The disease continued to take a heavy toll on Sarawak during the reign of the second White Rajah, Sir Charles Brooke, from 1868 to 1917. After one outbreak in 1856, Brooke wrote:

> Indeed, near the mouths of small streams the stench was almost offensive from the decaying bodies. When first taken with the unmistakable symptoms, they were left to look after themselves. The consequence was the disease proved fatal in almost every case . . . but where inoculation was practiced, the average amount of deaths did not exceed one per cent. The inhabitants (particularly the Dyaks) have an extraordinary fear of this disease, and never speak of it without a shudder. On making inquiries after a person's health, the question is put in a whisper for fear the spirit might hear, and it is termed by various names, the most usual being jungle flowers or fruits. (Roth 1968, 1: 290–91)

Roth (1968) observes the Dyaks were usually inoculated by Malays, who often had use for inoculation themselves. When and how the Malays first learned of inoculation, I do not know. In the Malay city of Penang, founded in 1786, smallpox is first mentioned in official records in 1805, and the city experienced full blown epidemics in 1813 and 1824. Smallpox became endemic in Singapore during the first decade of its existence, starting in 1819, according to Lee (1973). Epidemics were recorded in 1838, 1849–50, 1859–60, 1899–1900, 1902–3 and 1910–11, and were perhaps due in part to the city's frequent commercial traffic with India and China. Buckley (1965) estimates the outbreak of 1838 claimed over three hundred lives within three months. On the eastern end of the Indonesian archipelago, New Guinea also suffered severe epidemics of smallpox and dysentery in the second half of the nineteenth century.

Australia's isolation from regular traffic with Europe ended with the arrival of settlers from England at Sydney in January 1788. Fifteen months later, a massive epidemic characterized by a rash and high mortality began among aborigines near Sydney and spread throughout Australia, especially the southeast coast. Few, if any, of the white colonists were affected. Cumpston (1914), who chronicled the history of the disease in Australia, believed that this outbreak was indeed smallpox, but not all writers agree. A Frenchman who landed at Botany Bay soon after the outbreak began, described the epidemic's impact on the aborigines:

> Then a disaster happened. In April 1789 black bodies were suddenly seen to be floating in the harbour and washed up in the coves. Smallpox had struck. . . . by May the disease had swept through all the harbour tribes. A few of the sick who were too feeble to protest were brought into Sydney for treatment, but the majority, comprehending nothing of this mysterious enormity that had struck them down, quickly succumbed by their campfires. (Moorehead 1966, 145)

Other outbreaks of a similar illness were recognized among aborigines in about 1829–30 and again sometime in the 1860s. The latter outbreak was probably introduced into the northern territory by Malay or Chinese fishermen. During these early outbreaks, which reduced the population of the terror-stricken aborigines considerably, "normal funeral rites were suspended, and in large mounds of earth, communal graves, scores of human skeletons have been found arranged in rows " (Dixon 1962, 206). A few Europeans were infected in the outbreak in 1829–30, and Cumpston considers them to be the first recorded cases of smallpox among Europeans in Australia.

The first real outbreak among Europeans in Australia occurred in October-November 1857, after the *Commodore Perry* brought the disease to Melbourne from Liverpool. Four of the sixteen persons infected died.

After the outbreak in 1857, there were at least nine other epidemics in Australia up to the end of the nineteenth century, all due to importations by passengers on ships. Cumpston noted that Australia was most likely to be affected when smallpox became epidemic in other parts of the world.

An outbreak of forty-three cases with ten deaths occurred at Melbourne in 1868–69. Three years later, the *Nebraska* left San Francisco, California, and discharged infected passengers at Hawaii, New Zealand, and Australia. Some passengers who transferred to another ship when the *Nebraska* called at New Zealand carried the infection to Sydney. In Victoria, the infection brought by the *Nebraska* caused seven cases of smallpox.

The *Nebraska* did not bring smallpox to New Zealand for the first time. It made its premier appearance there shortly before, via a ship from London. Smallpox had broken out on board the *England* early in the voyage, and was still uncontrolled when the ship arrived in New Zealand (the disease was rife in Europe as a result of the pandemic following the Franco-Prussian War). Later, an official inquiry into the voyage praised the *England*'s captain, but censured the shipowners for "insufficient light and ventilation," and noted that "the medical inspection [was] loosely conducted." The report went on to state that "the [ship's] doctor was subject to epileptic fits and defective memory, even forgetting the previous day's treatment and the sex of the patients, and on January 15 the passengers declined the doctor's treatment" ("Smallpox in New Zealand," 334). Nineteen years before the *Nebraska* arrived, another ship from San Francisco brought smallpox to Hawaii for the first time; when the disease killed eight percent of the inhabitants within eight months (Hirsch 1883; Windley).

The most destructive outbreak ever to occur among Europeans in Australia erupted in Sydney around May 1881 and lasted about nine months. Its origin is uncertain, but the first known case was a Chinese man. When the outbreak was over, 154 cases, including 40 deaths, had been recorded. Two of the cases were unvaccinated constables who had been assigned to quarantine houses of earlier victims. Cumpston reported that some physicians concealed cases from the authorities during this epidemic: "The probable reason . . . was that the first two medical men who reported cases were quarantined against their will for some months" (1914, 14).

Three separate importations led to a total of 123 cases in Australia in 1884–85, but only 10 of those victims died. Several medical students on hospital wards in Melbourne were infected during one of these outbreaks. Two years later, smallpox was imported into Tasmania, where it killed 11 persons. Australia's final outbreak in the nineteenth century occurred in the spring of 1893, when a Singhalese passenger on the SS *Saladin* brought the disease from Singapore to Perth, where 52 persons were infected and 9 died.

Six years after Jenner's publication, vaccine virus first arrived in Java from Mauritius. By 1816, vaccinators were employed on the island, paid with allotments of land, but organized efforts to maintain regular arm-to-arm vaccination only began forty years later. Still, only a small fraction of

Java's population had been vaccinated by the end of the nineteenth century, when a central vaccine institute was established at Batavia (Jakarta).

A year after vaccination was first practiced in Java, it was introduced into China at Canton by Dr. Alexander Pearson. Pearson used the vaccinia virus the Spanish king's famous Balmis-Salvany Expedition had brought to Canton and Macao from Spain, via South America and the Phillipines. At Macao, many persons were vaccinated during an epidemic in 1805–6.

Around the same time as the seaborne Balmis-Salvany Expedition introduced vaccination into China from the south, an overland expedition sent by the Russian tsar carried vaccine into Siberia. At Irkutsk, where Catherine the Great had founded an institution for smallpox inoculation just north of the Mongolian border, "several children were vaccinated, in order that a fresh and certain supply of virus might be had for transmission to China" (Baron 1838, 2: 93–94). According to Ball (1904), the expedition also introduced vaccination into northern China and Peking at this time, long before the practice was reintroduced in Peking in 1828. (These efforts did not prevent a Mongolian "living Buddha" from dying of smallpox soon after he arrived in Peking during the reign of Tau Kwang [1821–50]). A Chinese pamphlet on vaccination published at Canton in 1817 ascribed the discovery of vaccination "to a Western Barbarian Doctor named Chan-na" (Dudgeon 1871).

Owing largely, it appears, to the country's geographic isolation, its entrenched bureaucracy, and a traditional suspicion of all things foreign, China adopted Jennerian vaccination very slowly compared to other major nations. It might have been accepted more rapidly if the common Chinese method of inoculation had been in the arm, rather than up the nose. Between 1821 and 1833, vaccination was extended to a few other provinces of China near Canton, but according to Ball (1904), some Chinese doctors (i.e., inoculators), vigorously opposed it. During the last half of the nineteenth century, vaccination spread gradually to the different classes and areas of China. It was introduced into Shanghai in 1861. By 1864, there were three vaccination "establishments" in Peking. In Canton, the Customs Medical Report for 1877–78 estimated that at least ninety-five percent of the children in that city were vaccinated. But in view of China's enormous population, the numbers of people vaccinated in most of these early campaigns were miniscule.

Even more isolated than China was Tibet, where vaccination seems to have had no impact during the nineteenth century. Waddell (1906), who undertook an expedition to Tibet in the early twentieth century, believed that decimating epidemics of smallpox were partly to blame for Tibet's declining population. Two mid-nineteenth-century explorers, Huc and Gabet (1928) described the arrival of smallpox in Lhasa from Peking in a caravan (theirs). Because of it, they were obliged to postpone their visit to the Dalai Lama. They noted that as soon as smallpox became known in a Tibetan household, all of the inhabitants were forced to move to remote mountain tops or valleys, where they sometimes died of hunger. After one particularly devastating epidemic of smallpox, Lhasa was said to have "remained unpeopled, a city of the dead, for three years" ("Smallpox before Jenner," 1876, 1264). In 1882 S. C. Das found smallpox raging all over central Tibet, including Lhasa, and noted that villagers along the way were afraid to have anything to do with him and his fellow travelers, because of fear of the disease. Das stated that of all deaths in Tibet "death for smallpox is the most dreaded, since the victim is believed to be immediately sent to hell." (1902, 193). Wessels (1924) estimated that during an epidemic in Lhasa in 1900, one out of every ten of the inhabitants died.

Huc and Gabet realized of course that vaccination would be a valuable measure against the yearly epidemics in Tibet. But they also dreamed of using vaccination in Tibet as a tool for advancing Christianity: "The introduction of vaccination into Tibet would most probably be a signal of the downfall of Lamanism and of the establishment of Christian religion among these infidel tribes" (1928, 2: 250). Incredibly, vaccination is said to have been finally introduced into Tibet only shortly before 1944 by doctors with the British Trade Agency Hospital (MacDonald 1944). If this is true, it must have been due to that region's extreme isolation. Even Japan, which at the time was hardly in the mainstream of western ideas and commerce, preceded Tibet by almost a century.

After several unsuccessful attempts earlier in the nineteenth century, vaccination was finally introduced into Japan in August 1849 by Dr. Otto Mohnike, a German doctor employed by the Dutch, using crusts imported from the Netherlands East Indies. A Japanese historian, Matsuki (1970), attributed the delay partly to Japan's geographic remoteness from England and to the dominant influence of Chinese medicine, but the most important factor was undoubtedly the national policy of isolation since early in the seventeenth century.

Between 1850 and 1860, vaccination clinics were started all over Japan and these sites also served as meeting places for students and teachers of Western science. Once vaccination had been admitted, its undeniable success and rapid popularity helped to erode the very prohibitions against Western learning that may have delayed its introduction. In the opinion of Miyajima, another student of Japanese medical history, "In any history of the progress of Western civilization in Japan, the influence exerted by the introduction and spread of vaccination should be particularly noted" (1922–23, 23–26).

Commodore Perry sailed into Edo Bay four years after vaccination arrived in the country and initiated another aspect of Japan's reopening to the outside world. Between 1857 and 1859, the shogunate signed treaties opening Japan to trade with the United States and several European countries. Emperor Komei was finally induced to ratify these treaties in October 1865.

The Shogun Iemochi died in September 1866, although not of smallpox, and was succeeded by Keiki, who was the fifteenth Tokugawa shogun. Less than five months later, thirty-seven-year-old Emperor Komei died of smallpox on 13 February 1867, after twenty years on the throne (plate 21). Unlike earlier Western counterparts, Komei did not help lead his subjects into the vaccination era, an error that cost him his life. The fifth Japanese emperor to die of the disease, Komei was succeeded by his fifteen-year-old son, Mutsuhito.

Some Japanese believed the deaths of shogun and emperor in such a short time were divine retribution for signing the treaties with foreign devils. Whatever their ultimate cause, the timing of these two deaths had important consequences for Japan. "The death of Komei and Iyemochi," wrote Davis, "seems to have acted as an incentive in regard to the most progressive spirits of the age" (1916, 252). In November 1867, the new shogun, Keiki, agreed to resign and end the shogunate, thus restoring the full power for administering the empire to the emperor. Having caused the Japanese people and the imperial house of Japan so much anguish over the years—more than sixty-five great epidemics and the deaths of five emperors, says Miyajima—smallpox helped restore the imperial power.

Mutsuhito took the throne name of Meiji in 1868 to signal the new "Era of Enlightenment" and shifted the imperial capital from Kyoto to Tokyo (formerly Edo). This did not signal the end of smallpox in Japan. Dudgeon (1871) records that barely a year later, a fierce epidemic raged along the entire eastern coast of China, killing Westerners and Chinese alike. The following winter, the epidemic got even worse, spilling over into Japan, where there were more severe outbreaks.

Six years into the Meiji era, a vaccine institute was established at Tokyo. The twenty-three-year-old emperor and his empress were vaccinated a year later, and the year after that, a compulsory vaccination law was enacted, although the vaccination law only began to go into effect after about ten years. Wong and Wu (1936) argue that the Japanese emperor and empress were persuaded to be vaccinated not by the new vaccine institute at Tokyo, but by news from Peking that another Son of Heaven had died of smallpox.

T'ung Chih had been crowned emperor of China in 1861 or 1862, with his widowed mother, Empress Dowager Tzu-Hsi, as regent. He married in 1872 and terminated the regency the next year, but had continued to live a life of debauchery. Late in 1874, the emperor became ill, and according to Dr. Chen the illness "was treated as smallpox for 33 days without any effect." The official announcement of his illness began, "We have had the good fortune this month to contract smallpox . . ." (Bland & Blackhouse 1910, 77). He seemed to be improving around 19 December, when some of the lesions on his skin began to "desquamate," and were "scratched to bleeding." A week later, about seventy percent of the scabs were said to be falling off, but three days after that, serous fluid was discharged from the lesions in his lower back, and the emperor became restless. "Large ulcerations," and "two holes" (apparently bed sores) were soon noted in his lower back. A day or two later, Chen says, "his appetite became poor, and diarrhea set in." The nineteen-year-old T'ung Chih emperor died around 8:00 P.M. on 12 January 1875.

Because of T'ung Chih's life style and the unusual course of his illness, it was rumored that he had succumbed to syphilis. However, the protracted clinical course described is similar to that of a few smallpox victims I saw in India and Africa whose rashes became secondarily infected, subjecting the patient to a painful, lingering death.

The Shuh-Chih emperor's death from smallpox in 1661 had turned out to be a blessing in disguise, placing the nation in the capable hands of one of its greatest emperors, K'ang Hsi. But by allowing T'ung Chih's mother to come to power, the death of this second Chinese emperor was even more of a disaster than it first appeared to be. T'ung Chih left no son, but his wife, A-lu-te, was well along in pregnancy when he died. His mother was not unhappy that he had died childless, since that meant that she, and not T'ung Chih's widow, was still the Empress Dowager. Some of the princes and clansmen believed they should await the imminent birth of the late emperor's child, who if male, could ascend the throne. Tzu Hsi, however, "insisted on the election of another infant Emperor at all costs and in violation of the sacred laws of Dynastic succession" (Bland & Blackhouse 1910, 119). She arranged the selection of her infant nephew, with herself and the new emperor's mother as coregents. The infant emperor was vaccinated and given the reign title Kuang'Hsu, meaning "glorious succession." T'ung Chih's widow committed suicide over the insult to her unborn child (some suspect she was poisoned by Tzu Hsi), and at the time of the formal funeral ceremony for the late emperor four years later, a prominent court censor also committed suicide, near T'ung Chih's grave, leaving a long memorandum detailing his own fears and reservations about the unprecedented succession of 1875.

Skillfully brushing aside her sister coregent and eventually her nephew emperor, Tzu Hsi remained the effective ruler of China until her death in 1908, except perhaps from 1889 to 1898 when her nephew attempted to govern. She was a moving force in the coup d'etat of 1898 that blocked her nephew's attempt to reform China, in the Boxer Rebellion, and she appointed the last emperor of China. By diverting funds from the Imperial Navy to the rebuilding and decoration of the Summer Palace, she contributed to China's humiliating defeat by the Japanese in

1894–95. When she died, her complete title was the "Empress Dowager, motherly, auspicious, orthodox, heaven-blessed, prosperous, all-nourishing, brightly manifest, calm, sedate, perfect, long-lived, respectful, reverent, worshipful, illustrious and exalted" (ibid., 56, 169).

Meanwhile, in Japan nearly one hundred and twenty-six thousand cases of smallpox were reported throughout the country between 1885 and 1887 (Amako 1909). In 1898 alone, Japan reported nearly one hundred and fifty thousand cases of smallpox, of whom more than forty thousand died (Irwin 1910).

Toward the end of the nineteenth century, Dr. John Dudgeon reported from Peking that "it is difficult to find a Chinaman entirely free from 'pits' [pockmarks]" (1871, 117). In 1894, Smith found that persons blinded by smallpox were still very common in China. Morse (1917) reported around the same time that many persons blinded by smallpox in Japan were making a living as masseuses. In Japan especially, where people through the ages cultivated an acute love of beauty, including, presumably, the exquisite complexions of some of their fellow human beings, the disfigurement caused by smallpox must have been a very bitter legacy for many of its survivors. Although I am aware of only one person—the mistress of a Nepalese king—whose pock-marked face drove her to suicide, one would expect that some Japanese women probably reacted in the same desperate, tragic way.

TWENTIETH CENTURY

At the turn of the twentieth century, smallpox was still highly endemic in China, Tibet, and the Philippines, but it was a less severe problem on most of the other islands of the region. Australia and New Zealand counted only intermittent outbreaks as a result of importation, and these were relatively easily controlled.[6]

Without a system for reporting infectious diseases or causes of death, nationwide statistics are still unavailable for China in this period. Even in the Treaty Port cities, smallpox was grossly underreported, but years when it was epidemic were clearly evident. Shanghai suffered epidemics in 1902, 1904, 1907, 1910, and 1913; Peking in 1910–11; and Hong Kong in 1907–8, 1912 and 1917.[7]

The disease was usually most widespread in China during the spring. Most of the cases occurred in children under five years old, and about one of every three persons infected died. One out of every three Chinese seen on the streets still had obviously pockmarked faces. Geil (1926), who visited China around this time, reported that the Chinese regarded smallpox as something every child must get sooner or later. In one area he visited, the local word for smallpox was "inevitable-pox."

In 1900, another great epidemic of smallpox ravaged Tibet. Among the most severely affected patients in this outbreak was the Dalai Lama, who barely escaped with his life and who suffered deep scarring of his face. Some of the Dalai Lama's compatriots explained to a visitor that many of the countless abandoned houses in Tibet were a result of frequent invasions by the Mongols, whereas other houses had been abandoned because of smallpox epidemics, "which come with even greater frequency than the Mongols" (Bell 1928, 53).

Vaccination efforts increased throughout China in 1913, under the First Republic. J. M. Korns, a Western physician practicing in China, found relatively little prejudice against vaccination among the Chinese by this time.

Japan, with a population about one-tenth the size of China's, was able to mitigate smallpox's impact by the beginning of the century. During the Russo-Japanese War of 1904–5, when smallpox was still endemic in Japan, 362 cases of smallpox (35 deaths) were recorded in the Japanese army of over a million men. In 1905, when smallpox was more prevalent than usual, the civilian population of about 48 million reported 10,704 cases with 3,388 deaths. (England and Wales, with a population of about 33 million in 1901, reported 2,466 deaths from smallpox during an epidemic in 1902.)

Some of Japan's epidemics still originated in China. In April 1907, smallpox was discovered in a Chinese girl in Kobe, Japan, a city of about three hundred and seventy thousand people. Prior to this discovery, no smallpox had been reported in that city for five years, and only twenty cases were recorded in the four years before that. Four months later, the daughter in another Chinese family who traveled frequently between Kobe and southern China became ill with smallpox. By the time the resultant outbreak was ended in September 1908, over nineteen thousand persons in Kobe had been infected, nearly five thousand of whom died.

Notwithstanding the terrible outbreak in Kobe, smallpox continued to decline in Japan, which by 1918 required all children to be vaccinated at one year of age and revaccinated when entering school. During epidemic years in the 1920s, far fewer cases (between 1,900 and 3,200 per year) were recorded than in previous epidemic years. The entire country reported only 3,245 cases from 1927 to 1940, and the disease ceased to be endemic in Japan around 1950.

Smallpox was still rampant in the Philippines at the turn of the century, causing over forty thousand deaths annually and a large share of the blindness. An investigation of 145 blind persons in Cebu Province in 1914 revealed that more than one-third of them had been blinded by smallpox. In addition to virulent smallpox, *V. minor* had also been occurring in the Philippines for some time, one of the mild strain's rare appearances in Asia. Unlike its effect in the Americas and parts of Eastern Africa and Europe, *V. minor* didn't replace *V. major* in the Philippines. As elsewhere, *V. major* typically provoked more vigorous control efforts in the Philippines than did outbreaks of *V. minor*.

Soon after the United States succeeded Spain as the occupying power in the Philippines in 1898, an intensive, systematic vaccination program was initiated, and inoculation was declared illegal. The impact of these intensive control efforts was even more dramatic than similar efforts in Japan. By 1914, a local Philippine official could boast: "We have performed more than 10 million vaccinations, with the result that the annual deaths from this disease have decreased from 40 thousand at outset to seven hundred for the year just ended. There is now less smallpox in Manila than in Washington"(Worcester 1914, 1: 424). (The estimated population of the Philippines in 1922 was 11 million.)

Following this early success, however, full responsibility for health was transferred from American to Philippine authorities. This was followed by a relaxation in control efforts. Whereas only 276 deaths from smallpox were reported in 1915, a gargantuan epidemic killed more than 64,000 Filipinos in 1918–19. Inquiries into this disaster cited various inefficiencies, including falsification of vaccination reports by local health officials and inadequate care of the delicate vaccine being used. But it is impossible to be certain whether 1918–19 would have still been epidemic years even if American authorities had retained responsibility for health. American efforts had helped control the disease, but it had not been eradicated from the islands, and it was still being imported by ships into the Philippines from other Asian ports.

Very little was reported in the Philippines in the late 1920s, except for an outbreak of 367 cases in 1929. The last known cases of endemic smallpox in the Philippines occurred in 1930–31.

The most significant early success in controlling smallpox in this region was achieved in the Netherlands East Indies, where the disease had claimed nearly three thousand lives on the west coast of Borneo alone in 1905. A year earlier, it had killed the sultan of North Borneo's favorite grandson, the grandson's new wife, and the sultan's second son. In 1913, over eighteen thousand cases of smallpox, with five thousand deaths, were recorded in East Java.

The antismallpox campaign in the Netherlands East Indies was reorganized in the 1920s. More important, around the same time, the Dutch began to employ a new vaccine they had just developed that maintained its potency in tropical conditions much longer than glycerolated lymph and hence could be used to vaccinate effectively persons living in areas remote from refrigeration. The secret, discovered by Otten, was to dry the vaccine at room temperature, then seal it in vials with a vacuum (Polak 1968). As a result, smallpox was nearly eliminated from the entire Dutch colony by the late 1930s. Only about two dozen cases were reported from 1937 to 1940.

Meanwhile, Australia and New Zealand also became testimonials to the effectiveness of vigorous containment efforts, since despite continued importation of smallpox by passengers on ships, the disease caused relatively little damage. In 1903 an outbreak of sixty-six cases in Tasmania resulting from ship passengers infected at Java was the last of *V. major* among Europeans in Australia. Five workmen hired to build a temporary isolation hospital for some of the earlier patients were among the victims, and one of them was among the nineteen who died. The next year, there was a small outbreak (eight cases) among Asiatic members of a pearling fleet just off the Australian coast.

Not all the importations were handled in exemplary fashion, however. When *V. minor* was introduced into Australia and New Zealand in 1913 by a vessel from the United States, the resultant outbreak in Australia lasted for four years, with about twenty-four hundred cases (but only four deaths) reported. In the New Zealand outbreak, which ended after about twelve months, 114 Europeans were infected, none of whom died, but nearly two thousand cases were reported among indigenous Maoris, of whom fifty-five died. Thereafter, Australia reported only five imported cases in 1929, two in 1930, and one each in 1932 and 1938. New Zealand reported one case in 1926.

While there had been many needless deaths in Australia from smallpox—the first European cases occurred over thirty years after Jenner's discovery of vaccination—only a high level of vigilance by Australian authorities prevented even greater disasters. Dixon credits Dr. Ashburton Thompson with realizing that smallpox spread primarily from person to person relatively slowly and for emphasizing a strategy of quarantine and vaccination of contacts of victims, rather than routine vaccination of infants. This strategy was well suited to nonendemic countries such as Australia and New Zealand faced with periodic imported outbreaks. It would also have been a conveniently expedient strategy if antivaccinationist sentiment had been nearly as strong in these two countries as it was in England at that time. Only about one-third of infants born in Australia after 1860 were vaccinated, and by 1936 less than one percent of the infants born in Australia and New Zealand were being vaccinated against smallpox. Inoculation was never an important factor in Australia. Over a period of seventy-six years (1828–1904), one hundred and seventy-five ships from at least seventeen different countries were quarantined for smallpox at ports on all of Australia's coasts.

The usual effectiveness of Australia's containment efforts was demonstrated spectacularly in 1886, when the *Preussen* arrived in Australian waters with crew and passengers who apparently had been infected at Port Said, Egypt. Twenty-nine of the passengers landed and gave rise to 4 cases at Adelaide, another 230 landed and yielded 29 cases at Melbourne, and 435 of the passengers produced 79 cases at Sydney. However, all of the cases occurred among the quarantined passengers themselves. There was no spread to Australians on land.

Early in World War II, Japanese military forces overran all of the archipelago in the region, except for southern New Guinea, Australia, and New Zealand. The occupying forces disrupted routine health services in most of the territories they controlled, and smallpox statistics are generally not available for the war years. When the war ended, the virus had reestablished itself in the Netherlands East Indies and was also prevalent in Korea, Southeast Asia, and Malaya.

The Dutch colony, which became the independent Republic of Indonesia in 1949, reported more than 52,000 cases of smallpox the next year, and over 100,000 cases the year after that. When the global smallpox eradication campaign began nearly two decades later, Indonesia was reporting over 10,000 cases of smallpox annually in the five years before 1971, with a peak of nearly 18,000 cases in 1969. The national eradication effort soon restricted the virus to smaller and smaller corners of the Indonesian islands, where it caused 2,100 reported cases of smallpox in 1971, 34 cases in January 1972, and none after that.

Japan also reaped more smallpox as a result of its disruption in the Second World War, recording more than 1,600 cases in 1945, and ten times as many cases, with nearly 3,000 deaths, the next year. However, that was its last large epidemic.

China, which over the centuries had shared many of its epidemics with Japan, was slower to bring the disease under control. The Chinese reported some 81,505 cases (11,784 deaths) between 1939 and 1947. Over 36,000 of these cases occurred in 1946–47. More than 67,000 cases were reported in 1950, and over 68,000 cases in 1951. But these relatively small numbers of cases, considering the size of the population, almost certainly reflect poor reporting rather than a real reduction of smallpox at that time.

Soon after establishing the People's Republic, China's new government launched a national campaign against smallpox in October 1950. By 1953, when 3,485 cases were reported, more than 500 million Chinese had been vaccinated, out of a population of about 560 million. Thirty of the 317 cases reported in 1957 resulted from "the practice of variolation by nasal inhalation," in Hunan Province (WHO 1979c, 2). The last cases of smallpox in China, 44 in all, occurred in 1960 in Hunan Province and Tibet, the former as a result of an importation from Burma.

In 1974, a forty-nine year-old travel agent returned to Japan, which had been free of endemic smallpox for a quarter century, after a brief visit to northern India, where a violent epidemic was underway. He complained of fever, chills, and headache on 22 January, and two days later a rash appeared. Smallpox was diagnosed on 28 January. It was the last time that diagnosis was made in Japan and in this part of Asia.

T'OU-SHEN NIANG-NIANG: CHINESE GODDESS OF SMALLPOX

A major testament to the antiquity and dread of smallpox in China is T'ou-Shen Niang-Niang, the Chinese goddess of smallpox. As noted earlier, tradition traces the origin of worship of this goddess to an

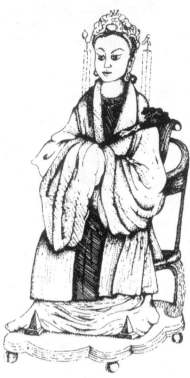

Fig. 8. T'ou-Shen Niang-Niang, Chinese goddess of smallpox. Drawing by Chris L. Smith.

eleventh century Buddhist nun who also is credited with introducing inoculation into China. Doolittle, who wrote a wide-ranging account of life in mid-nineteenth-century China, said the smallpox goddess then "ranked among the most popular objects of worship among all classes of the people" (1865, 1: 154). Religious affiliations were ignored as Buddhist, Taoist, and Confucian adherents paid tribute to "the Dame who controls Smallpox."

The Chinese goddess is "variously represented," according to the author of *A Dictionary of Chinese Mythology*, "sometimes wearing a large shawl to protect her infected skin from cold" (Werner 1932, 513). Apart from a standing figure portrayed in Doolittle's book, the only other surviving image of a Chinese smallpox goddess I have seen is reproduced here from a print in the National Museum of History at Taipei, Taiwan (plate 22).[8] The latter figure, in which Ch'uan Hsiang Hua Chieh ("One who hands on fragrant flower") is portrayed riding astride a horse, is strikingly reminiscent of the more familiar Indian goddess of smallpox, Shitala Mata, and may perhaps lend credence to the alleged Indian origins of smallpox inoculation and of worship of this goddess, in China. The relationship between the two Chinese goddesses is not clear.

T'ou-Shen Niang-Niang was feared more than she was loved. According to Doolittle (1865) and Bredon and Mitrophanow (1927), her mercy was sought to protect children from smallpox, to ensure a mild attack, or to secure recovery of those already ill with smallpox. She was believed to especially enjoy disfiguring children with pretty faces. The consequent pockmarks were considered so unsightly that Chinese children would wear ugly paper masks to bed on the last night of the year, hoping to trick the smallpox goddess into ignoring them. Others hung a vacant gourd, into which the goddess could "empty" the smallpox, near their beds on that night. Smallpox pustules, and the disease itself, were usually referred to euphemistically as "heavenly flowers," or by other names, to avoid offending T'ou-Shen Niang-Niang (Smith 1871).

Temples were erected to the smallpox goddess all over China. A member of a family affected by smallpox would be sent to take offerings at a local temple, a practice which no doubt helped spread the disease in some instances. More commonly, it appears, affected families set up a tablet or picture of the goddess to worship in their own homes. A well-known Japanese historian and novelist reported a similar practice in Japan when his grandchildren were attacked by smallpox in 1831: "As was the prevailing custom for smallpox treatment, red clothing, red playthings, red confectionaries and red pictures were prepared for the patients, and a smallpox-god was worshipped in their room" (Maekawa 1976, 391). The "smallpox god" referred to here was probably a red picture of Tametomo, the twelfth century Japanese archer whose image was hung in smallpox victims' rooms to aid their recovery.

Doolittle described a protocol for worship of the smallpox goddess in China. On the third day after the pustules appeared, bits of yeast were presented to the figure representing the goddess. This was repeated on the fifth and seventh days. On the ninth day, the offering consisted of fish, meat, fowl, and vegetables, but only if the child appeared to be improving. Otherwise, this more substantial offering was deferred, pending signs of recovery. On the fourteenth day, when most surviving patients would have been out of danger, the child sat on a large winnowing fan before the figure of the goddess:

> On the top of his head is then put a small piece of red cloth, and . . . parched beans are taken from before the goddess and laid upon this red cloth, whence they are allowed to roll off. . . . The name for the bean, pronounced in the dialect of this place, is identical in sound with the common name for the smallpox. This identity in name, and this similarity in appearance between the bean and the small-pox, have probably given rise to the ceremony above described, which *indicates the strong desire that the pustules should dry up, and become in appearance like the parched bean!* (Doolittle 1865, 1: 156)

Bredon and Mitrophanow (1927) reported that after the patient recovered, the temporary shrine to the smallpox goddess was escorted from the home in a specially made paper chair or boat and reverently burned—a practice which accounts for the scarcity of these figures now. If the sick person died, however, T'ou-Shen Niang-Niang was cursed off the premises.

Four

Kiss of the Goddess

ANCIENT MEDICAL WRITINGS, Hindu mythology, and Brahmin traditions provide evidence that India was one of the areas affected earliest by smallpox. The disease certainly existed in India for some time before the beginning of the Christian era. Despite India's long historical record, however, and the fact that smallpox had been present in India for two thousand years at least, there is only scant historical evidence of the disease before A.D. 1500.

From the beginning of this period, populous India was fertile ground for dissemination of smallpox. From the Himalayan barrier in the north, to the densely settled Indo-Gangetic plains and the southern plateau, by the fourth century A.D. all India was traversed by terrestrial and riverine trade routes, which increased opportunities for smallpox to spread within the subcontinent. Beyond the subcontinent itself, a coastal route had been established between India and West Asia by the end of the first century A.D., and Indian muslin was being traded for Ethiopian gold and ivory in East Africa. In the same century, there was increased contact with China, including export of Buddhism, and Indian culture began to be introduced into Southeast Asia (Thapar 1966). In 712, Arab armies added India's Sind Province to their variolous empire, which extended across West Asia and the Mediterranean basin to the Atlantic Ocean.

During the first fifteen hundred years after the birth of Christ, smallpox's presence in India is revealed largely by allusions to worship of the Hindu goddess of smallpox, Shitala mata. Raghavan (1969) states that the Lanka king Gajabahu of Ceylon inaugurated the cult of Pattini, goddess of smallpox and chastity, in his country, dedicating the first temples to her late in the second century, after witnessing ceremonies honoring the smallpox goddess in southern India. On the Indian mainland at Tanjore, just opposite Ceylon, an unusual bronze figure of Shitala dates from the thirteenth century. Further north, sculptured figures of the goddess have been found in a ninth-century temple in Rajasthan, a twelfth-century temple in Gujarat, and a site in eastern Bengal dating from the tenth to twelfth century (Majumdar 1965; Ions 1967; Nicholas 1981) (plate 23). This tangible manifestation of an ancient and strong belief in a theurgic explanation of smallpox survived to be beheld first hand by modern public health workers who struggled to eradicate small-pox in India during the 1970s.

The disease *masurika* (smallpox) is mentioned in the *Astangahrdaya-samhita* by the physician Vagbhata, which dates from about the seventh century, and in the *Nidana* by Madhava-kara, who described recom-mended treatments for measles, chickenpox, and smallpox in the early eighth century. According to Nicholas (1981, 26), Madhava provided "humoral and dietary explanations for the various forms of smallpox, measles, and chickenpox." Because fever was recognized to be a major symptom of smallpox, Indian treatment "emphasized continuous cooling of the patient throughout the course of the disease." This may explain the euphemistic references to Shitala as "the cool one" by those who believed in the goddess's ability to cure them. Thus, in addition to Ayurvedic humoral, dietetic, and theurgic explanations of smallpox, Indians also developed useful empirical knowledge about the virus including a mod-ernistic theory of infection by which they explained the principle of inoculation.

The reports of early explorers provide other hints of smallpox in India during this period. Vasco da Gama, the first Portuguese to reach the west coast of India, supposedly mistook a figure of the Indian smallpox goddess for the Virgin Mary when he visited one of her temples at Calicut in 1498. According to Edwardes (1969), when da Gama asked the name of the image, he thought he was told "Maria," but he was probably told "Mariamma," another name for the goddess in southern India. The well-known Moroccan traveler Ibn Batua visited India around 1340 and reported that the emperor of India was almost defeated in the revolt of a local emir because of "a pestilence" that "carried off the greater part" of his army (Lee 1829, 147). Unfortunately, he recorded no details of the illness.

One of the earliest specific accounts of an epidemic of smallpox in India derives from Goa, the small Portuguese settlement on the coast three hundred miles north of Calicut. In 1545, soon after the Portuguese established that enclave, a severe epidemic of smallpox broke out in which "eight thousand children alone succumbed within three months" (Pieris 1913, 1: 99). Emphasis on the mortality among children in this outbreak is consistent with the presumption that smallpox had long been endemic in India; thus, most adults were already immune. Nonetheless, the mortality in this early outbreak appears to have been typically staggering—despite the ancient knowledge of inoculation in India.

Among the victims of this epidemic were two princes from Ceylon who had come to Goa to complain to the Portuguese governor that his country's recognition of Don Juan Dharmapala as its vassal Christian king of Kotte—one of several kingdoms in Ceylon—had deprived them of their inheritance. According to Pieris (1913), the Portuguese were inclined to agree with the princes' suggestion that the Portuguese should help them win other kingdoms for themselves. But before either could act, smallpox killed both princes within a month of each other.

A generation before the outbreak at Goa, a prominent noble at the court of Sultan Sikandar Lodi in Delhi, Mian Bhowa, compiled a medical treatise called *Ma'dan-ul-Shifa Sikandar Shahi* (Mine of cures of Sikandar Shah) in 1512. Bhowa had "suggested to the Sultan that there was a need to have a book prepared in Persian that should contain the best of the Ayurvedic system and its drugs." Among the many topics covered was "small-pox, measles, their symptoms and treatment" (Jaggi 1977, 114, 117). Around the same time, another medical text authored by Bhava Misra, the *Bhava-prakasa*, "greatly elaborated the discussion of smallpox," evidence that by that time "there were two fully fledged interpretations of smallpox: one based on the biology of humors and diet of Ayurveda and deriving appropriate therapeutic procedures from it, the other based on the conception that the disease is a divine affliction and stipulating that the worship of Shitala is indispensable to treatment" (Nicholas 1981, 27).

Fourteen years after Bhowa published Sikander's *Mine of Cures*, the Delhi sultanate fell to India's first Moghul emperor, Babur. When Babur's grandson, Akbar, ascended the throne at mid-century, all Hindusthan was devastated by famine and an unspecified epidemic (Majumdar 1974). As Akbar expanded the empire, numerous small states in the eastern territory of Assam were caught up in a complex political cross fire, with ever changing alliances, between the Moghul emperors of Delhi and the Moslem rulers of Bengal. In addition to its strategic geography, this forested region of eastern India was coveted for its elephants, which the Moghuls needed for their armies. Among the most important of the small kingdoms in this area during the latter half of the sixteenth century were Ahom, Kachari, Koch Bihar, and Tripura.

In 1574 the kingdom of Ahom suffered a virulent outbreak of smallpox, which killed "many inhabitants" (Gait 1926, 102). At the time, Koch Bihar, which was ruled by King Nar Narayan and his brother Chilarai, was pre-eminent among the four neighboring principalities. Chilarai was commander-in-chief of the Koch army. During the previous decade, he had defeated Kachari, Ahom, Manipur, Jaintia and Tripura. After Chilarai helped Akbar defeat the Padshah of Gaur in 1576, the Padshah's kingdom was divided between Emperor Akbar and King Narayan. But in the course of another expedition "against the Mohammedans" a year later, General Chilarai caught smallpox and died, "on the banks of the Ganges" (ibid., 55).

After Chilarai's death, his son Raghu, who was heir to Narayan's throne, began to fear he might not be allowed to succeed his uncle. Raghu rebelled and raised an army, but rather than fight his nephew, Narayan agreed to divide his kingdom between them. Raghu thus became king of

Koch Hajo, the (eastern) half of a greatly weakened Koch Bihar, which "fell to pieces" after Narayan's death. (Marbaniang 1970, 29; Gait 1926).

Six years after General Chilarai died of smallpox, the disease claimed one of his former neighbors, the Maharajah Vijoy Manikya of Tripura. Vijoy had reigned for forty-seven years. His corpse "was followed to the pyre by a great number of women," according to the *Rajamala*, or *Chronicles of the Kings of Tripura* (Long 1978, 14). The *Chronicles* report that between the fifteenth and eighteenth centuries, five of sixteen maharajahs of Tripura died of smallpox (James 1909). Two of Vijoy's predecessors yielded their thrones to the virus in 1407 and 1462.

Other royal chronicles of the period, cited in Harvey (1925), also attest to smallpox's wide-ranging influence. King Thadominbya of Burma, the Lord of the Golden Palace at Ava, came down with smallpox during a military campaign in 1368 and died in the field at age twenty-five. Only four years earlier, soon after he succeeded to the throne, King Thadominbya had drained the swamps around Ava and built the city that remained his country's capital for five centuries.[1]

According to Varavarn (1930) and Wood (1926), the first definite mention of smallpox in Siamese history is in 1534, when the king of Siam, Boromaraja IV, succumbed to the disease after a five-year reign, leaving the throne to his five-year-old son Prince Ratsada. Within five months, Ratsada had been murdered by a relative and was succeeded by a half-brother of Boromaraja IV.

In Ceylon, the king of Kandy, his queen, and all his sons perished during an epidemic of smallpox that broke out among refugees in the port city of Trincomalee in 1582. King Karawliyadda and many of his subjects had fled to Trincomalee after a rival sacked his capital in the center of Ceylon. Pieris (1913) tells us that only the king's infant daughter survived, and she succeeded him. Many years earlier, long before the Portuguese arrived in Ceylon, the ancient kingdom of Lanka had also had to abandon its first capital, on account of war, famine, rats, and a depopulating epidemic of smallpox.

SEVENTEENTH CENTURY

Portuguese rule of Ceylon ended after a century and a half, when they were ousted by the Dutch in 1658. Numerous wars on the island early in the seventeenth century were associated with outbreaks of smallpox, which determined the outcome of some of those wars, which are chronicled in Pieris (1913) and De Silva (1972). In 1602, smallpox neutralized seven hundred men in the army of one local chieftain, Samarakon, but his foes' attempts to capitalize on this were unsuccessful. The following March smallpox became epidemic among besieged defenders of a fort at Talampitiya. In 1618–19, an outbreak in a Portuguese army commanded by General De Sa forced them to retreat. While retreating, De Sa set an ambush for his rebellious opponents and gained an important victory. Another smallpox epidemic and famine, followed wars that raged in the Ceylonese port of Jaffna until 1621. Two years later, following a war in which the Portuguese sought to subdue the Tamils on the island, the virus "caused havoc among now scanty inhabitants; whole villages were depopulated, entire families with numerous slaves killed off" (Pieris 1913, 2: 140).

Robert Knox, an English sailor who was held captive in the Kandyan kingdom of Ceylon for twenty years during the last half of the seventeenth century, observed:

> The smallpox also sometimes happens among them. From which they cannot free themselves by all their charms and enchantments, which are often times successful to them in other distempers. Therefore, they do confess, like the magicians in Egypt, that this is the very finger of Almighty God. (Ludowyk 1948, 172)

The "Finger of Almighty God" also pointed at seventeenth-century India, claiming another maharajah of Tripura, Chattra Manikyu, in 1666 or 1667. King Chattra had reigned seven years in alliance with the Bengali nawab of Murshidabad. Soon after Chattra's reign began, Emperor Aurangzeb's viceroy of Bengal, Mir Jumla, had invaded Assam and reached the capital of Ahom in March 1662, just as a dangerous epidemic, which may have been smallpox, broke out. The epidemic took a heavy toll of Mir Jumla's army. Infected refugees retreated to the Ahom capital, after which the disease spread all over Assam, killing an estimated 230,000 inhabitants (Majumdar 1974). Despite this calamity, or perhaps because of it, Mir Jumla's mission was a success.

A European visitor to India's east coast during the later part of the century reported that "smallpox invades the youth, as in all India" (Fryer 1909, 1: 285). On India's west coast, Calicut suffered a withering epidemic in 1675, of which another European witness said, "it carried people off as fast as the plague" (Fawcett 1936, 344). Fourteen years later, in the extreme south of India, the disease carried off another youthful prince, the rajah of Madura.

After he became rajah in 1682, Ranga Krishna Muttu Virappa of Madura had to reconquer large parts of his kingdom, including its capital. He was gradually restoring the power of his house when he died of smallpox in 1689 at age twenty-two. Virappa's pregnant widow was forcibly prevented from committing suicide immediately after his death, but she successfully poisoned herself shortly after giving birth to a son. The orphaned infant was crowned when he was three months old, with his paternal grandmother, Mangammal, as regent. As one historian reported, "Mangammal's reign was an enlightened one. She labored hard for public welfare, building chavadis (resthouses) and water reservoirs.

Down to this day her name is proverbial for charity" (Kalidos, 228). In the opinion of Professor R. Sathianathaier,

> Mangammal was a femme politique. Her vigour and diplomacy gave the Nayak Kingdom a longer tenure of life than it would have otherwise had. . . . Her prudent administration in an age of storm and stress marks her out as a ruler of high repute. (Ibid.)

Queen Mangammal campaigned successfully against Tanjore, Mysore, and Travancore, but tactfully acknowledged her kingdom's submission to Emperor Aurangzeb. Despite her vigorous efforts, however, the kingdom declined soon after her regency ended. Elsewhere in India, the British were preparing to gather up the remains of several such kingdoms.

EIGHTEENTH CENTURY

Among the most noteworthy aspects of Emperor Aurangzeb's reign over pre-British India was the compilation and translation of several medical texts. Hakim Muhammad Akbar-bin-Muhammad Muqin Arzani was the most famous medical writer of the Indian Moghul Empire during this period. Sometime between 1700 and 1707 he wrote the *Mufrih-ul-Qulub*, which included a record in Persian of "his own experiments about an unusual method of treatment adopted by him, to relieve the burning and throbbing sensation of the vesicles of smallpox":

> Muhammad Shukrullah, son of this humble servant, became ill with malignant type of small-pox. The eruption had been filled with discharge; burning was very severe and [he] was extremely restless. I had up to now never advised anyone to incise the vesicles, as it was not the custom in India. So I hesitated to undertake such a procedure. But being compelled by necessity, and in spite of the opposition of old women, I at last pricked the vesicles of my son with gold needles. As the discharge was drained out of them, immediately relief was felt by the patient. Working slowly and patiently for three *pahars* (nearly nine hours), I pricked all the vesicles and complete relief was the result of this procedure. I have, since, repeated this technique in several such cases and found it to be entirely satisfactory. (Jaggi 1977, 195–96)

Following Robert Clive's victory over the nawab of Bengal in 1757, which marked the beginning of formal British rule in India, increasingly detailed descriptions of smallpox's toll on the subcontinent began to be published in London. Ten years after the Battle of Plassey, Holwell, a British resident, described the situation in Bengal, a state nearly as large as France:

> Every seventh year, with scarcely any exception, the smallpox [occurs] in these provinces during the months of March, April, and May. . . . On these periodical returns (to four of which I have been a witness) the

disease proves universally of the most malignant confluent kind, from which few either of the natives or Europeans escaped that took the distemper in the natural way, commonly dying on the first, second, or third day of the eruption. The usual resource of the European is to fly from the settlements and retire into the country before the return of the smallpox season. ("Smallpox before Jenner," 1896, 1264)

A few years after Holwell described the cyclical epidemics in Bengal, the Bengali capital, Murshidabad, and surrounding parts of the Moslem-ruled state suffered a long drought, followed by disastrous floods. Ten years earlier, Clive himself described Murshidabad as being "as extensive, populous and rich as London, with individuals possessing infinitely greater property than those in the English metropolis. One of its palaces, situated on the western bank, was described to be big enough to accommodate three European monarchs" (Majumdar 1905, 7). Even allowing for exaggeration, Murshidabad must have been an impressive city.

The drought and floods of 1769–70 caused a great famine, at the height of which a calamitous epidemic of smallpox ravaged Bengal. Sixty-three thousand persons are said to have died of smallpox in Murshidabad alone, and Bengal allegedly lost one-third of its population in the epidemic. The mortality was so great, wrote an Indian historian, that "in and around the capital it became necessary to keep several sets of persons constantly engaged in removing the dead. Instances were not rare in which entire families became extinct" (Majumdar 1905, 9). One of the dead victims was a Dutch director at Chinsura.

Also infected during this epidemic was the twenty-year-old nawab of Bengal, Syefuddowla, who, though subject to British influence, was still the titular head of state. The head of the British East India Company sent a get-well letter from Calcutta on 5 March 1770, saying he was praying for the nawab's recovery (Govt. of India, Imp. Rec. Dept. 1919, 3: 27, 39). Syefuddowla, Ninth Nawab of Bengal, Nazim of Murshibadad, Syef-ul-Mulk (Sword of the Country), Shujandowla (Hero of the State), and Shahamat Jang (Arrow in War), died of smallpox that same month, after a four-year reign (plate 24).

Although Castiglioni (1941) reported that over three million persons died of smallpox throughout India that year, it was estimated by others that one-third of the population of Bengal died, which would have accounted for three million deaths in that state alone. This massive epidemic or one of its subsequent waves also killed the principal queen of Ahom and her daughter. In 1795–96, the virus punctuated its lethal tour of eighteenth-century India with a large epidemic in Calcutta, headquarters of the British East India Company.

That India and other neighboring countries in close contact with it continued to suffer so heavily from smallpox in the eighteenth century is ironic. Inoculation, which had been practiced in India for centuries, probably millennia, had finally been introduced into Europe and North America in 1721. It is particularly incredible that ruling princes of India who should have had access to the best possible protection against such a feared, dangerous, well-known disease, even if all their subjects didn't, were still vulnerable to smallpox. In Europe, Catherine the Great had recruited Dr. Thomas Dimsdale all the way from London to St. Petersburg, a four-week journey of over a thousand miles, to inoculate her two years before the nawab of Bengal died of smallpox.

Underused though it was, inoculation was said to be more common in Bengal than in other parts of India a decade and a half before Syefuddowla's demise (Ives 1773). In view of the 1770 epidemic's reported impact in Bengal, one can imagine how much more fiercely smallpox must have devoured other populations in India that terrible year. Or did it?

If inoculation was indeed more popular in densely populated Bengal, the epidemic of 1770 may in fact have been more severe there than elsewhere. Inoculation may have ended up spreading "natural" smallpox to more uninoculated persons than it protected. This would have been especially likely if only some of the susceptible persons in a community were inoculated. In the nineteenth century, inoculation was blamed for many such episodes. During an epidemic in Dinajpur, Bengal, in 1810, an Englishman observed inoculation being performed by Hindus, Moslems, and other Bengalis of all castes. Sengupta (1969) says the death rate there was about one per hundred among those inoculated. However, Gupta blamed ten to fifteen inoculators for keeping smallpox circulating in Calcutta, "from whence it spreads to every part of Bengal" (1959, 687–88).

In Burma, knowledge of inoculation with variolous material was reportedly introduced for the first time very late, in 1785. In February of that year, the Burmese king Bodawpaya captured the royal family and twenty thousand inhabitants of Arakan. According to Harvey (1925), the prisoners brought inoculation, already practiced in Arakan, into Burma. If this was indeed the first time the practice appeared there, it shows that the method did not necessarily spread to adjacent states any faster than to more remote countries. Meanwhile, both the British and inoculation were on the move in Ceylon.

Britain acquired control of Ceylon's maritime provinces around the turn of the century. In 1789–90, their colonial predecessor in Ceylon, the Dutch East India Company, was "harassed by repeated outbreaks of smallpox which caused much loss of life." But the king of Kandy's country in the interior of the island "was saved from infection by the great forests which guarded its frontiers" (Pieris 1918, 145).

After 1796, hospitals were established to inoculate susceptible persons and care for smallpox patients in parts of Ceylon, and Cordiner (1807) reported that the success rate of inoculations performed in those hospitals was comparable to that achieved in Europe. By April 1800, there were hospitals for treating smallpox patients at Jaffna, Trincomalee, and Colombo. Nevertheless, when the king of Kandy dispatched an embassy to meet the British governor in February 1799, they met at Sitavaka instead of at Colombo because of an outbreak of the disease in the latter city (De Silva 1953).

NINETEENTH CENTURY

The same year that Governor North met the king of Kandy's emissaries at Sitavaka, Edward Jenner began trying to get supplies of his vaccine to India. Unfortunately, no effective methods for preserving the sensitive virus against tropical temperatures were yet known. Jenner eventually succeeded by arranging for volunteers to be vaccinated in succession with cowpox during the voyage to the East. But before he did, vaccine sent by Jean de Carro in Vienna arrived at Bombay in June 1802 via Baghdad. Dr. Helenus Scott performed the first successful vaccination in India on 14 June 1802. She used the vaccine lymph sent by de Carro, who had obtained it from Luigi Sacco in Italy, who, as we have seen, recovered the original strain from a herd of Swiss cows at a county fair on the Italo-Swiss border in the autumn of 1800 (Bowers 1981). From Bombay, the practice was introduced into Ceylon in 1802. The supply of vaccine was sustained by arm-to-arm vaccination around the island, was carried on to Madras, and from there was conveyed via the British fleet to Calcutta and other parts of the British Empire further east.

Vaccination was only introduced into Siam in 1840, when vaccine scabs were first sent out by ship from Boston, Massachusetts. Similar shipments from Boston followed in 1844, 1846, and 1861.

Vaccination threatened the interests of inoculators, who naturally resisted it. According to Taylor (1971) and Bowers (1981), the fact that the vaccine derived ultimately from cows apparently was a negative factor in India, although one might have guessed that the vaccine's bovine origin would have favored its adoption among Hindus. Morgan observed in his 1898 article that Indian priests at Benares told of an old prophecy that India would expel the British through the leadership of a black child with white blood. Vaccination, the priests charged, was how the English intended to find that child to kill him. In Bengal, Gupta (1959) reported that inoculators spread propaganda that the English were using vaccination to exterminate Indians.

When vaccination was introduced into Burma, there were rumors remarkably similar to one encountered in India. According to the Burmese version, the queen of England had dreamed that a child existed in

Burma who would overthrow her dominion. Since it was impossible to know who that child was, the English were trying to poison the blood of the entire Burmese generation by vaccinating them (Ferrars 1900).

In Ceylon, rumor had it that vaccination meant taking an oath in favor of British rule. Cordiner found that Dutch residents on Ceylon favored vaccination neither for themselves nor for natives of the island. As in India, some priests of the local smallpox goddess's cult also resisted vaccination. One European resident found a priest who lived to regret his obstinacy:

> The next case I saw was that of a man lying near the door of his house; and even the strongly marked and well-known features of an inferior priest of the goddess Patine were so disfigured, that I could not recognize them in the blind, helpless, hopeless object whom I addressed, the same person who had a few days before been successful in preventing several of his neighbors from profiting by vaccination when I had visited the village with a medical practitioner. I turned the melancholy state of this man to the advantage of many, by contrasting the real security of those who now accompanied me, and had been vaccinated, with the hideous mass of disease—all that remained of this false teacher and factious opposer of authority. (Forbes 1841, 356)

The disease was still a serious hazard in Ceylon at the beginning of the nineteenth century, despite inoculation and vaccination. An epidemic in 1800–2 caused 2,110 recorded cases, of whom 473 died.[2] Cordiner visited the island three times between 1800 and 1804 and found many abandoned villages taken over by wild animals after panic-stricken villagers fled in the face of the epidemic. "On such occasions," he wrote, "the husband forsakes his wife, the mother her children, and the son his father" (1807, 1: 254).

Meanwhile, the First Kandyan War was in progress and the inhabitants of that kingdom, which by now was reduced to the forested center of the island without direct access to the sea, had not yet received the benefits of vaccination. Just prior to his retirement, Governor-General North planned a "decisive campaign" against the king of Kandy. North's assault never took place, however, because famine and smallpox attacked the Kandyans first. In February 1805, the king himself, Sri Vikrama Rajasinha, was infected, "a calamity which was said never before to have happened to a ruler of Lanka, and [which] was regarded as a token of divine displeasure" (Pieris, 82). De Silva says for a short while, after the king became ill, "Kandyan politics was in suspense" (1953, 1: 119–20). The king recovered, but the perceived display of divine disfavor induced him to seek peace—one of the few instances in which a nonfatal attack of smallpox was so significant. According to Ludowyk (1966), when North retired later that year, other native headmen chose to formally thank him above all else for his efforts related to cultivation of land and vaccination against smallpox.

Ten years after the First Kandyan War, King Rajasinha was seized by the British, who thereby completed their control of the island. They introduced vaccination into the kingdom during a widespread outbreak there in 1818. This epidemic continued into 1819, when 7,874 cases of smallpox, almost 3,000 of them fatal, were recorded during the first six months. Both the epidemic of 1818–19 and the next one in 1830–31 were caused by returning residents who had been infected in India. Over 1,000 cases, with 257 deaths, were recorded in the latter outbreak. Another epidemic in 1836–37 killed at least 303 persons.

In general, however, Ceylon's population was more receptive to vaccination than was India's, and the benefits of Jenner's discovery were soon apparent on the island. By the middle of 1805, thirty-three thousand Ceylonese had been vaccinated, mainly in the maritime regions. In some areas, smallpox hospitals were closed for lack of patients. By 1815, 278,000 Ceylonese had been vaccinated, and another 493,000 vaccinations were given between 1815 and 1836 (Ceylon's population totaled about 1.4 million in 1844). As early as 1821, endemic smallpox was claimed to have been almost eliminated from the island.

Unlike Ceylon, it was not until late in the nineteenth century that sufficient numbers of people were vaccinated to significantly reduce the severity of smallpox epidemics in India. Calcutta suffered four major epidemics of smallpox during the first half of the century. In the epidemic of 1832–33, 2,814 deaths from smallpox were recorded; in 1837–38, 1,548 deaths; in 1843–44, 2,949 deaths; and in 1849–50, 6,431 deaths. One writer estimated that more than 32,000 persons, or one out of every twelve residents of Calcutta, were infected in the latter outbreak. During one particularly bad week in 1850, the proportion of smallpox deaths in Calcutta in relation to its population was greater than the cumulative death rate from smallpox for any three months in London since 1837 ("Smallpox in Hindoostan," 1851).

Some inhabitants believed that vaccination had a significant positive effect in early nineteenth-century India, however. When smallpox raged at Lucknow in 1837, a British resident blamed the great loss of life in that outbreak on the economy measures imposed by the governor-general, Lord Bentinck, which allegedly included closing a vaccine department (*Wanderings of a Pilgrim*, 1850, 110).

One kingdom that did not benefit from vaccination early in the century was Ahom. In January 1811, a severe epidemic broke out in Jorhat and neighboring villages. According to one account, "The people were seized with a dire panic, and they refrained from visiting the houses of their friends, relatives, and neighbors" (Bhuyan 1933, 200–201). Chief among the victims of this outbreak was the sixteen-year-old maharaja of

Assam, Kamaleswar Singha, of the Tungkhungia dynasty. He was succeeded by his fourteen-year-old brother.

Another kingdom that suffered without vaccination was Eedur, in the
western Indian state of Gujarat. There, Crown Prince Oomed Singh, only
son of the reigning rajah, died of smallpox in May 1824, at the age of
twenty-seven. Two of the prince's wives, and one concubine, committed
suicide on his funeral pyre. In the *Ras-mala: Hindu Annals of Western India*
it is recorded that this prince was survived by two other wives "upon
whom the desire of accompanying their lord to Paradise did not come"
(Forbes 1973, 496–97). According to the *Ras-mala*, "a Brahmin of Eedur
was so deeply distressed when he heard of the prince's death, from
thinking of what would become of the state, that he dashed his head
against a grain jar, and dislodged a heavy weight lying on it, which fell
upon him and killed him."

The earliest references to smallpox in Nepal date only from the early
nineteenth century, although it is improbable that this Himalayan kingdom between India and China remained unaffected by the disease until
then. Shrestha (1972) observes that inoculation is known to have been
practiced there since at least the eighteenth century. We also know that
there were temples devoted to worship of the Hindu smallpox goddess in
Nepal at the end of the eighteenth century, since in 1800, when the king's
Brahman mistress "committed suicide because she lost her beauty after an
attack of small-pox," the rajah destroyed several temples dedicated to
Shitala "in the Nepal valley" (Crooke 1925, 120; Shrestha 1972, 108).
Among the shrines ransacked was the predecessor of the current temple
at Swayambhu in Katmandu.

Soon after the first British envoy arrived in Nepal in 1816, another
epidemic erupted, "and committed great ravages among the people"
(Wright 1877, 53–54). One of its victims was the twenty-one-year-old
rajah, Girvana Bir Bikram Shah, who died on 20 November 1816. A wife
and six female slaves of the dead king, whose father's mistress was the
unfortunate beauty who killed herself because of scarring from smallpox,
burned themselves to death on his funeral pyre. Girvana was succeeded
by his three-year-old son.

During the second half of the nineteenth century, when the British
government took over administrative control of India from the British
East India Company, authorities began to systematically compile statistical reports of smallpox and other illnesses in India. The figures were
known to be incomplete even for the areas reporting, and all areas of the
subcontinent were not included in the reports. Nevertheless, these data
still convey some idea of smallpox's toll. The disease, which was always
present or nearby, became epidemic every four to eight years throughout
British India. The statistical reports always ranked smallpox as one of the
leading causes of death, along with famine, cholera, malaria, and later,

plague. In 1869, after thirteen years' medical experience in India, Pringle said that if cholera victims numbered in the hundreds annually, and famine victims in the thousands, "these are but infinitesimal quantities besides the frightful amount of devastation caused in India by the small-pox" (Hirsch 1883, 1: 131).

The *District Gazetteers* for the United Provinces of Oudh and Agra include scattered accounts of health problems in the constituent districts during this period. Although the *Gazetteers* do not convey the anguish of individual families and ravaged villages as they mourned relatives and friends, the numbing litany of deaths does preserve some sense of the colossal mortality caused by smallpox in India:

> *Saharanpur District*: 20,942 reported dead of smallpox from 1867 to 1873 when registration of deaths was low. *Muzaffarnagar District*: Over 2000 smallpox deaths in 1868; more than 4332 died of smallpox in 1871. *Meerut District*: 4984 smallpox deaths in 1869. *Bulandshahr District*: 1873 is worst year on record, when 6967 died of smallpox; in 1869, there had been 6650 smallpox deaths. *Aligarh District*: A terrible epidemic early in 1850 was worsened by imperfect disposal of corpses; other epidemics followed in 1869, 1873, 1879 (8311 deaths) and 1884 (4851 deaths). *Buduan District*: In 1884 smallpox caused 8389 deaths, which was 29% of the total mortality for that year. *Shahjahanpur District*: 3835 smallpox deaths reported in 1878, 6307 in 1883, 2705 in 1897. *Cawnpore District*: 7428 died of smallpox in 1874. *Fatehpur District*: An epidemic in 1884–5 claimed 6067 lives. *Allahabad District*: 10,878 smallpox deaths in 1878. *Mirzapur District*: Over 4000 deaths recorded annually in 1878, 1879, 1884. *Jaunpur District*: Outbreaks in 1878–9 (6139 deaths), 1884 (5530 deaths), 1897 (7047). *Gorakhpur District*: Epidemics in 1879, 1881, 1884 (17,469 deaths), 1891 (11,117 deaths), 1897 (over 3000 deaths). *Basti District*: More than 19,000 smallpox deaths in 1884. *Azamgarh District*: 4330 smallpox deaths in 1884, 10,262 in 1891, 4780 in 1892, 11,270 in 1894, 4193 in 1895. *Sitapur District*: Earlier had the worst reputation for smallpox in Oudh; only 2753 smallpox deaths in 1897. *Hardoi District*: 9807 deaths in 1878, 13,256 in 1883, 7479 in 1889, 4918 in 1897. *Gonda District*: An average of over 3000 deaths from smallpox annually from 1872–1881, more than thirteen percent of all reported deaths for that period; 24,600 died of smallpox in 1885 epidemic. (Compiled from Nevill 1903–11, and Drake-Brockman 1903–11)

Massive epidemics were recorded all over India in 1868–69, 1872–74, 1877–79, and 1884–85. During these ten epidemic years, according to government estimates at least two and a half million of the estimated 180 million persons in British India were reported to have died of smallpox (Govt. of India 1932, 418). From twentieth-century experience in India and elsewhere, we know that for each such death that was reported, there were as many as ninety-nine others unreported (Basu et. al. 1979). Thus the projected number of actual deaths from smallpox in those ten epidemic years between 1868 and 1885 amounts to over ten percent of the estimated population of British India, a staggering number.

Even in "off years" for the country as a whole, smallpox killed tens of thousands of Indians.[3] During 1875–76, two nonepidemic years, 200,000 deaths from smallpox were reported for the whole country. In two months of 1865, seven thousand persons died of smallpox in Lahore. In Coimbatore District, where smallpox normally killed "only a few hundreds of people," it claimed 2,075 victims in 1882 and 2,676 in 1892.

In 1883, 75,588 deaths from the virus were reported for Oudh Province, 2,114 of which occurred in Lucknow, the provincial capital. Smallpox was also epidemic in Calcutta in 1857 (3,177 deaths), 1865 (4,923 deaths), 1884, and 1894–95 (2,220 deaths in 1895).

Many of the Indian epidemics were associated with famine—as cause, effect, or both. Some were triggered by the disruption and population movements precipitated by lack of food. Other outbreaks hampered cultivation of crops by temporarily indisposing farmers at critical times in the agricultural season, or by killing numerous villagers outright. Widespread famine accompanied nationwide smallpox epidemics in 1878 and 1897. In Jhansi District, Northwest Frontier Province, in 1868–69, a smallpox epidemic that killed thousands of the inhabitants was preceded by famine, accompanied by many deaths from sunstroke in the dry season, and followed by epidemic "fever" (probably malaria) and cholera in the next rainy season.[4]

Other epidemics were started or intensified by factors related to India's crowding, poverty, or religious worship. During the outbreak of smallpox in Calcutta in 1894, for example, it was reported that "the beddings of the deceased were in several instances thrown on the street, picked up by rag-sellers, collected at the rag depots, and ultimately sent to the Bally paper mills" (Das 1895, 114–15)—practices guaranteed to spread the contagion. Bose (1890) described how the sickrooms of smallpox patients in Calcutta around this time were closed to air and light and crowded with visitors. Calcutta's deputy superintendent of Vaccination blamed some of the city's annual outbreaks on infected pilgrims returning by ship from Mecca. According to Das (1895) unknown numbers of others were infected by prior victims reporting for treatment by priests at one of Calcutta's thirty-two temples dedicated to the smallpox goddess.

The innumerable victims in these epidemics were largely young children, among whom mortality rates sometimes reached over fifty percent. The epidemic of 1867–68 reportedly killed eight out of every ten children in United Provinces' Hardoi District. Pringle records a popular saying that warned poor and wealthy Indian parents "never to count children as permanent members of the family nor make arrangements to leave them money, etc., until they have been attacked and recovered from smallpox" (1869, 44–45).

Death was the most severe, but not the only serious effect of smallpox in nineteenth-century India. "Smallpox in those days," wrote S. J. Thompson, "was a terrible scourge in [Oudh] province, not only carrying off great numbers of people by deaths, but also frequently leaving the victim, when he survived, totally blind or disfigured" (1913, 97–98). We have already noted the tragic consequences of one such disfiguring attack at the royal court of Nepal. In the Rajpootana area of India, a visitor estimated that eight out of every ten persons were pitted from smallpox, and ten percent of the persons he passed on the streets of Jondpoor and Pallee were blind in one or both eyes or had some other eye damage, mostly from smallpox. Earlier in the century, Ranjit Singh of the Punjab, the "last of the great independent Maharajahs of India," was obliged to wear his giant Koh-i-noor diamond on a band around his right bicep, where he could admire it, because his left eye was blind from smallpox (Lord 1971, 4).

After the great epidemic of 1884–85, the cumulative effect of steadily increasing vaccinations began to be reflected by decreasing death rates from smallpox in British India. Death rates in the next peak epidemic years (1889–90 and 1896–97) were less than half those recorded earlier. Rates in nonepidemic years were also diminished, compared to what they were before. *The Imperial Gazeteer of India* (1909) reports that during the last three decades of the nineteenth century, the average number of annual reported deaths from smallpox in India was cut in half: from 169,000 per year in 1871–80, to 81,000 per year in 1891–1900.

But vaccination was still not known universally in India. It didn't reach Kashmir until 1894. In some villages, Thompson (1913) observes, vaccinators had to prove the procedure was safe by vaccinating lower-caste persons first. Inoculation also was still practiced in many areas, where it may have contributed as much to smallpox's dispersion as to its control.

In Ceylon, vaccination had by the end of the century reduced the threat of smallpox to much lower levels than in India. During the decade 1880–89, the average number of deaths from smallpox per year in Ceylon was only 311. According to Low (1918), in the last decade of the nineteenth century, even that was reduced to an average of 81 deaths per year in a population of nearly four million.

In contrast to the rapidly improving situation in Ceylon, and the slower improvement in India, Indochina continued to suffer severely. MacGilvary reported that during an epidemic of smallpox in Siam (Thailand) and Laos in 1866–67, "hardly a household escaped, and many had no children left." McGilvary, who had resided in Indochina for fifty years, called another outbreak in the same area in 1884 "the worst epidemic of smallpox I have ever seen" (1912, 89, 250). During the same period, the French director of Saigon's Pasteur Institute, Dr. Simond, reported that the Laotians were decimated annually by smallpox. He also described villages in which an epidemic killed all the children, and left so disproportionately few females of marriageable age that it had an unusually long-lasting depopulating effect. In Annam, in 1888, epidemics in coastal villages caused such panic that dozens of victims' corpses were thrown daily into the sea instead of being buried or cremated. In Tonkin, ninety-five of every one hundred adolescents between fifteen and twenty years old who were examined in 1898 "bore the stigmata of smallpox," which was said to cause nine-tenths of all the blindness in Indochina (Hervieux 1899, 61).

That smallpox continued to ravage Indochina so late in the nineteenth century was due to insufficient vaccination, not absence of vaccination altogether. During the outbreak in Siam and Laos in 1866–67, Prince Chengmai lost one of his granddaughters to smallpox, and a grandson died of diarrhea after being vaccinated. Thirty years later, Cambodians were said to still prefer inoculation by Chinese or Malaysian practitioners and therefore resisted Jennerian vaccination. (McGilvary 1912; Hervieux 1899).

Twentieth Century

In India, death rates from smallpox in epidemic years fell from over 2,000 per million population to less than 500 per million between 1870 and 1930, as more and more Indians were vaccinated (fig. 9).[5] Epidemics continued to erupt at five to eight year intervals, however, and India remained the premier focus of smallpox in the world until 1975. Over a hundred thousand Indians were reported as having died of the virus in each of eleven years between 1902 and 1945. More than three thousand persons died of smallpox during an epidemic in Bombay in 1900, and nearly four thousand died in an epidemic in Calcutta nine years later.

In 1930, a nonepidemic year for the country as a whole (only 215,260 cases and 48,860 deaths were reported nationwide), all of the major maritime cities of India suffered from epidemic smallpox. That year India's suffering was compounded after cases occurring in ships that had called at Indian ports caused other countries to impose severe restrictions on Indian shipping worldwide.

Children continued to bear the brunt of these epidemics, despite a Vaccination Act that required Indian children to be vaccinated within six months of birth (the act did not apply to all jurisdictions or areas). During an epidemic in Bombay Presidency in 1924, 3,532 of the 11,152 deaths reported were infants less than one year old; while 5,606 of the remaining victims were children between one and ten years old.

The main reason Indian children continued to suffer so much from smallpox, albeit at a lesser rate than in years past, was that the nation's vaccination laws were incomplete and inadequately enforced. The annual

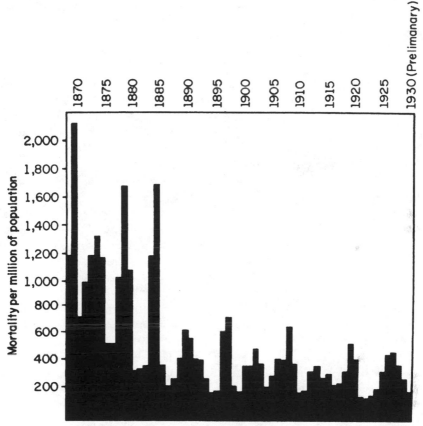

Fig. 9. Reported deaths from smallpox in British India, 1868–1930. From Govt. of India (1932). Note the steady decline in death rates as vaccination became more widespread.

report for 1928 of India's Public Health commissioner explained: "Vaccination in India is not compulsory. The Vaccination Act of 1880, as amended in 1909, is intended to give power to enforce compulsory vaccination in certain areas only. It has not been considered practicable to enforce this in India generally." By 1941, primary vaccination was legally compulsory only in about 81 percent of the towns and 62 percent of the rural areas in British India. At that time routine revaccination had been made compulsory only in the provincial area of Madras (1932) and Madras City (1936).

In Burma as in India, smallpox was partly but not completely, controlled between 1900 and 1960. An epidemic killed over a thousand persons in Rangoon alone (population about 290,000) in 1906. Six years later an outbreak in Bangkok claimed 2,368 lives. Still, the regional burden of smallpox was gradually becoming lighter. A physician at the court of Siam (Thailand) reported that pockmarked faces were a relatively rare sight there after the mid-1920s, compared to only twenty years before (Smith 1947). Thailand reported less than one hundred cases annually in the early 1930s.

Ceylon's natural insularity and vigorous vaccination efforts combined to reduce smallpox to an occasionally imported nuisance. By 1932, Ceylon had virtually eliminated the disease. Only seventy-six cases were recorded from 1928 to 1931. In November 1932, the disease was reintroduced from India, and caused an epidemic of 443 cases. The next three decades were marked by similar intermittent outbreaks.

World War II produced an upsurge in smallpox in several countries of the region. Thailand reported over 61,000 cases in 1945–46, and Ceylon over 1,100. In Thailand the epidemics resulted from infections introduced by prisoners of war, who had been brought to Thailand by the Japanese forces. In Burma, thousands of cases occurred annually but the worst year was 1950 when over 10,000 cases were reported.

India also recorded substantial, though diminishing epidemics in 1950–51 (105,781 deaths reported) and in 1957–58 (68,998 deaths). The latter outbreak was part of an upsurge of smallpox in several Asian and African countries, during which East Pakistan (Bangladesh) reported over 86,000 deaths from smallpox in a three-year period.

Thailand and Vietnam reported their last cases of smallpox in 1962, the year India began its National Smallpox Eradication Program. Laos had reported its last case in 1953, and Cambodia in 1959. Ceylon reported no cases in 1955 and 1956, but still had occasional small outbreaks following importations from India. Burma vaccinated nearly 90 percent of its population between 1963 and 1966, and suffered no more smallpox except for an outbreak of 250 cases in 1968–69, following an importation from East Pakistan.

Since 1895, over 8 million persons had been vaccinated annually in British India, whose 1911 population numbered about 315 million. By 1944, some 60 million vaccinations were being given annually in a population of about 435 million. Between 1962 and 1965, the Indian Smallpox Eradication Program vaccinated approximately 324 million of the country's 473 million persons, an incredible accomplishment. Yet over 65,000 cases of smallpox were reported in India in 1965 and 1966, and when the WHO's global Smallpox Eradication Program began in 1967, two-thirds of the world's smallpox was being reported from India. Clearly something was wrong.

A consultant to the National Institute of Communicable Diseases in Delhi, Dr. Henry Gelfand, evaluated the Indian program in 1963–65 and found that in spite of the massive numbers of vaccinations performed, large pockets of unvaccinated persons remained untouched—especially children under five, slum dwellers, and others. Certain easy-to-reach groups, such as school children, were being vaccinated over and over, while many of the floating population of pilgrims, beggars, itinerant tradesmen, and laborers, who often carried the disease from one locality to another, had never been vaccinated. Another contributing factor was the continued use of heat-sensitive, often impotent vaccine.

A vigorous program made East Pakistan free of the virus by August 1970. It had no smallpox in 1971, although West Pakistan reported nearly six thousand cases that year. Following the Indo-Pakistan War in December 1971, however, refugees returning to East Pakistan (now Bangladesh) from India in January 1972, reintroduced smallpox, which quickly spread again throughout the new country. In 1972, India reported 27,407 cases of smallpox, Pakistan 7,053 cases, and Bangladesh reported 10,754 cases.

Late in 1973, India, Pakistan, and Bangladesh intensified their eradication efforts, beginning with an "Autumn Campaign" in which I participated. Afghanistan had reported its last cases of smallpox in July that year. The only other countries in the world still reporting smallpox were Ethiopia and Nepal, the latter owing all its remaining smallpox to importations from India. During this final push, workers from several other national and local health programs, in addition to those in the respective Smallpox Eradication Programs, were mobilized to visit each village in the three Asian countries during one week each month in an effort to find any persons who had smallpox. In the three weeks before the next all-out search began again the following month, teams of workers from the smallpox programs sought to vaccinate everyone who had been exposed to those newly discovered cases. The Autumn Campaign was extended into the next year, and increasingly large cash rewards were offered to anyone who first reported a case of smallpox. Pakistan reported its final case in October 1974. But in India and Bangladesh, the disease made a startling comeback.

A century before the Autumn Campaign got underway, a British surgeon encountered a group of Bihari tribesmen while he was trying to control an outbreak of smallpox in Bengal. He found the Biharis to be particularly reluctant to be vaccinated; a characteristic that was still true in 1973.

> [They] absolutely refuse to have themselves and their children vaccinated. These people, therefore, suffer most; and when smallpox gets among them, it continues for a long time. They do not isolate the attacked . . . they buy, and sell, and wash, and go into the infected houses, utterly regardless of the result. One workman told me lately: "If Kali [Sitala, the smallpox goddess] takes my child, she will. It is not our custom to offend her by vaccination." (Hunter 1876, 242–43)

The Biharis came from the adjacent Indian state of Bihar, which possessed an unusual geologic feature that was believed to be especially revered by the goddess of smallpox. The *Imperial Gazetteer of India* described this sanctuary of the goddess, which was near Tilothu village in Sasaram subdivision of Shanabad District.

> Five miles to the west is a gorge by which the Tutrahi, a tributary of the Kudra river, leaves the hills. This spot is sacred to the Goddess Sitala. The gorge itself is a half mile long, terminating in a sheer horseshoe precipice from 180 to 250 feet high, down which the river falls. (U. K., H. M. Sec. of State 1908, 23: 360)

As Indian health workers and their international allies gradually closed in on smallpox early in 1974, cornering it in northeast India, the disease suddenly erupted in a huge, explosive outbreak, centered in Bihar State. It was as if the goddess herself angrily threw all her might into a fierce, indignant defense of her power and sanctuary.

> Victory! Victory to Sitala Bhavani
> Victory, Mother of the Universe, repository of all qualities,
> In every house is your power established,
> As beautiful as the full autumn moon.
> When the body burns with poisonous eruptions,
> You make it cool and take away all pain.
> Your auspicious name is Mother Sitala;
> You help everyone in time of trouble.
> You take away all sorrow, O Sankari Bhavani,
> You protect the lives of children, O giver of happiness.
> Adorned with a pure broom and a water vessel in your hand,
> The luster of your forehead is like the Sun.
>
> (from Prabhudas, *Sitala Calisa*)

Whereas 88,114 cases of smallpox had been reported in all of India in 1973, Bihar State alone (population 60 million) reported over 35,000 cases, with more than 10,000 deaths for smallpox in May 1974. Bihar recorded nearly 127,000 cases in all that year. Travelers carried smallpox from Bihar all over India.

In Bangladesh, the renewed eradication effort continued to progress satisfactorily up to the end of October 1974. But late summer floods that year led to widespread famine, which caused thousands of Bengalis to converge on Dacca, the capital, searching for food and work. Some were infected with smallpox, which reestablished itself in the slums of Dacca. From Dacca, it spread again all over Bangladesh.

Redoubled efforts by indigenous and expatriate health workers gradually overcame the reverses in India and in Bangladesh, Shitala's wrath not withstanding. After a thirty-year-old woman, infected in Bangladesh, became ill in Assam State on 24 May 1975, there was no more smallpox in India. Nepal's last case of smallpox was recorded one month before India's. In Bangladesh, *V. major*'s final victim was a three-year-old girl whose rash began on 16 October 1975 (plate 25).

SHITALA MATA: INDIAN GODDESS OF SMALLPOX

While it is known that a smallpox goddess has been worshipped in India for centuries, just how long she has been worshipped is not known. According to Holwell, the *Artharva veda*, dating from two to three thousand years ago, contains prayers and accounts of ceremonies for this goddess, but Holwell's report is disputed by some knowledgeable students of Sanskrit literature (Moore 1815; Nicolas 1981). The Bangs believe Shitala was a pre-Hindu folk goddess, thus antedating even the Vedas (Taylor 1971). Dudgeon (1871) and Wise (1845) postulate a later appearance of the goddess in India, coinciding with a change in the character of the disease from an older, milder form to a more dreaded, fatal type. Ralph Nicolas, in an excellent recent article (1981), theorizes that in West Bengal, Shitala was transformed from a minor to a major deity only in the eighteenth century. As mentioned above, the king of Lanka inaugurated worship of a smallpox goddess in Ceylon late in the second century A.D. after witnessing ceremonies devoted to a similar goddess in southern India, and sculptured figures of the goddess have been found in Indian temples dating from the ninth, twelfth, and thirteenth centuries A.D.[6] We can assume, therefore, that Shitala is at least two thousand years old, and probably older than that.

There are several traditional accounts of the origin of this smallpox goddess, which vary by geographic area and ethnic group. Moore (1815) and Elwin (1955) each quote two different accounts, all four of which portrayed the goddess as being ill-tempered and governed by desire for revenge. According to Ishwaran (1968), the fact that Shitala is female is believed to be significant in explaining how smallpox can be so vicious. According to the latter theory, Indian children were more severely affected by smallpox than were adults because by attacking children, the goddess was striking at the very roots of the community.

The two explanations recorded by Elwin and cited below are from an Indian tribe in Orissa State (1955, 286–87). The first emphasizes the goddess's close relation to the red gram, called *rogon*, which resembles a smallpox pustule, and from which the local name of the goddess, Rugaboi, is derived. Elwin believed Rugaboi was actually a tribal smallpox goddess who was gradually being replaced by the Hindu goddess of smallpox. Other observers believe the two goddesses are essentially the same. According to Elwin's first explanation:

> When the gods were born, each went to his own place and did his own business. Tupru Saora lived on Tamchaya Hill. He made a clearing and sowed red pulse. Under one of the shrubs Rugaboi was born; when Tupru went to see his crop he found her like a young girl and took her home. She worked for him, brought him water, cleaned the house. One day Tupru took his pulse and beans to the bazaar. The other villagers went on ahead, but Rugaboi lagged behind and on the way a Dom and a

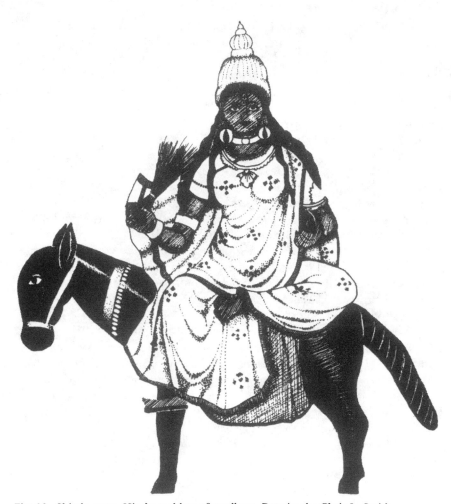

Fig. 10. Shitala mata, Hindu goddess of smallpox. Drawing by Chris L. Smith.

Saora caught hold of her and stole the pulse she was carrying. She was very angry and changed her appearance and took the form of a goddess. The Dom and Saora dropped their baskets and ran for their lives. Rugaboi went to Kittung and told him what had happened and he said, "You can have your revenge by giving them swellings like pulse and beans on their bodies. They will sacrifice to you and you will get all the food you want." Rugaboi went back and entered into the bodies of the Dom and the Saora and gave them smallpox. They called the shaman and he made a little chariot, put every kind of grain into it, took it out of the village and sacrificed a pig before it. Rugaboi was satisfied, and the pestilence ceased.

According to his second version of the goddess's origin:

> Rugaboi was the eldest and she was very beautiful. Her body was
> tender as fresh leaves, her breasts were bael fruit, the bun of her hair was
> a bulbul's nest. One day Ramma-Bimma called the sisters to divide the
> world between them. Uyungboi and Angaiboi went, but Rugaboi stayed
> behind. Ramma-Bimma, therefore, gave the night to the Moon and the
> day to the Sun, and each went to her own place. This made Rugaboi very
> angry. "I am the eldest," she cried, "and the most beautiful, yet I get
> nothing." And she went to Ramma-Bimma, intending to devour him.
> Now Ramma-Bimma was bringing out of his bins the twelve kinds of seed
> to give to men, and when Rugaboi came to attack him, he threw the seed
> at her. Whenever a seed hit her a sore broke out and soon she was
> hideous with pustules swelling like seeds all over her body. She abused
> Ramma-Bimma, but all he did was to hand her a mirror. When she saw
> how ugly she was, she went into the sky and devoured half the body of the
> Moon. When Ramma-Bimma saw this, he said, "I will give you all human-
> ity to eat, but leave the Moon alone." So Rubagoi left the Moon and now
> she attacks men instead, when she remembers how unjustly she has been
> treated.

In the Hindu pantheon, dominated by Brahma (the Creator), Vishnu
(the Preserver), and Shiva (the Destroyer), Shitala, Goddess of Smallpox,
is held to be a form of Shiva's wife. Crooke (1921) and Stevenson (1915)
report that she is said to be one of seven sisters, each of whom is responsible for a different exanthematous illness. In India, she is worshipped by
Hindus, Moslems, and Jains. In Nepal, Shitala was incorporated into the
Buddhist pantheon as "Ajima," or "Sitala ajima," and is revered as the
mother of Guatama Buddha (Sekelj 1959; Nepali 1965).

She has many names. Shitala, meaning "the cool one" or "the chilly
one," is a euphemistic title widely used in northern India, based on the
high fever and burning sensation associated with smallpox and her reputed ability to relieve them. She is called Mariyammai in the Tamil
country of southern India. Shitala mata, Shitala devi, devi mata, Thaku-
rani, Patragale, Mariatale, Rugboi, and Jyeshtha are some of the other
names by which she is known.

Whatever the local thoughts about her origin and the variety of
names by which she goes, the cult of this goddess is very popular, and her
wrath is feared. According to Morgan (1953) a medieval poet in southern
India complained in some of his songs that people were worshipping
Shitala when they should have been worshipping Vishnu. Mayer (1960)
listed forty-four shrines according to frequency of worship in a central
Indian village twenty years ago, and found that Shitala mata was second
only to the Mother Goddess in popularity. He also found that ceremonies
honoring the smallpox goddess were the only occasions when caste and
subcaste villagers simultaneously participated in the same activity, and

were the only circumstances in which Harijans (Untouchables) were permitted to enter the main village temple.

Classically, and especially in Bengal, Shitala is represented by a woman riding an ass, with a broom in one hand (to sweep the disease along or to sweep away nonbelievers), a waterpot in her other arm (to hold the germs or to soothe feverish victims), a winnowing fan on her head (to sift the smallpox germs), and dressed in red clothes, sometimes with polka dots.[7] Sometimes she is "more Brahmanized, a four-armed figure, like that of Durga." Elsewhere she is sometimes represented by a simple stone, by a piece of stone or wood studded with nails to imitate the pustules, or simply by a pot of water (Crooke 1925). Crooke (1906) observed that some faithful followers wear an image of the goddess on a medallion around their neck. Whenever possible, her shrines are located near a Nim tree (*Melia azadirachta*), and devoted only to her, but often her image is included with that of other deities in multipurpose temples.

Temples dedicated to Shitala are found all over India. Individual homes or villages may have shrines patronized only by their own inhabitants. Other highly respected shrines attract pilgrims from long distances away and are the scenes of large periodic festivals. According to Tupp (1877), in March 1875, an estimated fifteen thousand persons attended a service in homage to Shitala in Farukhabad District, near Agra. The *Imperial Gazetteer of India* (1909) records that a temple dedicated to this goddess in the Punjab was visited annually by fifty to sixty thousand people early in this century. In Coimbator District, Travancore State, there is a temple dedicated to Shitala at which continuous worship for eight weeks was believed to cure blindness caused by smallpox (Aiya 1906). At Benares, most sacred of all Hindu cities, there are four temples devoted to worship of the smallpox goddess.

An annual festival is held on the goddess's feast day. In Gujarat, cooking and all other activities that require contact with "hot" things are avoided on Shitala's feast day. Only cold food and drink are taken for fear of annoying the goddess, who is believed to wander among the ovens on that day. Some of these festivals last up to ten days. Whether Shitala will continue to be worshipped so fervently years after smallpox has been eradicated only time will tell. Although she was also worshipped sometimes for other communicable illnesses, smallpox was by far the worst and most awe-inspiring.

Shitala is felt to have both a benevolent and a terrible aspect. On the one hand, she is worshipped, especially by mothers on behalf of their children, as a preventive measure for those who have not had smallpox and to secure a cure of others suffering from the disease. E. W. Hopkins wrote that in one area worshippers prayed on behalf of adults, "O kind goddess of smallpox, Keep away from us," whereas for babies they prayed, "O kind smallpox, come soon to this baby and treat it gently"

(1901, 322). On the other hand, as Mather and John (1973) observe, when smallpox was in the immediate area, it was thought to be useless and even dangerous to attempt to prevent an attack. In this latter belief lay part of the difficulty of controlling outbreaks in areas where belief in the goddess was strong. Some believers took no chances. MacMunn reported that in some areas, the smallpox goddess "is at all times and in all parts, most properly worshipped, dreaded, glorified and propitiated, but the vaccinator is also accepted lest the goddess be not listening or be in a persnikety and malevolent mood" (1933, 233).

When smallpox actually struck, devout believers were pleased that the goddess had "deigned to visit their humble dwelling" (Biscoe 1922, 63). When a child was infected naturally, or as a result of inoculation by priests of the cult, Shitala was believed to have entered the child, who then was "sacred, treated with respect, and spoken to as *devi* the goddess" (Govt. of India 1885, 8: 224–25). Gurdon (1914) reports that among the syntegs, the infection was an honor, and pockmarks were said to represent the "Kiss of the Goddess": the more violent the attack, and the deeper the scars, the higher the honor. During the illness, taboos were numerous:

> the temples of no other gods other than those of smallpox are visited for fear of exciting the jealousy of the smallpox god; guests or visitors cannot be courteously received or dismissed or given a special dinner; family disagreements and quarrels and wailings are forbidden; journeys are put off; both festive and mournful ceremonies are avoided; sexual intercourse is forbidden; . . . no article of food can be fried in a pan or otherwise seasoned; and among the lower classes liquor and flesh are avoided. (Govt. of India 1901, 9: 370)

Patients were fed a diet of cooling food and drink. Morgan (1953) says that ass's milk was believed to be especially propitious because of its connection with the goddess's mount. Offerings were made to an image of the goddess in the home, or a family member was sent to worship at a village shrine. Cold water was poured on the image; rice, flowers, and red powder were thrown on it, and other gifts were sometimes made. Water that had annointed the goddess's statue was sometimes used to bathe or sprinkle the patient. The patient himself was sometimes taken to a village shrine during the illness. Leaves of the Nim tree were put on or around the bed or used to fan him. Victims were cared for by family members, or priests attendant to the goddess.

If the patient died, the corpse was not supposed to be cremated according to the usual Hindu tradition, since to do so would be to set fire to the goddess herself (Sleeman 1915).

Five

The Spotted Death

WITH INDIA AND CHINA, AFRICA is the third area where smallpox was apparently endemic before the birth of Christ. Indeed, the evidence of smallpox in ancient Egypt—rash-bearing mummies dating from the sixteenth to twelfth centuries B.C.—is the oldest and most convincing proof of the disease's existence in the ancient world. Despite that shared pre-Christian heritage, however, Africa differed from India and China in two important respects. First, unlike the rich written historical legacies of the two Asian civilizations, after the collapse of ancient Egypt there are relatively few historical records in Africa for the next two thousand years, until Europeans began to explore the continent around 1500 A.D. Second, except for the lower Nile valley and parts of West Africa near the Gulf of Guinea, most of Africa was relatively thinly populated until quite recently.

Geography and climate were two major determinants of the distribution of early African populations, and hence, of smallpox. The arid Sahara Desert in the north, and the smaller Kalahari Desert in the southwest, were virtually uninhabited in historical times. Midway between these two great deserts, dense tropical rain forest in the Congo River basin formed a third, very sparsely inhabited region across the middle of the continent, broken only in the east, by the Great Rift Valley and East African highlands. Subject to these geographic barriers, and a coast nearly devoid of natural harbors, most medieval African states arose in the interior. One group of states evolved in the band of hospitable grasslands just south of the Sahara: from Ghana, Mali, and Songhai in the west, to Kanem-Bornu and Darfur in the center, and Funj and Ethiopia in the east. South of the Congo River, Kongo, Lunda, and Luba formed a second group of states, loosely linked to Zimbabwe in the southeast and several closely packed smaller kingdoms along the western shore of Lake Victoria. Linked as they were inland, and later to the coast, by caravans, these states, kingdoms, and empires were vulnerable to smallpox despite the great distances between them.

The first trace of smallpox in Africa after Ramses V appears in the sixth century A.D., south of the crowded lower Nile valley, where the disease had probably already been endemic for over a thousand years.

Other ancient states in Northeast Africa, especially Nubia, Kush, and Axum, had considerable commercial ties and variable political connections with Egypt. Egyptian Queen Hatshepsut's well-known maritime mission to "Punt" (located possibly beyond the horn of coastal East Africa) was but one example of the regional links. Although details from the brief reign of Ramses V are rare, his name has been found inscribed at Buhen, near the second cataract of the Nile, in northern Sudan (Cerny 1975). Thus smallpox could easily have spread among these Northeast African states long ago.

Early in the sixth century, soldiers from the Ethiopian kingdom of Axum attacked the southern Arabian kingdom of Yemen and established Ethiopian rule there. In 570, Abraha, the Christian Ethiopian prince who was then viceroy of Yemen, led a large army of Ethiopian soldiers to besiege another Arabian stronghold, Mecca. During this conflict, known as the "Elephant War" because Abraha arrived mounted on a white elephant, a severe illness, characterized by a rash, broke out among the Ethiopian soldiers and "miraculously" saved the day for their vastly outnumbered enemies. The illness almost totally destroyed Abraha's army, although the viceroy himself escaped back to Ethiopia (Moore 1815, 45). Abraha's defeat invited Persian intervention, which ended Ethiopian rule in Arabia.

The Elephant War was allegorized in the Koran, which states that "Large birds appeared, which dropped stones the size of a pea on to the persons, and they were killed" (Dixon 1962, 189).[1] According to another translation of the relevant passage from the Koran:

In the name of Allah, the Beneficent, the Merciful.
Hast thou not seen how thy lord dealt with the possessors of the elephant?
Did He not cause their wars to end in confusion?
And send against them birds in flocks?
Casting at them decreed stones-
So he rendered them like straw eaten up?

(Willis 1971, 139).

Centuries later, the Scottish physician-explorer James Bruce (1805, 2: 440–43) found Ethiopian chronicles that confirmed the destruction of Abraha's army by a pestilence at Mecca. This outbreak is generally considered to be one of the earliest known epidemics of smallpox, although it should be noted that the direct clinical evidence for that conclusion is slim. Only fifty-two years later, however, Aaron's clear description of smallpox in Alexandria proves that smallpox was very well known in that part of Northeast Africa by then.

It is not certain where the Elephant War epidemic originated. Dixon (1962) believes that it most likely was carried to Arabia from Ethiopia by some of Abraha's troops. According to Pankhurst (1965), Ethiopian

(Aksumite) soldiers had also carried smallpox into Arabia around 370. But the Elephant War epidemic could also have spread to Mecca from Syria, where it may have arrived overland from Persia early in the same century during the invasion of Chosroes. In fact, Bishop Eusebius had described an epidemic of smallpox in Syria as early as 302:

> [It] was characterized by a dangerous eruption which unlike the true plague spread over the whole body and which also affected the eyes and often resulted in loss of sight, which had the effect of protecting against a second attack of the same disorder, and whose eruption was, according to a later writer, accompanied by a very offensive smell. (Dixon 1962, 189)

Richter (1912) argues that the Elephant War epidemic might also have arrived at the southern coast of Arabia by sea, from India. Axum and southern Arabia had both traded with the Orient for hundreds of years and by the sixth century, Axum was a busy commercial center, exporting gold, ivory, and slaves from the African interior to Arabia, Persia, India, and China. Richter cited the decimation of the Ethiopians and relative sparing of the Arabians as evidence that the disease must have spread from Mecca's defenders to the Ethiopians. He assumed smallpox had been present among the Arabians for a long time, and many of them were immune, whereas the Africans were encountering it for the first time. But even if his assumption is correct, it does not necessarily follow that the Arabians were the source of the outbreak.

Whatever its source, and it seems most likely that it originated in Ethiopia, the epidemic that saved Mecca was carried by the defeated Ethiopians back to their homeland. Abraha himself died of smallpox in Axum soon after he fled Arabia. We know nothing of the disease's impact on sixth-century Axum, which was then a kingdom of about four hundred thousand persons.

Saved by the Elephant War epidemic and united by Mohammed's teachings, Arab armies erupted from Arabia early in the seventh century, accompanied by wives, children, slaves, and inevitably, smallpox. Even a "private in the Syrian Army," wrote the historian Philip Hitti, "had from one to ten servants waiting on him" (1964, 235). Consequently, the Moslem army was an excellent breeding ground for the disease. According to Penna (1885), Mohammed's armies took smallpox to the Persian Gulf coast of Arabia and to Mesopotamia during the Prophet's lifetime. Wernher believed epidemics of smallpox in Egypt actually facilitated the Arab conquest of that state around 641 (Lersch 1896). That there was still smallpox in Egypt at the time we can be sure. Aaron, a Christian priest who had lived in Alexandria for thirty years before the Arab conquest, left clear descriptions of smallpox and measles, written in 622. Aaron described the symptoms, and distinguished mild and dangerous varieties of smallpox, which must have been quite common in Alexandria during his lifetime.

> When the smallpox pustules are white and red, they are healthy; when green and black, malignant; and if after a time, the eruption of smallpox and measles changes to a *saffron* colour, and the fever moderates, good hopes may be entertained; but if these eruptions appear during a frenzy fever, they are fatal (Moore 1815, 115)

After Alexandria, the Arab armies swept across western Asia, North Africa, and conquered Spain before they were stopped at Constantinople in 717, and at Poitiers, France, in 732. Smallpox went with them, into Syria, Palestine, Sicily, Mauritania, Spain, and France. Only a century after Mohammed's death, the Arab Empire stretched from the Atlantic Ocean to China.

As the Arabs consolidated their conquests, smallpox began raiding the royal palaces of Baghdad and Damascus. Moore (1815) and Hitti (1964) provide us with several examples. In 754, the caliph Abu-al-Abbas, who only five years before had overthrown the Umayyad dynasty, slaughtering all but one of its members—he called himself *al-saffah*, "the blood-shedder"—died of smallpox while still in his early thirties. Abu-al-Abbas was succeeded by his brother al-Mansur, the caliph of *A Thousand and One Nights*, who built a new capital at Baghdad.[2] Al-Mansur, says Hitti (1964, 290) "rather than al Saffah, was the one who firmly established the new [Abbasid] dynasty," which lasted for five hundred years.

Three of the early caliphs were deeply pitted from smallpox: Yazid (r. 680–683), who earned the title Yazid al-Khumur, "the Yazid of Wines," and trained a pet monkey to drink with him; al-Walid (r. 705–715), "the greatest Umayyad builder," who erected schools, built hospitals for lepers and blind persons, and converted the Cathedral of St. John the Baptist in Damascus into the Umayyad Mosque, fourth holiest mosque in Islam; and al-Mutamid (r. 870–92), "the only real caliph musician." Al-Mutamid's reign is also remembered for a bloody fourteen-year-long rebellion of East African slaves employed in mines south of Baghdad. Two other early caliphs, al-Mahdi (r. 775–85) and al-Wathiq (r. 842–47) were partly blinded by smallpox.

In the tenth century, Moslem learning began to counter the virus's ravages when Rhazes (al-Razi, 850–925), the Persian-born physician-in-chief of the hospital at Baghdad, published *A Treatise on the Small-pox and Measles*. Rhazes was widely traveled, having visited Jerusalem, Africa, and perhaps Spain. He was already over forty when he began to study medicine. Later, Prince al-Mansur urged him to put his knowledge in writing. Rhazes' treatise became a medical landmark. It was translated into Latin and Greek, and influenced the treatment of European smallpox patients until the seventeenth century.

He distinguished the clinical symptoms of smallpox and measles for the first time in the "Western" world. The Chinese alchemist Ko Hung had distinguished smallpox clearly five centuries earlier, and it is intriguing to wonder whether Rhazes knew of the Chinese observations when he wrote his own treatise. According to Needham (1954), for a year (exactly when is not clear), Rhazes had as a houseguest a Chinese scholar who was interested enough in medicine to translate Galen's works from Arabic into Chinese.

According to Rhazes,

> The outbreak of small-pox is preceded by continuous fever, aching in the back, itching in the nose and shivering during sleep. The main symptoms of its presence are: backache with fever, stinging pain in the whole body, congestion of the face, sometimes shrinkage, violent redness of the cheeks and eyes, a sense of pressure in the body, creeping of the flesh, pain in the throat and breast accompanied by difficulties of respiration and coughing, dryness of the mouth, thick salivation, hoarseness of the voice, headache and pressure in the head, excitement, anxiety, nausea and unrest. Excitement, nausea and unrest are more pronounced in measles than in smallpox, whilst the aching in the back is more severe in smallpox than in measles. (Arnold 1931, 323–24)

Rhazes also recognized the seasonal variation of smallpox epidemics, although he misunderstood the cause of the disease, attributing it to the need of children's new blood to ferment. The fact that smallpox was mainly a disease of childhood in Rhazes' time, however, is further evidence that it had by then been endemic in West Asia for some time. He made many recommendations for the treatment of smallpox, including his "heat treatment," an admonition to wrap patients up in order to increase perspiration and facilitate the eruption.

Two generations after Rhazes' death, another great Moslem physician, Avicenna (980–1037), was born in Persia near Bukhara. Known among the Arabs as the "sheik and prince" of the learned, Avicenna wrote some ninety-nine works on philosophy, medicine, geometry, astronomy, theology, philology, and art, including the *Canon of Medicine*, which was translated into Latin in the twelfth century. In *Canon of Medicine*, which became pre-eminent among medical textbooks in European schools, Avicenna improved on Rhazes' treatment for smallpox by reducing the recommended amount of bleeding. In the same era, Haly Abbas (d. 994) noted that proximity to previous victims seemed to be one of the causes of the illness, thereby suggesting the idea of contagiousness, and Constantinus Africanus (1020–87), who translated some of the Arabic medical treatises into Latin, used the term "variola" for the first time to denote the disease described by Rhazes.

Two generations after Rhazes produced his masterpiece, smallpox blinded a four-year-old Syrian boy in the town of al-Ma'arratu, near

Aleppo. As if in compensation, the youth developed a "prodigious memory," committing to heart his favorite manuscripts from the local library. Abul-Ala al-Ma'arri (973–1057) eventually wrote nearly sixteen hundred poems, some of which reportedly influenced the Persian poet Umar al-Khayyam, who died sixty years after him, and Dante's *Divine Comedy*. Acclaimed as a "philosopher of poets and poet of philosophers," al Ma'arri "closed the period of great Arab poetry" (Hitti 1964, 459). The period of Arab-transmitted pox was just beginning.

Mamelukes are said to have introduced inoculation into Egypt "at the time of the Crusades," in the thirteenth century (*History of Inoculation*, 1913, 25). They could well have learned about it from Moslems in India or from Arabs previously resident in China, perhaps via western Asian intermediaries. From Egypt, Arabs reportedly carried knowledge of inoculation to African countries bordering the Red Sea. Whether they also carried that knowledge into Moorish Spain centuries before inoculation was introduced into Europe is an interesting question, though I know of no evidence that they did.

According to Johnston, smallpox "commenced its ravages on the East Coast of Africa" in the thirteenth or fourteenth century (1908, 553). He presumably meant the east coast lowlands south of the Horn of Africa. Coastal Arab merchant settlements at Mogadishu, Malindi, Mombasa, Zanzibar, Kilwa, Sofala, and elsewhere were frequently visited by trading vessels from India, China, Arabia, and the Red Sea coast of Northeast Africa, any one of which could have been the source of smallpox. The first specific mention of the disease along this more southerly coast of East Africa dates from a little later.

Portuguese traders had replaced Arab merchants in many of the East African coastal settlements by the last half of the sixteenth century, when warriors of the cannibalistic Wazimba tribe emerged from the Southeast African interior to terrorize Africans and Portuguese along the coast at Kilwa and Mombasa (fig. 11). The Wazimbas were followed by locusts, famine, and in 1589, by smallpox:

> The fourth affliction and trouble that overtook this Kaffraria was a severe outbreak of smallpox, of which a great number of people died. This disease along the whole of the coast is like a subtle pestilence, as it kills everyone in a house where it appears, men, women, and children alike, and very few escape who are attacked by it, as they do not know of a cure. Those who [are] bled freely die, and also those who will not be bled, but the most certain remedy is to be bled immediately the malady shows itself. This smallpox is not infectious to Portuguese, except to children of tender-age, even though they hold intercourse with Kaffirs suffering from it. (Theal 1903, 7: 319)

In addition to establishing the time and place of this early outbreak, the account also suggests that smallpox was more common in Portugal

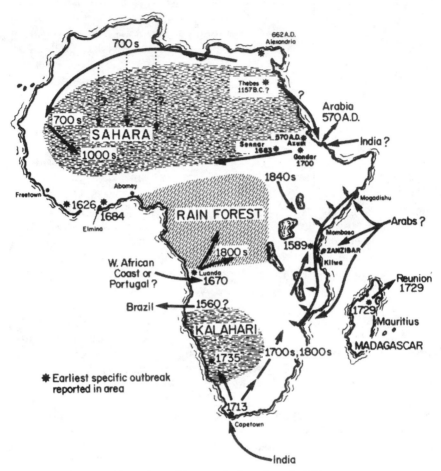

Fig. 11. Early outbreaks and possible spread of smallpox in Africa

than in that part of East Africa. The disease was clearly not yet endemic among the Africans, since it attacked natives of all ages. The report does not mean, however, that this was necessarily the virus's first appearance in the area. It almost certainly wasn't. There is also a strong suggestion that this generation of coastal Africans knew nothing about inoculation. Thus, the epidemic probably was imported from somewhere else along the coast or even farther afield, since if the Wazimba had brought it from the interior, they themselves probably would have been disrupted by it, rather than pillaging the coast for two decades, as they did.

We saw above that Arab armies carried smallpox across North Africa as far west as Mauritania in the eighth century. Long before the Arabs appeared, traders from North Africa were regularly exchanging salt for gold with black tribes south of the Sahara. These goods were transported across the Sahara in caravans, along well-established, north-south trade routes. Islam and black slaves were soon added to this older commerce. Thus, if smallpox was not already present in subsaharan West Africa by the eighth century, it very likely arrived there soon after, via one of the transsaharan caravans.

Smallpox might also have spread into West Africa along a popular east-west trade route, from East African kingdoms in Nubia or Ethiopia. Mansa Musa, the emperor of Mali, made a spectacular pilgrimage to and from Mecca along the latter route in 1324, and the emperor of Songhai made an equally famous pilgrimage from Timbuktu to Mecca in 1497 (Bovill 1968). It is not surprising therefore, that Johnston (1908, 553) says smallpox was known "in the valley of the Niger" river by the eleventh century, although he doesn't disclose the basis for his statement.

It is tantalizing that more is not known about smallpox's first appearance in relatively densely populated West Africa, which must have been catastrophic. Even such well-known Arab travelers as Ibn Batua and Leo Africanus, who described much of what they saw on visits to this region in the fourteenth and early sixteenth centuries, do not mention it. Another sixteenth-century Arab writer refers to an outbreak called *gafé* (? "dry season") which killed "many persons," including Sheik Mahmoud ben Omar, in ancient Mali in 1463–64, but it is not known what disease this was (Kati 1913, 175). Since West African slaves carried malaria, and probably yaws (another infectious tropical disease), to Portugal in the fifteenth century, a search of contemporary Portuguese records might yield further evidence of smallpox in medieval West Africa (Hudson 1964).

Distant proof of smallpox in this part of Africa derives from the New World, where the disease was introduced repeatedly by slaves from West Africa. Brau attributed the epidemic of smallpox that began among slaves in mines on Hispanola in 1518 to illegal slave traffic from West Africa. According to Wiedner (1962), virtually all such slaves at that time were taken from Senegambia. Penna (1885) records that in Brazil, slaves imported probably from Angola caused one of the earliest outbreaks on the South American mainland in 1560.

Whenever smallpox first appeared in West Africa, it probably became endemic there early. By the time direct accounts are available, from the seventeenth century, the disease was already very widespread, inoculation was well known and practiced widely, and Yoruba-speaking tribes of modern Nigeria and Dahomey (Republic of Benin) had incorporated a god of smallpox into their indigenous pantheon, as we shall see. That such a strong religious cult of smallpox did not develop, or spread, elsewhere in Africa as in India and China may have been due to stronger Christian and Islamic influences in other regions, or to lack of as old a tradition of endemic smallpox as that in West Africa.

SEVENTEENTH AND EIGHTEENTH CENTURIES

The transatlantic slave trade was a dominant feature of African history from the sixteenth century. It is important to our story for two reasons. First, the disruption that resulted from expeditions to capture and transport slaves was often associated with outbreaks of smallpox. Second, the arrival of infected slaves in the New World provides much of the early evidence of smallpox in West Africa.

Although the slave trade provided excellent conditions for spreading the disease in East and West Africa in virtually all its phases, the overland caravans were especially notorious for doing so. Accounts of these processions illustrate how other caravans must have helped spread smallpox in Africa much earlier. Slave caravans probably posed an even greater risk than did caravans transporting nonhuman cargo or those that accompanied European explorers in the nineteenth century, simply because of the larger numbers of potential victims. However, most accounts of smallpox in African caravans were written by European explorers, since slave caravans were less likely to include autobiographers or journalists.

One such witness was the American journalist Henry M. Stanley. In *How I Found Livingstone,* Stanley wrote:

> But the great and terrible scourge of East and Central Africa is the small-pox. The bleached skulls of the victims to this fell disease, which lie along every caravan road, indicate but too clearly the havoc it makes annually, not only among the ranks of the several trading expeditions, but also among the villages of the respective tribes. Some caravans are decimated by it, and villages have been more than half-depopulated. (1872, 533–34)

The British explorer Richard Burton had found smallpox on the same slave route nearly twenty years earlier:

> The most dangerous epidemic is . . . the small-pox, which, propagated without contact or fomites, sweeps at times like a storm of death over the land. . . . The ravages of this disease amongst the half-starved and over-worked gangs of caravan porters have already been described; as many as a score of these wretches have been seen at a time in a single caravan; men staggering along blinded and almost insensible, jostling and stumbling against every one in their way; and mothers carrying babes, both parent and progeny in the virulent stage of the fell disease. (1860, 2: 318)

The problem of disease-carrying caravans was not, however, peculiar to subsaharan Africa. In 1600–1790, "slave caravans sometimes carried contagious diseases: the Fezzan [southern Libya] suffered from smallpox brought in this way, but desert nomads, encountering such caravans less frequently, were better protected" (Fisher 1975, 102).

Plate 1. Smallpox patient at height of rash. Photo courtesy World Health Organization.

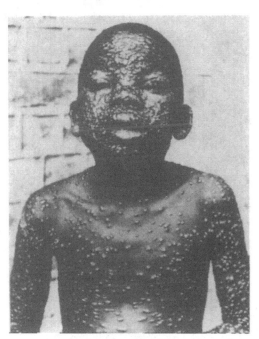

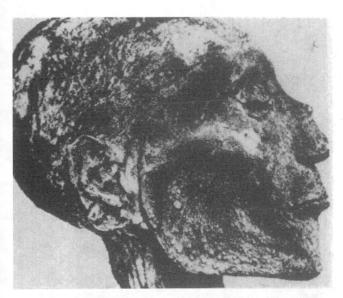

Plate 2. Mummy of Ramses V. Photo courtesy World Health Organization. The pharaoh died in 1157 B.C., apparently of smallpox.

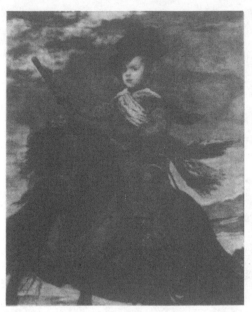

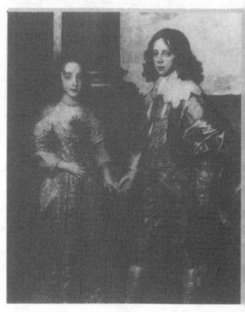

Plate 3. Portrait of Balthazar Carlos by Diego Ro-
dríguez de Silva y Velásquez. Copyright ©
Museo del Prado, Madrid. All rights reserved. The Spanish prince died of smallpox in 1646.

Plate 4. Portrait of William II of Orange and his
wife, Princess Mary Henrietta of England,
by Anthony Van Dyck. Courtesy Rijks-
museum-Stichting, Amsterdam. The
prince and princess both died of smallpox, as did their daughter-in-law Mary II
of England.

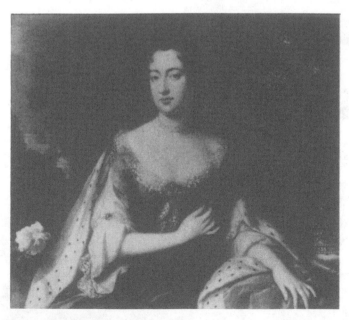

Plate 5. Portrait of Queen Mary II of England, after William Wissing.
Courtesy National Portrait Gallery, London. Mary died of
smallpox in 1694.

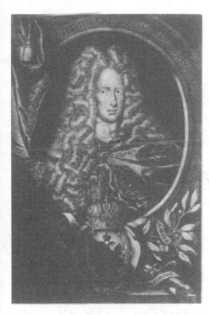

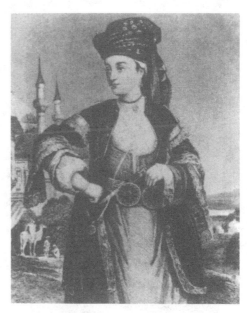

Plate 6. Portrait of Emperor Joseph I of Austria. Courtesy Bild-Archiv der Österreichischen National-bibliotek, Vienna. Joseph and three other European monarchs (plates 8–10) died of smallpox within a span of thirty years (1711–41).

Plate 7. Portrait of Lady Mary Wortley Montague by J. B. Wanderforde. Courtesy The Boston Anthenaeum. Lady Montague learned of inoculation when her husband was ambassador to Turkey. She helped introduce the technique into England in 1721.

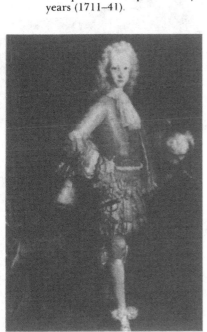

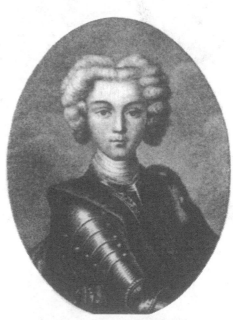

Plate 8. Portrait of Luis I of Spain by Houasse. Copyright © Museo del Prado, Madrid. All rights reserved.

Plate 9. Portrait of Peter II of Russia. Courtesy The Illustrated London News and Sketch, Ltd.

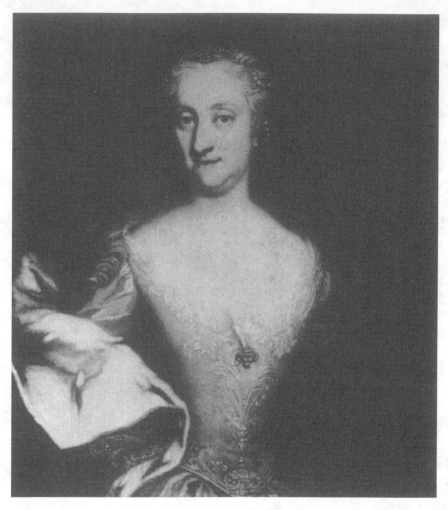

Plate 10. Portrait of Ulrika Eleonora d.y. (1688–1741), queen of Sweden, Grips-
holm Castle. Photo: Swedish Portrait Archive, Stockholm.

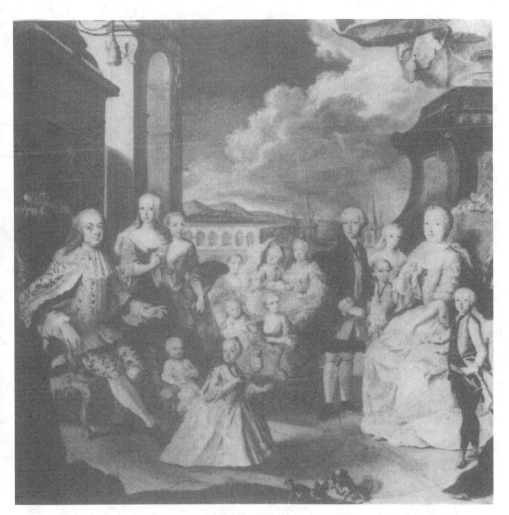

Plate 11. Portrait of Emperor Francis I and Empress Maria Theresa with thirteen of their children by Martin van Meytens d.y. Courtesy Bild-Archiv der Österreichischen Nationalbibliotek, Vienna. *Middle foreground*: Maximillian, Marie Antoinette; *left side group*: Francis Stephen, Marianna, Maria Christina; *right side group*: Joseph (II), Charles Joseph, Elizabeth, Maria Theresa, Leopold (II); *Background, first row, left to right*: Maria Carolina, Maria Josepha; *background, second row, left to right*, Joanna, Ferdinand, Amalia.

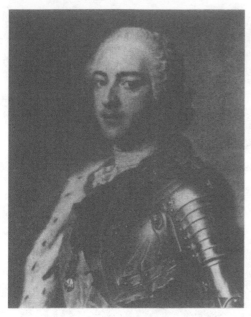

Plate 12. Portrait of Louis XV of France by Maurice Quentin de La Tour. Courtesy Musée du Louvre, Paris. The king died of smallpox in 1774.

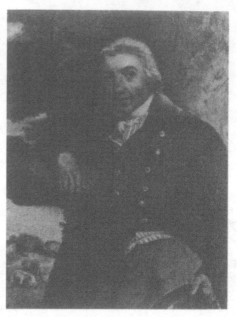

Plate 13. Portrait of Edward Jenner in the Jenner Museum. Courtesy The Jenner Trust. Jenner discovered vaccination in 1796.

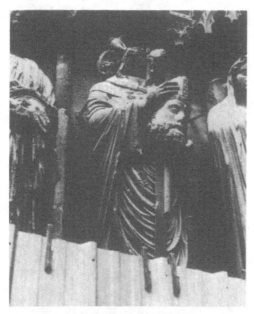

Plate 14. St. Nicaise. North portico, Rheims Cathedral. Photo by author. Nicaise died in 451 and subsequently became the Catholic saint of smallpox.

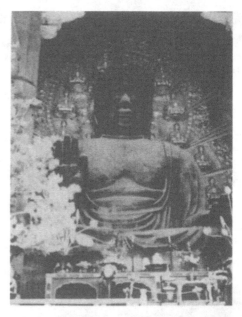

Plate 15. *Nara Daibutsu*. Photo courtesy Japan Air Lines. Fifty-three-foot statue of Buddha erected at Nara, Japan, in 748 in an effort to halt a smallpox epidemic.

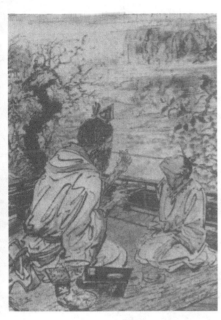

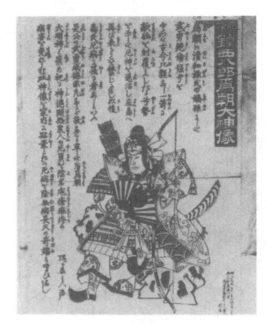

Plate 16. Chinese inoculator and patient. Courtesy National Library of Medicine. Immunity to smallpox was induced by blowing powdered smallpox scabs up the patient's nose.

Plate 17. Nineteenth-century print of Chinzei Hachiro Tametomo, legendary Japanese archer. Courtesy of Professor Teizo Ogawa, Jutendo University, Tokyo. Red images like this one were often hung in Japanese homes in the belief that they could prevent or cure smallpox.

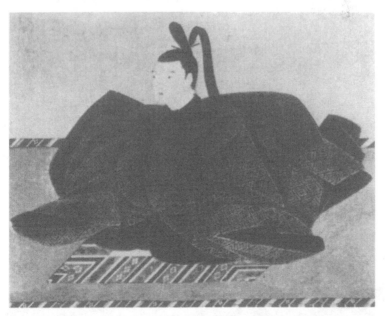

Plate 18. Portrait of Emperor Gokwomyo of Japan. Courtesy Senyū-ji Temple, Kyoto. The emperor died of smallpox in 1654.

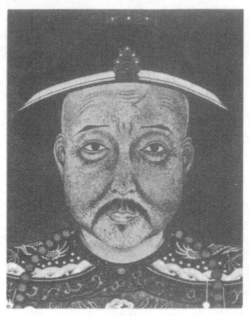

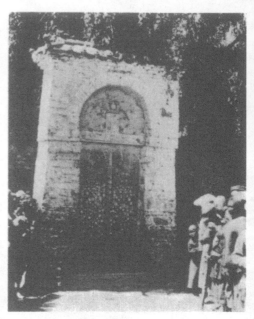

Plate 19. K'ang Hsi, emperor of China. Detail from nineteenth-century portrait. Courtesy Metropolitan Museum of Art, New York. All rights reserved. K'ang Hsi became emperor in 1661 after his father died of smallpox, because he had already had the disease and his older brother had not.

Plate 20. Tablet erected in eighteenth century on road outside Lhasa, Tibet, instructing travelers what to do when smallpox broke out in the city. From Waddell (1906).

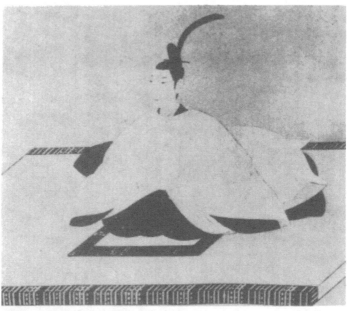

Plate 21. Portrait of Emperor Komei of Japan. Courtesy Senyū-ji Temple, Kyoto. Komei died of smallpox in 1867.

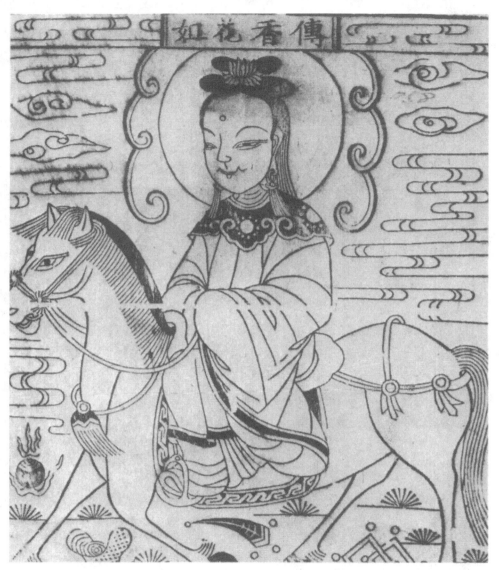

Plate 22. Ch'uan Hsing Hua Chieh, Chinese goddess of smallpox. Courtesy National Museum of History, Taipei, Taiwan.

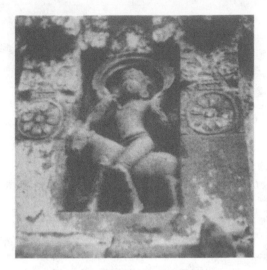

Plate 23. Shitala mata, Hindu goddess of smallpox, from a ninth-century temple in Rajasthan, India. From Majumdar (1965).

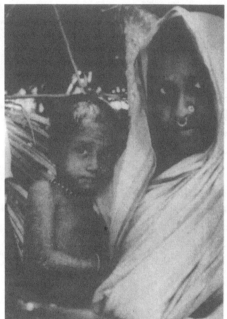

Plate 25. Rahima Banu of Bangladesh, the
world's last case of naturally occurring *Variola major*. Photo courtesy
World Health Organization. Rahima's rash began 16 October 1975.

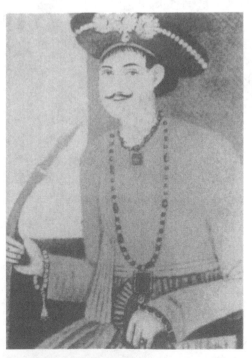

Plate 24. Syefuddowla, nawab of Bengal. From
Majumdar (1905).

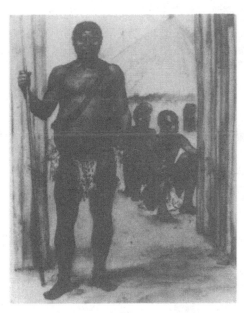

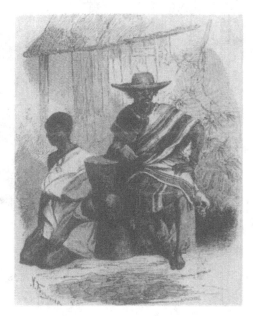

Plate 26. Chief Lobengula of the Matabele. Portrait by Ralph Peacock adapted from a sketch by E. A. Maund (1889). Courtesy National Archives of Zimbabwe and Dr. E. Burnett Smith.

Plate 27. Prince Badahun (King Glele) and King Guezo of Dahomey, 1856. From Burton (1966). Photo courtesy Library of Congress.

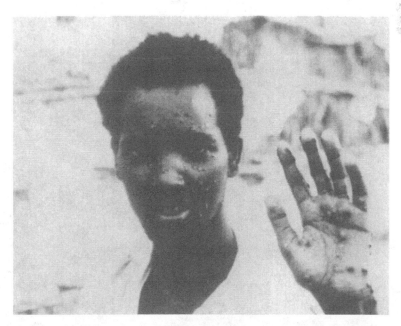

Plate 28. Ali Maow Maalin, the world's last case of naturally occurring smallpox. Photo courtesy Dr. Jason Weisfeld. Maalin's rash began on 26 October 1977 in Merka Town, Somalia.

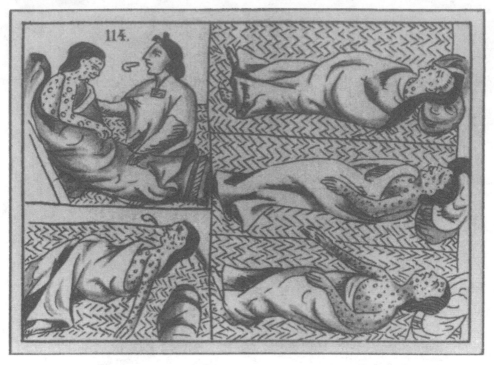

Plate 29. Sixteenth-century Aztec drawing of smallpox victim in the Códice Florentino. Courtesy Peabody Museum, Harvard University.

Plate 30. Portrait of the Reverend Cotton Mather by Peter Pelham. Courtesy National Library of Medicine. Mather helped to introduce inoculation into North America, having learned of it from his African slave.

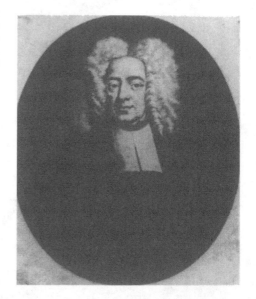

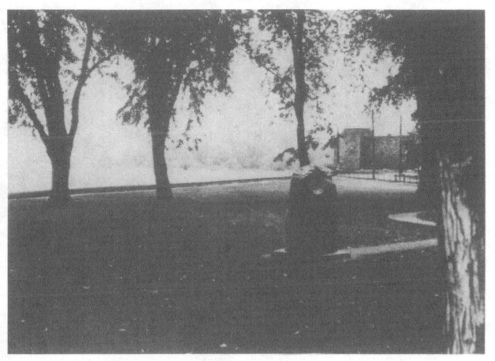

Plate 31. Mass grave near Montreal of Continental army soldiers who died of smallpox during 1776 Canadian campaign in Revolutionary War. Photo by author. But for the epidemic, the Continental troops would have captured the city, and hence, control of Canada. A solitary headstone at Fort Chambly marks the grave of their commander, General John Thomas, who died in the same epidemic.

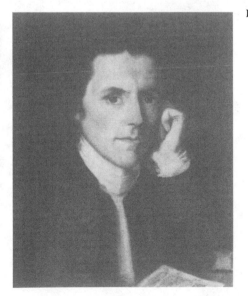

Plate 32. Portrait of Benjamin Waterhouse by Gilbert Stuart. Courtesy of Boston Medical Library in Francis A. Countway Library of Medicine. Stuart painted this portrait of his friend when they were students in London.

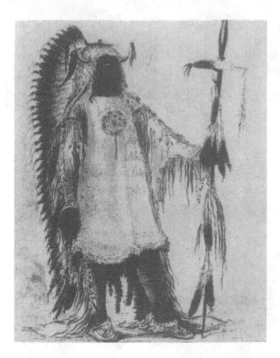

Plate 33. *Four Bears, Second Chief, in Full Dress* by George Catlin (1832). Oil on canvas, 29 × 24 inches (73.7 × 60.9 cm.). National Museum of American Art (formerly National Collection of Fine Arts), Smithsonian Institution. Gift of Mrs. Joseph Harrison, Jr. After he finished this portrait of Ma-to-toh-pah, Catlin described the chief's death in a smallpox epidemic in 1837.

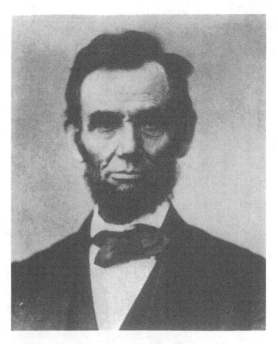

Plate 34. Alexander Gardner's well-known photograph of Abraham Lincoln. Courtesy Library of Congress. The president may have caught his smallpox infection the same day he sat for Gardner. He became ill a few hours after delivering his Gettysburg Address eleven days later.

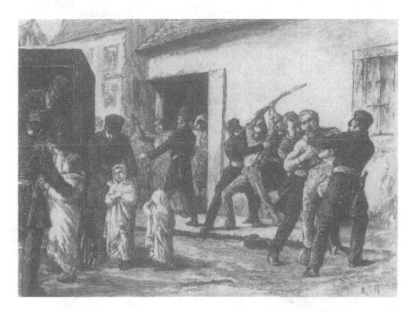

Plate 35. "An Indident of the Smallpox Epidemic in Montreal." From *Harper's Weekly*, 28 November 1885. Many families in Montreal violently resisted control measures during the deadly 1885 epidemic. Similar riots erupted in Norfolk, Virginia, in 1768–69 and in Milwaukee, Wisconsin, in 1894–95.

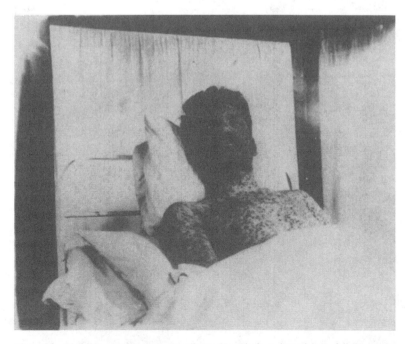

Plate 36. Physician at Boston's Smallpox Hospital undergoing red-light treatment for smallpox in the hospital's "Red Room." Photo courtesy Boston Medical Library in the Francis A. Countway Library of Medicine. The doctor became infected while treating others during the 1902 epidemic.

Because of their repeated long journeys, the porters in caravans were at particularly high risk of getting smallpox and of spreading the disease further when they did. On one expedition, of Stanley's ten porters who were susceptible, "five had died at the time of his writing, and five more were seriously ill" (Hartwig 1979, 668). Those who came down with the virus were no longer welcome in the caravan, no matter where they happened to be. A German explorer described the pathetic attempts of one of his guides to conceal his smallpox infection, since he knew he would be driven off when it was discovered (von Höhnel 1894, 2: 214). Stanley summarized this aspect of the problem:

> Members of a caravan attacked by the small-pox are excluded from the society of the healthy, and have special sheds set apart for them outside of the camp. But the succeeding caravans contain several reckless young fellows, who thoughtlessly enter within, and in a few days afterwards begin to feel ill . . . and before long we know they have become victims, and are in their turn ostracized, and if unable to walk are left to die, for no settlement will permit them to approach their gates, and a caravan cannot halt in the wilderness. (Hartwig 1979, 663)

Slaves who survived the trek to the coast were still subject to outbreaks. Lawrence (1963) records that in 1789 an epidemic was reported among slaves awaiting shipment at Cape Coast Castle, near El Mina on the coast of modern Ghana. Others who developed smallpox aboard ship were sometimes thrown overboard while still alive by captors vainly attempting to prevent the disease from spreading. In 1769 the *Cato* carried 210 slaves, "all of whom have had the smallpox" from Benin to South Carolina. Fourteen years later, another ship sailing from Benin to Santo Domingo lost more than a fourth of its 390 slaves to the disease during the voyage. As early as 1695, more than a hundred of the 700 captives on the slave ship *Hannibal* contracted smallpox before they arrived in Barbados from the "Guinea coast." So severe was the threat to Bahia (and to valuable human cargo) by infected slaves from Angola during severe epidemics in that part of Africa in 1687, that shippers in the Brazilian city almost suspended the slave traffic (Ryder 1969; Creighton 1965; Verger 1964).

Accounts from eighteenth-century America provide what was perhaps most unexpected evidence of smallpox in early West African history. In 1706, Reverend Cotton Mather of Boston, while routinely interrogating his new slave, Onesimus, asked whether he had had the disease. Onesimus described how he had been inoculated against smallpox in Africa, and therefore was immune, though he had not really had the disease. When Mather questioned Onesimus further, and made similar inquiries of several other slaves in Boston, he discovered that "they, too, had had the operation in Africa," and "had the marks to prove it"

(Herbert 1975, 539–40). Onesimus, whom Mather described as a "Guru-mantese," probably belonged to the Gurumanche tribe of eastern Upper Volta rather than to the Garamantes of Fezzan, in southern Libya, as is often stated. More important, the other slaves whom Mather surveyed in Boston and found to have also been inoculated were from many different parts of West Africa. Asked how long inoculation had been practiced in their homelands, Mather's informants stated "only that it had been done since long before they were born." (ibid., 541).

Lawrence (1963) and Schram (1971) tell us that inoculation was also employed in an unsuccessful attempt to stop the epidemic among slaves waiting to be shipped from Cape Coast in 1789, about the same time that Mongo Park heard of inoculation being used near the Gambia River. By then, however, inoculation had become widely known and used in Europe and North America. (Mather and Zabdiel Boylston introduced the practice in Boston during an outbreak there in 1721, the same year Sir Hans Sloane and Lady Montague introduced it in London.)

Smallpox is said by Johnston (1906) to have been already established in that part of West Africa later known as Liberia by 1626, though as we have seen, there is good reason to believe it was widely endemic long before that date. The first specific reference to the impact of smallpox in West Africa I have found is by a Dutchman, who described the inhabitants at Elmina a century before the outbreak among slaves at nearby Cape Coast:

> 15 to 16 years ago [1684–85] Elmina was very populous, eight times as strong as present . . . and could under a good general succeed in great undertakings . . . tis hardly to be believed how weak it is at present. When I first came, I frequently saw 500–600 canoes fishing each morning, now scarce 100 appear, and all people are so poor that their miserable case is very deplorable. (Bosman 1958, 84)

He attributed the dramatic change to an epidemic of smallpox, which had "swept so many away" around 1685, to wars, and to a "tyrannical government." By the end of the eighteenth century, British officers living at Cape Coast felt obliged to found a smallpox hospital, apparently West Africa's first.

Not much is known about the kingdom of Dahomey, located between Lagos and Cape Coast, before its fourth king, Agadja, whose face was pitted from smallpox, extended his kingdom to the sea in 1727. He took over the already-flourishing slave trade there, and established contact with European traders. It is known that Dahomeyans who died of small-pox were buried without ceremony the same day, since an attack of the disease was interpreted as signifying the displeasure of the gods. During what was probably a slave raid in 1786, Dahomeyan warriors captured over eighty canoemen on the coast near Porto Novo, more than thirty of whom soon died of smallpox (Herskovits 1938; Ronen 1975; Dalzel 1793).

Three years later, a large force of Dahomeyans attacked the nearby kingdom of Ketu, but was repulsed. Soon after Adahoonzou II, Dahomey's sixth king (also known as Kpengla), returned from this unsuccessful expedition, his entourage became unusually agitated. Dahomeyan authorities claimed that "their oracle had forbidden them to attack Ketu and that it had warned them that whenever they did so, their King would die of smallpox" (Akinjogbin 1965, 324). This may have been only retrospective rationalizing. Dalzel describes the scene in his *History of Dahomey*, published in 1793:

> The conquest of Ketoo was the last remarkable transaction that happened during the reign of Adahoonzou. The time drew nigh that was to rid the earth of this scourge of the human race. Messages had been frequently brought from the King to the European governors, for some time after the Ketoo victory; but now it was a month since any messenger had arrived at Grigwhee, either from the King or his Caboceers. A certain gloom was apparent over the whole Dahoman empire. A mysterious silence prevailed. Every countenance betrayed a secret which the tongue durst not reveal. The truth at last came out—Adahoonzou *was dead of the small-pox!*
>
> This disorder had not been attended with any unfavourable symptoms; but the King, impatient under confinement, was desirous to convince his people that all was well with him. The *Gong-gong-beater* [public herald or crier] had been commanded to summon all his subjects to the King's door, in order to see him; and he was actually on his way, from an inner apartment to the gate, accompanied by some of his women, when he was seized with a giddiness, fell down, and expired. This happened on the 17th of April, 1789.
>
> The women retired; the Tamegan made a speech to those who were assembled at the gate, informing them, "That the King had intended to play a little in public, but was prevented by some particular business; that he designed, however, very shortly to see his people, when he would put in execution his purpose of diverting them."
>
> The minister had scarcely concluded this short address, when a loud shriek was heard from within the palace. This was quickly communicated from Agoonah, where the King then lay, to Calmina and Pahou. The whole kingdom was immediately in an uproar, the people beating their breast, tumbling down, and exhibiting such marks of frenzy, that one would have thought the whole country had been seized with the same disorder. Confusion and anarchy, as usual on such occasions, universally prevailed; every body was armed, and frequently robberies were committed.
>
> The Caboceers, nevertheless, attended to the main business, which was the conveyance of the corpse to Abomey. They had it on the way three hours after the breath departed. The man called the *King's Devil*, was killed on the path, between Agoonah Dawee; and on the arrival of

the corpse at the gate of Dahomey-house, at Abomey, sixty-eight men (all Ketoos) were massacred, before it was carried into the house.

The butchery now began among the women, who immediately proceeded to destroy one another; and this scene continued for two days and a half. Human nature shrinks at the recital of such horrible facts. The simple narration is sufficiently shocking, without the detail of the particular circumstances that marked this bloody scene. Suffice it to observe, that *five hundred and ninety-five* women were murdered by their companions on this occasion, and sent, according to the notion that prevails in this unhappy country, to attend Adahoonzou in the other world. (203–5)

The king and people of Adra-Allada, which the Dahomeyans had over-run in 1724, celebrated Adahoonzou's demise for a week.

Adahoonzou was succeeded by his son, Agonglo. Gourg, the commander of the French fort at Porto Novo, reported:

His son, a young man of twenty-two or twenty-three years, has succeeded him; we are going to be forced to go and offer him the usual presents which are the same as for the customs . . . I am quite fearful that this change will be harmful for our projects, and as this young man is surrounded by people who are looking to harm trade, it can be feared that our position will not improve. (Verger 1976, 189)

One of the new king's first acts was to expel Gourg.

Dahomey's continuing political subjugation to the Yoruba kingdom of Oyo and an economic depression resulting from local slackening of the slave trade on which Dahomey depended heavily caused "a widespread dissatisfaction among the Dahomeans against their rulers" (Akinjogbin 1965, 315). Against this unhappy background, Agonglo alarmed some of his relatives and subjects by receiving, on 23 April 1797, two Roman Catholic priests "sent by the queen of Portugal, Dona Maria, to try to convert the King of Dahomey to Catholicism" (Verger 1976, 199). Thus, when the king unluckily fell ill with smallpox later that same week, plotters at court seized the opportunity provided by his illness and poisoned him. "Since then," observed a Nigerian historian, "all the kings of Dahomey had been wary about which European ideas to accept" (Akinjogbin 1965, 320).[3]

Across the continent, in Northeast Africa, other kings and their subjects had to contend with smallpox imported by pilgrims traveling to and from Mecca, as well as that stirred up by wars or brought by trading caravans. Even in the early twentieth century, the location of the Anglo-Egyptian Sudan's westernmost province of Darfur "on the major east-west route for pilgrims and labor migrants" was noted to expose the province to "smallpox and other epidemics" (Hartwig 1981, 18). Toward the end of the nineteenth century, Egyptian authorities began requiring pilgrims to present proof of vaccination before entering the Sudan and established a quarantine station at the Red Sea port of Suakin soon after, to check on the health of pilgrims traveling to and from Mecca. Poncet, a French adventurer who visited Gerri, the political center and crossroads of northern Sennar (Funj) on the Nile about forty miles (66 km) north of present-day Khartoum, confirms that infected travelers had long been regarded as a menace in this part of Africa. At the time of Poncet's visit in January 1699, Gerri was the residence of "a governor, whose principal employ is to examine whether in the caravans which come from Egypt any one has the smallpox" (Crawford 1951, 65).

Sennar's attempts to protect itself derived from first-hand knowledge of what an epidemic of smallpox could do. According to Budgeii (1907) and Bayoumi (1976), the disease swept the Moslem kingdom in 1683, and returned in 1687–88, when Sennar was "devastated by a serious combination of famine and smallpox." In 1719, smallpox killed several local notables in Sennar, including former king Ounsa III, who had recently been deposed, but who was "the last of the line of Funj kings who belonged to the royal family." That year is known as *Sannat el Gidri*, "the smallpox year," in the historical tradition of Sennar (Crawford 1951, 328, 237).

Moslem Sennar and the Sudan formed a continuous epidemiologic region with adjacent Christian Ethiopia. This relationship was repeatedly manifest in the nineteenth and twentieth centuries, and was periodically enhanced by wars between the two states. Ethiopia imported an unspecified "epidemic" from Sennar during their first war in 1618–19. The year before Sennar's "smallpox year," many Ethiopian nobles perished during an epidemic of smallpox in their country (ibid.; Pankhurst 1965).

In 1700, King Nagassi of Shoa, the founder of the modern ruling family of that Ethiopian kingdom, died of smallpox soon after his investiture by the "King of Kings," Emperor Iyasu I. Nagassi's illness may have been part of a severe epidemic that affected the Moslem Galla tribe in Ethiopia for the first time during the reign of Iyasu I (1682–1707)(Levine 1965; Pankhurst 1965). Nagassi's successors in the kingship of Shoa eventually won leadership of the empire for themselves.

As in ancient times, Arabia may have been the source of an outbreak that struck the port city of Massawa, on Ethiopia's Red Sea coast, in 1768. The effects of this epidemic were witnessed by the Scottish physician-explorer, James Bruce: "It was feared the living would not be sufficient to bury the dead. The whole island was filled with shrieks and lamentations both night and day" (1812, 136). The epidemic spread inland to Adowa, and later reached the Ethiopian capital, Gondar, where Bruce was again a witness to its destructiveness a year later. In Gondar, the Queen Mother ordered Bruce to care for several royal children and grandchildren who were suffering from smallpox. Two of them, the son (Welled Hawaryat) and granddaughter of the most powerful man in the empire, Ras Michael, died. Another granddaughter, Ayabdar, was "very much marked."

Bruce blamed Arabia for periodic epidemics that occurred every twelve or fifteen years in Sennar, where he says the disease was "not endemial." He attributed that route of infection to "the constant intercourse they have with, and merchandizes they bring from Arabia" (Bayoumi 1976, 1). He also described a common "pseudo-inoculation," called "the buying of the smallpox," at Sennar.

> The women [of Sennar] from time immemorial, have known a species of inoculation which they call Tishteree el Jidderee or, the buying of the smallpox. . . . Upon the first hearing of the smallpox anywhere, these people go to the infected place, and wrapping a fillet of cotton cloth about the arm of the person infected, they let it remain there till they bargain with the mother how she is to sell them. . . . One piece of silver or more be paid for the mother. . . . This being concluded, they go home and tie the fillet about their own child's arm; certain, as they say, from long experience, that the child infected is to do well, and not to have one more than the number of pustules that were agreed and paid for. (Ibid., 8)

By Bruce's time, African tribes further south along the eastern coast had apparently learned, or relearned, inoculation in the two hundred years since the Wazimba invasion, perhaps from the Arabs or the Portuguese. In a letter dated 3 March 1776, a Frenchman on a slave ship wrote to the French minister of the Navy, describing how he had bought seven hundred slaves at Zanzibar the previous year, but arrived at Mauritius with only about five hundred, having lost the others en route because of smallpox. The writer said he would have lost even more had he not inoculated 430 of them. "Even in the interior of the country," he wrote, "they know of inoculation" (Freeman-Grenville 1965, 120). Another slave ship carried smallpox from Madagascar to Réunion in 1729 (Hirsch 1883, 1: 129).

The southern third of Africa was apparently free of smallpox until relatively late—perhaps because of its scattered population and relative isolation. Potential sources of infection were the southward-migration of Bantu tribes starting before 1000; the Arab settlement established on the east coast at Sofala, terminus of the gold trade from Zimbabwe in the interior, in the thirteenth century; and the Portuguese settlement established at Luanda, on the west coast, in 1484.

It may well have been the Portuguese who introduced smallpox into Angola and the lower Congo basin for the first time, perhaps from further up the West African coast, or from Portugal. As we have seen, in 1560 an outbreak among freshly arrived slaves in Brazil had probably originated from this part of Africa. The earliest direct report of smallpox in Angola dates from 1620, when according to Curtin's 1978 history, "the Tio country and all Portuguese Angola" were affected by it. In 1670, a Jesuit priest remarked on the virus's decimation of the native population around Luanda (Wheeler 1969, 353). By the 1680s, wars and devastating epidemics in Angola were blamed for that area's depopulation. Slavery was another probable cause of the depopulation. As we saw above, authorities in Bahia, Brazil, threatened to suspend the slave trade because of an epidemic of smallpox in Angola in 1687. The patent of a slave ship from Bahia stated that "because of the news received from the Kingdom of Angola, that small pox disease is so rampant there, it could be feared that the country may not be able to recover from the loss of so many Negroes who are dying there" (Verger 1976, 577). A century later, a Brazilian described conditions in Luanda during the period 1782–99 and noted that the Africans there were attacked by the "horrible epidemic of smallpox, which freely spreads and kills a majority" (Wheeler 1964, 353).

According to Johnston (1908), smallpox didn't penetrate the interior Congo basin until around 1808. When it did appear, its impact among a family or small cluster of families struggling to feed and shelter themselves in an isolated, precarious clearing in the bush, must have been a calamity. The death of even one or two adults could make survival for the others nearly impossible, even if they remained healthy. The inhabitants of the Congo basin, scattered deep in the forest, were much more isolated from Europeans and Arabs, as well as from other native Africans, than were the tribes nearer the coast. They could very conceivably have existed in blissful ignorance of smallpox for centuries, like the Hottentots.

Bantu migrants pushing southward from eastern Africa began to arrive at the southern tip of the continent around the same time the first Dutch settlers arrived at Capetown in 1652. Both groups displaced sparsely settled Hottentots and Bushmen. The southward-migrating Bantus and northward-migrating Dutch first collided at the Fish River in 1775. By that time, the Portuguese had had settlements along the southeast coast (Mozambique) and the southwest coast (Angola) for more than two hundred and fifty years.

Smallpox made its first appearance in South Africa in March 1713, when a ship returning from India docked at Capetown. The sailors who had been ill during the voyage had already recovered, but their laundry was put ashore and infected several African washerwomen. Nearly every white family on the Cape was affected by the epidemic before the end of July. Capetown was paralyzed. After July, there were no more coffins in which to bury the dead. Census figures revealed a fourteen percent reduction of the white population two years after this outbreak (Burrows 1958).

Although the whites at Capetown suffered severely, the Hottentots, who were meeting smallpox for the first time, suffered more. Gie (1963) says that entire clans of Hottentots were wiped out in this initial epidemic. Hottentots fleeing the epidemic were killed by other hostile tribes, perhaps in futile attempts to prevent their own contamination: "With the

Hottentots, to be ill and to die were synonymous" (Theal 1969, 1: 428). How far this epidemic spread and whether it persisted among the tribes in the interior are not known.

An even worse outbreak followed the second introduction of smallpox at Capetown by ships from Ceylon in 1755. Between May and October that year, Theal (1969) estimates that nearly a thousand European settlers and over eleven hundred blacks died. Although farmers in rural areas were relatively spared, "Capetown suffered heavily, the property market crashed, even plate and jewels became unsalable, and for months the frightened farmers refused to bring their produce into the stricken capitol" (Walker 1928, 92). When the epidemic subsided nearly a year later, residents of Capetown held a day of thanksgiving, fasting, and prayer on 7 April.

The epidemic of 1755–56 also spread inland among the Hottentots, this time as far as South-West Africa. According to Burrows (1958, 64), this second epidemic "wiped out the identity of the individual Hottentot tribes, and remnants of these people were henceforth always referred to merely as 'Hottentots.' "

A third importation occurred in 1767, brought by a Danish ship returning from Europe. This outbreak lasted until April 1769 and infected nearly two thousand European settlers, of whom 179 died. Four hundred and forty slaves also died (ibid.). At Capetown,

> a placart was issued which ordered . . . the bodies of those who died from the disease were not to be undressed but to be coffined immediately and buried within forty-eight hours, meals were not to be provided at the deceased's house for those attending the funeral. (Laidler & Gelfand 1971, 57)

The whites in South Africa began using arm-to-arm inoculation of smallpox virus for the first time during this outbreak, which may account for their lower mortality rate. Bantu tribesmen reportedly also learned how to inoculate from the Dutch during this epidemic and so suffered less than the Hottentots (Roberts 1967). Most of the Bantu were also farther away from Capetown than the Hottentots had been during the earlier epidemics. The Bantu may conceivably have brought knowledge of inoculation, and some immunity from smallpox, with them from eastern Africa.

For the Hottentots, who had no knowledge of inoculation and no prior immunity, the three eighteenth-century epidemics were an unmitigated disaster. While they were probably never strong enough to stop the white settlers' expansion from the Cape, they did go to war intermittently, until smallpox greatly reduced their numbers and demoralized them.

NINETEENTH CENTURY

Only in the nineteenth century did smallpox complete its invasion of interior tribes in eastern and southern Africa, bringing death, dislocation, and depopulation to areas of the continent that heretofore had apparently remained untouched. During the early part of the century, the disease continued to be associated with the slave trade at sea and on land. But the increasing communication and wars that accompanied European establishment of colonial states in Africa, succeeded the slave trade in stimulating destructive epidemics. Caravans, however, continued to be a dangerous source of smallpox into the twentieth century. Although Jennerian vaccination came to be used in Egypt and South Africa by the second decade of the nineteenth century, its use elsewhere in Africa appears to have been very limited before 1900.

The Atlantic slave trade was sharply curtailed in the early nineteenth century and was later halted altogether, but it and the more persistent Arab-dominated trade in East African slaves continued to be important factors in the spread of smallpox.[4] Slave ships from Madagascar introduced the virus to the island of Réunion three times during the nineteenth century. During an epidemic in Mozambique early in 1812 in which great numbers of people were reported to have perished, a Portuguese slave ship from East Africa brought the infection to Capetown again, triggering an outbreak that lasted from mid-March until May.

Slave ships intercepted by the British navy also sometimes brought smallpox into "safe" African ports. Fifty-seven of 424 captives on board the *Perpetuo Defensor* died of dysentery and smallpox before they could be landed at Freetown, Sierra Leone, in 1826. Following the capture of an East African slave ship, the *Escorpao*, in 1840, infected slaves brought the disease into Simon's Bay, South Africa, starting another outbreak that killed over 2,500 inhabitants of the Cape Colony. The same year, another slave ship captured off the East African coast caused Mauritius to suffer its first epidemic in over thirty years. At first, wary authorities at Mauritius wouldn't even let the ship come into the harbor. They eventually relented, but instituted strict quarantine measures, permitting no one to come ashore. A man on a barge that carried water to the vessel became ill about two weeks later. By January the next year, a hospital set up especially for smallpox victims on the island had already received 702 victims, of whom 150 died.

Ordinarily infected former slaves were merely a local hazard to port cities where they were liberated. After the British government contracted with a private company to transport volunteer captives from Sierra Leone and St. Helena for work as free men in the West Indies, however, their health ceased to be only a local concern. Asiegbu (1969) describes one particularly embarrassing incident in 1850–51, which caused a barrage of international criticism. In December 1850 the Hodge Company demanded reimbursement from the British government for over eighteen hundred pounds expenses incurred while the *Atlantic* was detained in quarantine at Trinidad. The ship had embarked over 560 emigrants at St. Helena and Sierra Leone that summer and hastily departed for the West Indies, even though it was known that the passengers from both ports had recently been exposed to smallpox. Over seventy of the liberated slaves died of smallpox after the ship left Africa. Her Majesty's Government was held liable for the company's loss, and the subsequent contract was modified to remove the financial incentive to immediate embarkation.

According to Peterson (1969), in the cosmopolitan Crown Colony of Sierra Leone itself, indigenous Mende and Sherbro tribeswomen took advantage of the local outbreaks of the disease in the 1850s to mount a successful drive for new members of their Bundu Society among the gullible freed African women of the colony. Fourah Bay, then the site of the only institution of higher learning in West Africa, suffered one such epidemic in 1859, two years after a similar outbreak in nearby Aberdeen. Some of the new recruits were persuaded that membership in the secret society would protect them from smallpox.

Caravans were as dangerous as captured slave ships. While searching for Livingstone in 1871, Stanley found the corpse of a smallpox victim beside a caravan trail. Later in the century, smallpox-infected porters or principals turned up in Stanley's sensational "relief expedition" that rescued Emin Pasha in the Sudan in 1887, in the first European mission to climb Mount Kilimanjaro, and in a British military caravan during the last Ashanti war (Shorter 1972; Harke 1891; Meyer 1891; Willcocks 1904).

At least once, in 1892, porters of an East African caravan were infected deliberately. Hinde (1897) describes how during the struggle for control of Nyangwe, terminus of one of the slave routes from the East African coast, Arab slavers gathered up smallpox victims from surrounding districts and sent them into the town, creating an epidemic among the townspeople that soon spread to porters for the Congo Free State, as intended. About two-thirds of the two hundred porters from the lower Congo were infected, of whom sixty-five died.

The Arab slave trade in East Africa was transformed in 1840, when the sultan of Oman moved his capital to Zanzibar, introducing clove trees to the island and expanding the slave trade on the mainland. Of the three main caravan routes used by Arab traders, one led from Pangoni to Mwanza on Lake Victoria, another from Kilwa to Lake Nyasa, and a third from Bagamoyo to Ujiji, later extending on to Nyangwe in eastern Congo. With the expansion of the slave trade, these and other such routes were heavily traveled trajectories, through which smallpox apparently reached some tribes in the East African interior for the first time, even as it returned to affect other populations who already knew it well.

According to a Ugandan oral tradition, smallpox and syphilis arrived in Uganda in the 1840s from Unyoro, where smallpox had been brought by Nubian slave and ivory caravans (Roberts 1967). Apparently reflecting this belief about the disease's origin, some Ugandan Bantus worshipped a smallpox spirit, Ndaula. The practice derived from worship of the founder of the Unyoro-Chwezi dynasty, whose army was believed to have been decimated by the virus (Johnston 1902; Curtin et al. 1978). Roberts notes that smallpox and syphilis were soon reportedly brought to Uganda again by "Zanzibar trading caravans from Unyamwezi." Gerald Hartwig (1979), a historian with a special interest in African medical history, cites oral evidence from the Kerebe tribe that led him to believe that smallpox reached the area around Lake Victoria from the East African coast even before 1800, probably brought by ivory hunters.

If not established already among the scattered interior tribes of Southeast Africa, smallpox was becoming a familiar epidemic pestilence by early in the nineteenth century. Most of these populations may not have been large enough for the disease to remain among them endemically, however. Some tribes may have been infected by epidemic waves moving northeastward after one of the introductions at Capetown in the eighteenth century. As we have seen epidemics could spread at least as far away as South-West Africa. In addition to panic-stricken Hottentots trying to escape infection, nineteenth-century migrants and war expeditions also spread smallpox northward from the southern tip of Africa. However, Theal (1892) states that an outbreak among the Griques and Koranas north of the Orange River in 1831 was thought to have been caused by persons who traveled overland from Delgoa Bay in Mozambique.

Smallpox was allegedly present among the Mashona people of present-day Zimbabwe by 1822. Around 1832, smallpox broke out at the court of the Lunda king, Kazembe, in the northern part of present-day Zambia, and according to Livingstone, it reached the Makolo tribe at Linyanti on the Chobe River, about the same time (Herbert 1975, Wheeler 1964).

The havoc wrought by the virus among many inland tribes in the nineteenth century was extreme. Though the disease may only have been absent for several generations, the ferocity of many of these East African epidemics supports the assumption that some of the tribes were encountering smallpox for the first time. Laidler and Gelfand (1971) report that mortality rates among the Griqua people in 1831 may have been reached as high as eighty to ninety percent of the total population. In 1876, Stanley described an outbreak at Ujiji in which, in a population of only three thousand persons, between fifty and seventy-five people were dying daily:

> The arabs were dismayed at the pest and its dreadful havoc among their families and slaves. Every house was full of mourning and woe.

> There were no more agreeable visits and social discourse; each kept
> himself in strict seclusion, fearful of being stricken with it. Khamis the
> Baluch was dead, his house was closed, and his friends were sorrowing.
> Mohammed bin Gharib had lost two children, Muini Kheri was lament-
> ing the deaths of three children. (1878, 2: 62)

In his *Uganda Memoirs*, A. R. Cook remarked that when smallpox descended on a Ugandan village, it "swept through it like a destroying
pestilence, killing many, blinding others, and leaving a trail of disfigured
faces behind it" (1945, 49). After one such outbreak in the latter part of
the century, a Waganda villager told a visitor, "If we stayed here much
longer, there would be none of us left" (Colville 1895, 212).

In northern Kenya, an ivory trader found half a dozen villages
depopulated by smallpox in 1899 and observed that the Rendile tribe had
been nearly exterminated. In some villages, the few survivors had inherited so many sheep, goats, and camels that there were not enough people
left to drive all the animals to water in one day (Hardwick 1903).

One notable exception to invasion of interior East African tribes by
smallpox were the Masai, whose militancy, by discouraging Arab slave
traders, apparently also delayed their first encounter with the disease.
Johnston (1902) reports that as late as the mid-nineteenth century, smallpox seems to have been unknown among the Masai of Kenya. But by the
time the British, at the end of the century, decided somewhat cautiously to
construct a railroad on the edge of Masai territory, they discovered that
the warriors had been "weakened partly by war, but more especially by
cholera and smallpox" (Mungeam 1966, 39). Even then, the Masai were
said to have been extremely wary of travelers coming from the coast,
because they feared smallpox, which they called the "White Illness" and
associated with the arrival of the Europeans. Johnston believed that
without vaccinations to control epidemics of smallpox and cattle plague
and the consequent famine the Masai would have become extinct.

To a lesser extent, a pattern similar to that in East Africa was also seen
in Central Africa as smallpox spread inland from the west. The virus
caused severe epidemics among tribes in the eastern Congo basin during
the nineteenth century, decimating the populations of some districts.
According to a 1906 report by the Congo government, with yellow fever,
it completely depopulated some areas along the Congo River. Many
victims were simply abandoned in the forest. Others couldn't be isolated
effectively because of crowds in their huts demanding to know whom they
had bewitched, since members of some tribes believed smallpox only
attacked persons who had bewitched someone else. One contemporary
claimed that "before the Belgians came, smallpox was as great an evil as
the slave trade and [the Congolese's] own internecine wars" (Wack 1905,
266). Mary Kingsley, an intrepid Englishwoman who traveled in the

French Congo at the end of the nineteenth century, reported that small-pox was then "common" in that area and that local tribes called it "the spotted death" (1897, 401).

Even as the disease extended its range to new parts of nineteenth-century Africa, however, it continued to exact tribute from areas where it had been known for hundreds or thousands of years. On six occasions smallpox was epidemic in Ethiopia and adjacent Sudan in the same or successive years: in 1811–13, 1838–39, 1865–6, 1878–79, 1885–7, and 1889–90. In Ethiopia, the outbreak of 1889-90 was accompanied by a great famine, as were epidemics in Sudan in 1813 and in 1824–25 (Bayoumi 1976; Pankhurst 1965). Even without coincident natural disas-ters, the mortality from these epidemics was substantial. Describing an epidemic that struck northern Sudan in 1814, a European witness wrote:

> About one-third of those who were attacked recovered. . . . Of the large
> family of Temsah (our landlord's), fifty-two persons died within a few
> months and while I am writing this (at Cairo, December 1815), I hear
> from some traders, that the same disease has again broken out, and
> that almost the whole family, including Edris, have perished. (Hartwig
> 1981, 7)

In his 1965 report, Pankhurst refers to mortality rates of fifty percent among nineteenth-century Ethiopian children who caught smallpox, and up to eighty percent among affected adults.

Late in the century, the nationalist Mahdist movement in Sudan (1885–98), with its tribal uprisings, wars with Egypt and Ethiopia, and mass migrations, set the scene for several more severe epidemics. A subordinate of General Charles "Chinese" Gordon, who tried in vain to defend Khartoum for the British, reported that "smallpox and dysentery carried off many of my troops." Another of Gordon's officers cut short an exploratory mission, for fear of infecting his Sudanese escort, after hear-ing that "the smallpox was raging" (Hartwig 1981, 11). After the Mahdi's successful siege of Khartoum in 1885, the disease rapidly increased to epidemic proportions. Hundreds died daily in the suburb of Omdurman. The outbreak there caused many people to flee to Kordofan, Darfur, and elsewhere, spreading the disease over the whole country. At Obeid, capital of Kordofan Province, a British prisoner of war observed that

> while waiting till huts should be made for us we were housed with slaves
> suffering from smallpox . . . these unfortunate sufferers had no one to
> help them, and they were left to die either of the disease or of hunger;
> they lay about under the trees in the market place shunned by everyone;
> often, when still living, they were dragged off by men, who tied ropes
> around their bodies, and pulled them along the ground till they were
> beyond the Outskirts of the town, and there they were left to be devoured
> by the hyenas . . . ("Smallpox in the Soudan," 1898, 1003–4).

New recruits, especially blacks from southern Sudan, where the slave trade was still rampant, posed a special danger. Hill (1970) observes even in 1839, it was reported that nearly all the blacks conscripted into Ahmad Pasha's army died of smallpox, in spite of inoculation. In 1887, reports Bayoumi, "smallpox appeared among the Mahdist forces mobilized near the Egyptian frontier for a prospective invasion of Egypt," whereupon "numbers of deaths took place daily" (1976, 6). According to Wingate's 1893 memoirs, the Mahdi himself told his followers that the disease was punishment by Allah for their evil-mindedness and appropriation of booty.

In neighboring Ethiopia, the Mahdi's contemporary, Emperor Menelik II, who was busy expanding his empire to the southeast and southwest and preparing to defend it successfully against would-be Italian colonists, also had problems with smallpox.[5] Menelik's own fierce face was pitted by smallpox. While returning from Tigre in the first year of his reign (1889), the Ethiopian emperor lost fifteen percent of his army to smallpox, dysentery, typhus, and bronchitis. Mindful, perhaps, of these and other such episodes, the emperor issued an edict proclaiming vaccination to be obligatory in his new capital on 12 May 1898, coupled with a stern warning: "And those who are found in Addis having smallpox, things will not go well for them" (Fasquelle 1971, 741). Vaccination had only reached Ethiopia during the reign of Emperor Menelik's predecessor, sometime after 1871.

Although Ethiopia was apparently one of the last African territories to benefit from Jenner's discovery, one of the most remarkable aspects of smallpox's impact in nineteenth-century Africa is the relative lack of effective systematic efforts, whether by isolation, inoculation, or vaccination, to protect threatened communities. Isolation of some type was practiced in many areas, though often only as a result of the panic induced by an outbreak. Burckhardt reported that in Sudan, "their only cure for the smallpox is to rub the whole body with butter three or four times a day and to keep themselves closely shut up" (Bayoumi 1976, 7–8). He also noted that "great numbers of the inhabitants emigrate to the mountains, to fly from the infection" (Hartwig 1981, 9). Another observer of epidemic smallpox in early nineteenth-century Darfur reported, "As soon as a person is attacked by it he is immediately removed to a hut built in a lonely place—a kind of hospital, in fact, where there are servants who have already had the disease" (ibid.,10). In Ethiopia, eighteenth-century Gallas had incinerated smallpox victims, living and dead, with their houses in attempting to halt further outbreaks. During one nineteenth-century epidemic, the king of Shoa, Sahle Sellassie, isolated himself in a village near his capital to avoid infection. Less well guarded was the governor-general of the Sudan, Musa Pasha Hamdi, who Bayoumi says died of smallpox in his palace in Khartoum in 1865.

Thus the idea that smallpox was contagious and spread somehow from person to person was recognized and acted upon in some nineteenth-century African societies. The practical implications of immunity following inoculation or a previous attack were also understood. Although some members of a cannibalistic East African tribe drew the line at eating persons who had died of smallpox, others did not, but took care to depute relatives who had had the disease to perform the mourning ceremonies (Kitching 1912; Roscoe 1924).

Although there is evidence that inoculation was used by various groups in all regions of the continent, only rarely does it appear to have been applied to protect communities, as opposed to individuals, even in areas where it had been known for a long time. In Ethiopia, the practice of inoculation was reportedly common in Tigre and Shoa after 1820, before Emperor Yohannes IV (r. 1871–89), during whose reign vaccination was introduced into that country, outlawed it. According to Burckhardt (cited in Bayoumi 1976) inoculation was unpopular in northern Sudan and southern Egypt, perhaps because it was believed to spread the disease more than it helped prevent it. At Wad Medani, Sudan, in 1839 an anonymous medical officer reported in his diary:

> It is asserted that smallpox did little harm before the Turks came whereas it now makes serious ravages. The Turks brought with them inoculation which was unknown before them but is now widely used. (Ibid., 4)

Livingstone reported in 1860 that the Bakwains, a Bechuana tribe in southern Africa, practiced inoculation for smallpox "at a time when they had no intercourse, direct or indirect, with the southern missionaries" (1860, 142). That same year, the Lunda king, Kazembe, is said to have granted a foreign advanturer permission to trade in Katanga in gratitude for sharing the "secret" of inoculation with his tribe during an epidemic (Curtin et. al. 1978).

Jennerian vaccination apparently was first practiced in Africa either at Capetown, where it was already in use before the epidemic of 1812 and where it was widely employed by the time the next outbreak occurred there in 1840, or in Egypt, where it was made legally compulsory in 1819. Vaccination is said to have been introduced into the Sudan sometime after 1820, and into Madagascar before 1828. It was used to protect the king of Calabar, in Nigeria, during an epidemic in 1847 and to combat epidemics in Freetown, Sierra Leone, in 1859. In Uganda, vaccination helped to preserve the Bugandan royal line: a missionary doctor vaccinated King Mutesa in 1878, and during an outbreak in 1899, A. R. Cook vaccinated the boy-Kabaka (King) of Buganda, the Queen Mother, and another prince arm to arm.

Among the reasons vaccination arrived so late in most parts of Africa and was so little used before the twentieth century despite the need were the hot climate and the long distance from sources of vaccine in Europe; cowpox did not occur naturally in Africa. Often, repeated shipments had to be made before vaccine arrived in viable condition. After the first potent vaccine finally arrived safely on Madagascar there was yet another short delay before it was used. A recent outbreak of smallpox in King Radama's (r. 1810–28) family had been exacerbated by careless inoculation efforts, and the king was persuaded only with some difficulty of the distinction between vaccination and inoculation (Coulanges 1976, 133). For their part, King Radama's subjects were accustomed to much more draconian action to stop smallpox.

When the virus was first introduced into Madagascar remains a mystery. Ellis, in his *History of Madagascar*, says it was already there when the first missionaries arrived in the sixteenth or seventeenth century. The large island soon became a popular stopover for ships traveling between Europe and the Orient, and its people were in frequent contact with groups on the east coast of Africa long before the Portuguese sailed around the Cape. Hirsch 1883 states that the earliest specific report of smallpox dates from 1729, when a slave ship carried the infection from Madagascar to Reunion. Much of the following account of smallpox on Madagascar is based on the work of Clarac and Coulanges.

During the reign of King Andrianampoinimerina (r. 1787–1810), smallpox epidemics occurred all over the island, especially on the central plateau, which the king controlled. One probably apocryphal legend claims the king used the virus as a biologic weapon to assist him in conquering Analamanga (Tananarive). Although he liked to boast that "the sea is the limit of my rice field," King Andrianampoinimerina's domain never extended to the sea in his lifetime.

Andrianampoinimerina took drastic measures to try to eliminate smallpox. He established a policy that all persons who had the disease were to be buried alive as soon as the diagnosis was made. Anyone caught trying to save them would be enslaved. Unlucky patients with chickenpox, syphilis, or other rashes sometimes paid dearly for a mistaken diagnosis. Convinced of the danger, if not of the inefficacy of such measures, his nobles implored the king to change this policy:

> We ask you, Andrianampoinimerina, on condition that this request entails neither the reduction into slavery of our wives and our children, nor the loss of our lives, grant us to take the smallpox patients far away in order to care for them, for cured, they will not be less your subjects; if they succeed in dying, they will be buried very deeply by us, following the laws of the kingdom. (Coulanges 1976, 148)

The king finally agreed that some patients could be isolated instead of buried alive, so long as they were kept far from his other subjects for a long time. His successor, King Radama, abolished the burial law altogether.

James Hastie, a British envoy who visited King Radama's court between December 1817 and February 1818 following the signing of an Anglo-Merina treaty, recorded a deadly epidemic that was apparently worsened by inoculation. The king himself was inoculated that December and recovered, but his sister died on 23 December. By 5 January, five of the king's captains, all of whom were members of the royal family, had died of smallpox, and thirteen of the persons who had accompanied Hastie from the coast were also dead. After hundreds of moribund victims were cast into graves in old abandoned villages, the king warned that henceforth such crimes would be punishable by death. A packet of Jennerian vaccine arrived at court on 12 February, and Hastie eventually persuaded the king to permit vaccination.

Malagasy funeral customs enhanced smallpox's spread among the island's population. Corpses were exposed for several days while the family mourners held a feast nearby, and the bodies were wrapped in expensive shawls before burial. Prosperous families sometimes transferred deceased loved ones after a few weeks from hastily prepared temporary tombs to more elaborately constructed ones befitting their status. Some smallpox outbreaks were caused by exposure of persons to the corpse at the funeral ceremonies themselves or by exposure of others to contaminated shrouds sold by grave robbers.

King Radama's successor, Queen Ranavalo (r. 1828–61) reinstituted some of King Andrianampoinimerina's control measures during a large epidemic at the beginning of her reign. Other severe epidemics were recorded in Madagascar in 1864, 1869, 1878, 1892, and 1898–99. According to Little (1884), one particularly severe outbreak along the east coast of the island in 1876–77 was started by a shipment of old uniforms from Mauritius.

Ships en route to Europe or North America from Madagascar, Mauritius, or Mozambique continued to introduce smallpox into South Africa in the late nineteenth century. As we saw earlier, vessels carrying slaves from Mozambique caused two major outbreaks in Capetown in 1812 and 1840. The third major outbreak to strike the Cape peninsula in the nineteenth century also began in Capetown harbor, in May 1882, courtesy of the *Drummand Castle*, exact origin unknown (Mathews 1887). Since the city's previous outbreak, however, diamonds had been discovered at Kimberley, some 400 miles (666 km) inland, where a large African labor force was employed to work the mines. When this latest epidemic got underway at Capetown, therefore, there was great concern that "if it broke out among the native labourers [in Kimberley], a general stampede from the mines might result that could cripple the industry"—which is exactly what had happened when smallpox appeared in the coppermining areas of Angola seven years before (Burrows 1958, 259). In September, a quarantine station was established south of Kimberley at which all travelers into the area were obliged to present proof of vaccination and to undergo disinfection with burning sulfur in a closed shed for three minutes. The alternative was six weeks of quarantine. While over four thousand persons died of smallpox in Cape Colony, the disease did not spread to Kimberley before the epidemic ended the following March. Before it ended, however, this epidemic of 1882 "practically exterminated" Capetown's Moslem Malay population, who for religious reasons still refused to be vaccinated (Balfour & Scott 1924).

Even as the satisfaction of having mounted such a successful southern defense was savored, however, there was a similar scare at Kimberley's unguarded rear, toward the north. In October 1883, smallpox was reported in a group of Africans heading toward Kimberley from Portuguese territory. After being examined by a delegation of three doctors, who diagnosed them as suffering from "aggravated chicken pox," the Africans were permitted to resume their journey. Only a few of them made it to Kimberley's outskirts. The others were too ill, too tired, or dead. Rumors of smallpox began to fly as the disease started spreading.

The medical profession split into two opposing groups: those who declared the disease was smallpox, and others, mindful of the profitable industry at stake, who insisted the illness was anything else but smallpox. A favorite diagnosis of members of the latter group was "a bullous disease allied to pemphigus" (Burrows 1958, 261). By the time the outbreak ended at the end of 1884—it was indeed smallpox—there had been about two thousand three hundred cases, and seven hundred deaths in Kimberley. One physician accused of deliberately misdiagnosing a case in the "Kimberley Mines Scandal" was arrested and charged with murder but was acquitted. Because of this outbreak and the one that immediately preceeded it, vaccination and reporting of infectious diseases were made compulsory in the Cape Colony.

British authorities reportedly took advantage of the outbreak at Capetown in 1882 to delay returning the Zulu king Cetewayo to his homeland following a three-year exile. Cetewayo had been captured a few months after his warriors inflicted a humiliating defeat on a British force at the Battle of Isandhlwana. After the British agreed to restore Cetewayo to his kingdom, it was rumored that he was deliberately landed at Capetown so that he could be detained there for several more months in quarantine (Cox 1888). He died a year after returning to Zululand.

Barely a decade after Cetewayo's death, smallpox intervened more directly in the rapidly changing political landscape of southern Africa. Gold had recently been discovered in the Witwatersrand, and a smallpox epidemic was getting underway at Johannesburg (nearly three thousand six hundred cases reported between 1893 and 1895) in the heart of the gold mining area. Meanwhile, Europeans raced to gain control of Matabeleland and Mashonaland further north in 1893.

During a major skirmish between the Matabele and soldiers of the British South Africa Company, the army of the Matabele chief Lobengula, including his best regiments, was not at full strength because of smallpox in their ranks. Since the British South Africa Company's soldiers were now using machine guns, however, the collapse of Matabeleland's defense cannot be attributed to smallpox alone. Wilmot (1889) reports that the disease also broke out among the British African allies, who were pursuing Lobengula's army along with the British soldiers. The Africans retired, leaving the British to pursue Lobengula alone.

Early in 1894, Chief Lobengula, successor and son of the founder of the Matabele nation, died of smallpox near Victoria Falls while fleeing the British South Africa Company's forces (plate 26). As a result, "Matabeleland, by virtue of conquest and royal death, was now legally a province within the Rhodes Company Charterland" (Wiedner 1962, 289).

In West Africa, Dahomey was at the height of its power when a visitor to that kingdom in 1845 reported that leprosy and smallpox were the most common diseases there, (Duncan 1968, 2: 214). Smallpox was also epidemic at Warri, in neighboring Nigeria, that year. During a long reign that began in 1808, the king of Dahomey, Guezo, had freed his country of paying tribute to Oyo, established diplomatic relations with his powerful neighbor to the west, Ashante, and refused to abandon the slave trade, which brought him guns. Two envoys brought Guezo a note from Lord Palmerston of the British Foreign Office in 1850 deploring the Dahomeyan's attitude:

> The Queen of England takes a great interest in favour of [Abeokuta] and its people, and, if you value the friendship of England, you will abstain from any attack upon and from any hostility against that Town and People. . . . With respect to what you have written about the slave trade, the British government is much disappointed at your answer, for they had hoped and expected that you would have complied with their very reasonable requests accompanied as it was by a handsome offer of full compensation for any temporary loss which you might sustain by putting end to the Slave Trade. But as you have declined to consent to what the British government has asked upon you to do, the British government will be obliged to employ its own means to accomplish its purpose, and, as England is sure to succeed in any object which it is determined to attain, the result will be that the Slave Trade from Dahomey will be put an end to by British cruisers and thus, you will sustain the temporary loss of revenue without receiving the offered compensation.(Verger 1976, 503)

Guezo attacked British-armed Abeokuta with an army of about sixteen thousand men and women less than six months after receiving Palmerston's letter, but Dahomey was defeated, with many losses (Akinjogbin 1965). An epidemic of smallpox forced Guezo's heir, Gelele, to abandon one attempt to avenge his father's defeat, and the fabled Dahomeyan army was crushed during a second attempt a year later. The later defeat, wrote Herskovits, signalled the beginning of the decline of Dahomey's power.

Guezo himself, who a French missionary described as a "great soldier and great king . . . no doubt because of his noble spirit, his worth, and his military talents" had died of smallpox in 1858 (Ronen 1975, 28; Herskovits 1938, 1: 21) (plate 27). According to one authority, however, Guezo was supposedly killed by a "point-blank gunshot wound" while returning to Abomey from a raid (Cornevin 1962, 125). By this latter account, the story attributing Guezo's death to smallpox was allegedly contrived to cover up the "true" version of his death and thus preserve the myth of the king's invincibility. Without specific evidence one way or another, it seems at least as likely that the king encountered smallpox virus as an assassin. Even if it is not true, however, the existence of this second version of Guezo's demise is noteworthy in revealing that the idea of an otherwise invincible king who could not be expected to survive smallpox, was so acceptable.

West of Dahomey, the disease played an influential part in several wars waged by the powerful inland kingdom of Ashante against the Fante and other coastal tribes, and later against the British, in generally unsuccessful attempts to gain secure access to the sea. Twice, in 1807 and 1824, outbreaks of smallpox in the Ashante army forced the ruling Asantehene (king) to withdraw to his capital, Kumasi, from the coast. The Asantehene's sister also died of smallpox in 1807, and four years later, he lost one of his principal vassals, the Okyenhene Ata Wusu Yiakosan, to the virus (Crowder 1977; Wilks 1975).

During the Sixth Ashanti War in 1873, fighting, famine, and disease, including smallpox, drove an estimated fifteen to twenty thousand refugees to Cape Coast Castle. By June that year, smallpox was raging in Cape Coast itself, as well as the "surrounding country." The historian Claridge speaking of the Ashanti army, said the ravages of smallpox and dysentery that year "disheartened them and made them miserable" (1964 3: 34, 36). Isichei (1976) notes in Onitsha, Nigeria, the same year, an epidemic of smallpox "carried off many of the inhabitants," including the Obi, or king, of Onitsha. Kumasi suffered yet another epidemic during the final Ashanti War, which completed the British conquest of Ashante in 1900. Between the Sixth War and the British conquest, Asantehene Kwaku Dua II died during another epidemic in 1884 only forty-four days after his enthronement on 10 or 11 June.

Funeral rites for smallpox victims helped to amplify many epidemics in Africa during the nineteenth and twentieth centuries at least, not just in Madagascar. To what extent this was due to lack of understanding about how the disease spread or perceived social pressure to take part in such rites despite known risks is not clear. During the smallpox eradication campaign in Sierra Leone in 1967–69, I investigated a few epidemics among faithful secret society members who were infected while attending the sickbed or funeral of a fellow member who had been attacked by the disease (Hopkins et al. 1971b). Similar outbreaks were also reported during the eradication campaigns in twentieth century Dahomey and Ethiopia (WHO 1969; C. DeQuadros, personal communication). Malays who attended funerals in Simonstown allegedly carried smallpox into Capetown itself after the disease was imported into Simonstown in 1840 (Laidler & Gelfand 1971).

In the area of modern Gabon, a French traveler encountered a large epidemic triggered by funeral ceremonies for a smallpox victim in 1864–65. He reported the outbreak "was not to be wondered at considering their style of mourning, the relatives and neighbors all surrounding the corpse, touching and embracing it" (du Chaillu 1871, 124–25). A local ruler, King Olenda, was among the victims who died in this outbreak, which occurred around the same time as an even more important epidemic just to the south.

The outbreak in Gabon may have been related to what Wheeler (1964, 356) described as "the most serious smallpox epidemic in the 19th century history of Angola." The outbreak followed the arrival of a ship, probably from Europe, at Ambrizette around February 1864. This devastating epidemic, which lasted into 1865, ultimately affected about a third of the Angolan population, killed over twenty-five thousand persons, and because of its more severe effect on the northern part of the country helped shift the balance of population in Angola towards the south. According to Wheeler, who described this outbreak in detail, "It was months or perhaps a year before the economy could recover from the dislocation" (ibid., 359).

> The *variola* epidemic by mid-1864 was on the rampage. It spread inland to the east with many caravans of trade, and spread south along the coast by contact with vessels in the ports. Two of the most famous explorers of Central Africa residing in Angola died as a result of this epidemic in 1864. Joaquim Rodrigues Graça died in April 1864, in Golungo Alto district on his farm; he led an expedition which reached Lunda country 1843–46. Ladislau Magyar also died in this wave of sickness and famine in 1864 somewhere near Bié. Thus Angola lost two illustrious settlers.
>
> The negroes fled in all directions to avoid the epidemic. . . . entire populations would migrate from their villages. . . . Luanda was on the verge of anarchy as people died in great number. . . . Great quantities of wax, ivory, gum, and copper, indeed the sinews of trade, stayed in piles along the roads and paths or abandoned in heaps at such inland stations as Malanje. (Ibid., 238)

Wheeler reported also that "the important trade *entre pot* town of

Cassange in eastern Angola was said to have broken direct communications with Malanje in this period for fear the dread disease would spread eastward" (ibid., 359). In addition to spreading inland from Luanda, which was the epidemic's focal point, the disease was carried by sea to Sao Tome and Novo Redondo. It reached Angola's Bié plateau, and the Herero tribe in South-West Africa, in 1865, a year known in Herero oral history as *Ojotjukoroka*, "the year of the smallpox." Another epidemic interrupted commercial activities, especially copper mining, in northern Angola again in 1875 by contributing to a severe decline in population.

TWENTIETH CENTURY

By the turn of the twentieth century, smallpox was entrenched throughout Africa and the Middle East.[6] Here and there some Africans who had not had smallpox were protected by vaccination, and others by inoculation, but the majority were not protected by either method. Outside the cities, especially, inoculation with smallpox virus was still widely practiced and persisted into the second half of the twentieth century in several countries, despite legal sanctions against it. It was reported from Northern Rhodesia (Zambia) in 1900, from Mozambique in 1912, from Tunisia in 1918, from Gold Coast (Ghana) in 1930, from Tanganyika in 1951, Sierra Leone in 1957, Mali and Dahomey in 1967, and Togo in 1968. It was even practiced in the city of Accra during an outbreak in 1920. I observed it in rural Ethiopia in 1971.

The fact that inoculation was known to spread smallpox and cause fatal illness made some people, who had difficulty perceiving any difference between inoculation and vaccination, reluctant to be vaccinated. One observer, describing an outbreak in Sudan in 1939, reported: "Backward people still think that the same result would attend vaccinating as attended their home method [inoculation] and they naturally resent any attempt to introduce the disease into a 'clean' family or village" (Hartwig 1981, 28). This confusion of the two methods was abetted in a minor way in Ethiopia during the eradication campaign in the early 1970s, after well-meaning health workers issued vaccine and bifurcated needles to traditional inoculators in an attempt to enlist their cooperation in the vaccination program. According to C. DeQuadros (personal communication, 1980), some of the inoculators used the modern bifurcated needles to inoculate smallpox virus.

For susceptible Africans who were neither vaccinated nor inoculated, the next best alternative was to get the new type of mild smallpox, *V. minor*, which was described in South Africa in 1895 and soon appeared in other parts of Africa. Known locally as "Amaas" in South Africa, *V. minor* behaved and looked exactly like the usual severe virus, except that it killed only one percent or less of its victims. Hartwig (1981, 11) states that a European referred to a "mild kind" of smallpox occurring in Sudan in "very few instances" in 1815, but it is difficult to know whether those outbreaks had mortality rates as low as one percent.

The fact that *V. minor* also tended to cause less scarring than *V. major* provides further evidence that most if not all of the smallpox in Africa up to the early twentieth century was caused by the more virulent virus, since scarring was so common. According to Pankhurst (1965) in the late nineteenth century, it was reported that few Ethiopians in northern provinces were without smallpox scars, and about one-fourth of the Shoan population was pockmarked. Around the same time, a British observer in Ashante reported that men and women encountered in that country were "constantly fearfully pitted" (Musgrove 1896, 109). Dixon records that among the Bantu, smallpox was sometimes called *Ngqakga*, which means "face is spoilt."[7]

In 1916, there were an estimated two thousand cases of "Amaas" in South Africa's Natal Province, and some twenty thousand more in Bechuanaland (Botswana). Five years earlier, the mild smallpox spread into northern Sierra Leone from adjacent French territories. In 1932, an apparent outbreak of *V. minor* caused eighty-nine cases of smallpox, but no deaths, at Banrenda, British Cameroons. *V. minor* was reported in the Belgian Congo a few years later, and sporadically from other countries in East and West Africa after that. By the 1960s and 1970s, *V. minor* had become the prevailing type of smallpox in Ethiopia and the Sudan.

In most areas of Africa, however, it was the familiar *V. major* (and the more recently distinguished *V. intermedius*) that continued to predominate, killing a large percentage of its victims. Against a background of nearly universal, constant, low-level endemicity, devastating smallpox epidemics recurred with deadly regularity, usually at intervals of five to ten years. Nationwide smallpox epidemics appeared for example in Ghana in 1901, 1925–26, 1930, 1941–42, 1946–48, 1953, and 1956; in Sierra Leone in 1932–35, 1945–46, 1956–57, and 1967–68; in Kenya in 1916–19, 1934, 1943–47, and 1956–59; in Egypt in 1904, 1909, 1914–15, 1919–20, 1926, 1933, and 1943–44; in Sudan in 1929–30, 1936–40, 1947–48, 1952–56, and 1971–72; and in Zambia in 1927–30, 1945, 1955, and 1963–64.

Except for coastal areas and regions of year-round rainfall, the epidemics were usually worse during the dry season. This marked seasonal variation of smallpox incidence, observed in virtually all endemic countries with sharply defined rainy and dry seasons, was attributed in part to the greater mobility and social activities of rural inhabitants during the dry season. But it was also partly due to increased survival of the virus when ambient humidity was relatively low (Harper 1961).

By and large, all age groups were affected during epidemic periods, although adults who were immune from previous infection were spared. In Sudan and in some other Moslem countries, religious barriers caused women to be even less well vaccinated than men, and the women suffered accordingly. During an outbreak in a village of Blue Nile Province in 1938, eighty-one percent of the sixty-four persons dying of smallpox were females. The impact of these sudden, thorough catastrophes was felt all over the continent as improved communications outstripped improvements in vaccination and smallpox control.

In Togoland and Cameroon, German colonizers considered smallpox the most dangerous disease of all, as far as the African population was concerned. Between August and December 1904, smallpox killed nearly a third of the two thousand residents of the village of Tschambi, in Sokode District, Togoland; and after surveying sixty villages in Togoland in 1905, Külz calculated that each year one percent of that country's population died of smallpox! If Külz's calculation of a one percent annual mortality rate is even approximately correct and if it applies, as one might reasonably expect, to the rest of densely populated West Africa, it would mean that smallpox's toll in that region alone over the years (population about 60 million in 1960) must have rivalled the loss due to the entire transatlantic slave trade, which Wiedner (1962) estimated at about 4 to 6.5 million persons between 1441 and the 1880s.

In addition to inoculation and isolation, many Africans continued to simply flee their villages when smallpox appeared, to try to ensure their personal safety. Apart from disrupting communal activities, many terrified villagers carried the infection into other areas. In the first two decades of the century, reports by colonial administrators and missionaries often referred to "abandonment" of villages or regions and "depopulation" of whole districts or countries as a result of the disease. A traveler in Angola reportedly came upon a stretch of the Coanza River where all the villages along the right bank had been abandoned because of severe epidemics a year before his arrival (Statham 1922, 85). It was in Kenya, however, at the turn of the century, that villagers fleeing smallpox had its most fateful consequences.

Early European explorers had found the Kikuyu reluctant to sell their fertile land in the Kenyan highlands, all of which was occupied and cultivated—a "vast garden," according to one description. Toward the end of the nineteenth century, the idyllic pastoral countryside was transformed by several poor harvests due to drought and locusts, burning and looting of Kikuyu crops and cattle, and a devastating epidemic of smallpox. The worst of the smallpox epidemic was illustrated in Kiumbu District where, according to Sorrenson's estimate (1967), seventy percent of the population perished. Kjekshus (1977) states that in some areas of neighboring Tanganyika, the smallpox epidemics in 1897–99 were so severe that collections of the Hut Tax were postponed, or entirely forgiven, for a year. Survivors of the epidemic in Kenya retreated to the forest of the Kikuyu escarpment or to Fort Hall. "Many of these poeple," wrote one researcher, "had not returned to their own land by 1902 when the alienation of land [by British settlers] started" (Sorrenson 1967, 17). Thus, the Kikuyu abandonment (temporary they thought) of their land to escape smallpox and famine was an important contributing factor to British settlement in the highlands of Kenya (Montafakis 1966).

Some areas, beyond the reach of fleeing villagers, could still be infected by a caravan. All over Africa, caravans on waterways and overland routes continued to spread smallpox, whether in French Equatorial Africa, Cameroons, or Ethiopia. Over a thousand caravan porters passed through the Cameroonian town of Lolodorf, an important point on the Kribi-Yaounde caravan route, daily in 1908. In Cameroon, government authorities attempted to control smallpox by quarantine and vaccination of persons traveling in caravans. The traders however, fearing losses and their competition, did not welcome any such actions which slowed their progress or threatened their porters. In Egypt and Sudan, massive numbers of pilgrims in transit to and from Mecca continued to pose special problems in smallpox control.

Meanwhile, railways added new routes for spreading smallpox. An outbreak along the railway line from Dakar to St. Louis, Senegal, infected both Africans and Europeans in 1913–14. Nearly four hundred persons lost their lives in an epidemic at Morogoru, a railhead in Tanganyika, in 1909. In the western Congo, corpses of Africans dead of smallpox, dysentery, and beriberi were strewn along the track even before the line from Matadi to Stanley Pool could be completed in 1892. Johnston (1908) says the survivors, who were demoralized by fear, had to be forced to work.

Both caravans and railways converged on seaports, the hubs of all external traffic early in the century. Smallpox arrived in port cities from all directions. As we have seen, Luanda was the focus of the powerful epidemic that battered Angola in 1864–65. In Kenya, the disease was frequently imported into Mombasa from India, especially in the late 1920s and early 1930s. Eighteen cases of smallpox were removed from ships in port and quarantined at Zanzibar in 1916. In Cameroon and Morocco, on the other hand, outbreaks usually spread from the interior toward the coast. At the seaport of Berbera in British Somaliland, a large annual fair that attracted thousands of visitors from the interior virtually guaranteed fresh importations of smallpox even when the virus wasn't imported by sea. Epidemics were recorded at Berbera in 1904–5, at Lorenço Marques in 1907–8, at Dar es Salaam in 1906–7 and 1909–10, at Zanzibar in 1910–11, at Mombasa in 1912, and at Algiers in 1918. Smallpox was almost always present at Alexandria between 1898 and 1916.

During the 1930s major epidemics were reported across Africa. A large epidemic in Ivory Coast spilled over into neighboring Gold Coast (Ghana) in 1930. Nigeria recorded over 22,000 cases, with nearly 6,000 deaths, in 1932–33. In Sierra Leone nearly 8,000 cases of smallpox were reported in 1932–35, while Kenya reported almost 1,800 cases in 1934, Cameroon over 1,000 cases in 1936, Tanganyika over 3,000 cases in 1936–37, and Belgian Congo (Zaire) over 6,000 cases in 1939. In Ethiopia, a political crisis during this period gave rise to more smallpox.

When Italy invaded Ethiopia in 1935–36, the Italian army had been vaccinated and had no smallpox, but many Ethiopian troops were affected. The author of a letter written in Addis Ababa in 1936 claimed that smallpox "decimated" the army of the Ethiopian general Mulughieta on the Northern Front (Scott 1939, 2: 60). It is unlikely, however, that the virus influenced the outcome of the Italo-Ethiopian War. Refugees from this conflict in Ethiopia also caused a small outbreak in Kenya in 1937.

As the twentieth century progressed, improvements in vaccination and smallpox vaccine made control efforts increasingly effective. Those systematic vaccination efforts that did exist early in the century were usually limited, and were usually only conducted to halt epidemics. Thus some 56,000 persons were vaccinated at Zanzibar in 1910–11 during an epidemic of smallpox. In 1918, the recent relative freedom of Lagos, Nigeria, from smallpox was attributed to increased vaccination efforts, and an estimated 70,000 persons were vaccinated during an epidemic at Accra, Gold Coast, in 1920, the first major vaccination effort in that country. Nearly two decades later, two million persons were vaccinated in northern Sudan. Similar vaccination campaigns made Madagascar free of smallpox after 1922, the first African country to achieve that distinction. Still, in some countries, the quality of the vaccine itself was a serious problem.

Because nearly all the vaccine used was sensitive to heat, and adequate refrigeration was scarce and mainly limited to the cities, many Africans were "vaccinated" in the first half of the century with impotent vaccine and hence were not successfully protected against smallpox. In the Gold Coast, an assessment of the results of a vaccination campaign during an epidemic in 1930 revealed that of 413,000 vaccinations given, only about one out of every five was successful. Vaccine institutes were established in Africa to avoid some of the problems of lost potency inherent in shipping vaccine via the long voyage by sea from Europe. In Sudan, which set up a facility to produce vaccine locally in 1936, the medical staff made imaginative attempts to keep vaccine lymph cold during trips to rural areas in the 1920s, including packing it in watermelons (Hartwig 1981).

The most successful attack on the problem of vaccine potency in Africa was made by the French, who had begun serious efforts to control smallpox in their colonies early in the century and conducted research to develop a vaccine better suited to tropical climates. The first of these experimental vaccines were tested in Guinea in 1909 and in Ivory Coast in 1911–12, with encouraging results (Fasquelle 1971). The much more stable "dried" vaccine that resulted from these and other studies began to replace the old glycerinated lymph in French Somaliland as early as 1929, in Sudan in 1930, and in Ghana in 1937. Nevertheless, the older type of glycerinated vaccine lymph was still used widely in West Africa into the late 1960s.

The end of World War II was followed by the largest recorded upsurge in smallpox on the African continent in the half century before the disease was eradicated. This pandemic was probably fueled by movements associated with the war, and perhaps also by the colonial powers' relative neglect of control measures, "owing to their preoccupations elsewhere" (Tulloch 1980, 408). Ninety-nine thousand cases of smallpox were reported for the whole continent in 1944 and 1945, with major epidemics in Egypt, Kenya, South Africa, Sierra Leone, and Guinea. Smallpox was still endemic in at least thirty-two African states, but vaccinations began to be conducted systematically among large populations, with better vaccine. When highly stable freeze-dried vaccines were developed in the early 1950s, they began to be used in Africa after a few years' delay.

By 1963, all of North Africa, from Egypt to Morocco, was free of indigenous smallpox, as was Saudi Arabia, Iraq, Syria, and Iran, which had started its program to eradicate smallpox in 1955. Sudan began a national campaign in 1962. This momentum toward freedom from smallpox soon spread to countries south of the Sahara. Portuguese Guinea became smallpox-free in 1962, followed by Mauritania (1963), Senegal (1964), Gambia (1966), and Ivory Coast (1967). Ivory Coast had undertaken an eradication campaign with French assistance in 1961, the same year it achieved political independence. Angola detected no smallpox cases in 1960 and 1961, then reported 73 cases, apparently due to reintroduction of the disease in 1962–63. In the Sudan, smallpox was apparently eradicated by 1963, and reported cases again fell to zero rapidly after a brief importation, probably from Ethiopia, in 1965. But in 1968, the disease became re-established in Sudan after being reintroduced from Ethiopia, and this time it could not be eliminated immediately, because of a civil war. Smallpox was finally eradicated from the Sudan in 1972, several months after the civil war in southern Sudan ended.

At the beginning of the global eradication campaign in 1967, nineteen West African countries accepted an offer of assistance from the United States. About the same time, the World Health Organization began providing assistance for smallpox eradication programs in twenty other countries of eastern and southern Africa, except for the Congo (Zaire), which started a little later, and Ethiopia, which began its program in 1971. As a result of these programs, the West African region was completely freed of smallpox in May 1970, when Nigeria reported its last case.

By December 1973, Ethiopia was the only country on the continent that still had smallpox. Less than three years later, Ethiopia, which had reported 43,000 cases of smallpox in the first two years after its eradication program began (only about 1 in 10 of the actual number of cases was discovered) reported its last known case of smallpox in August 1976. The onus of harboring the last cases of smallpox in Africa then passed to Somalia, where a small outbreak, traced to a person infected in Ethiopia, was discovered in Mogadishu in late September 1976. This outbreak of *V. minor*, smallpox's last appearance in Africa, proved much more persistent than expected. It was crushed only after a difficult thirteen-month-long struggle. The final patient, Ali Maow Maalin (plate 28), was a cook at the hospital in Merka Town. He developed a rash on 26 October 1977 and recovered.

Shapona: Yoruba God of Smallpox

In West Africa as in India and China, smallpox's pronounced impact was manifest by its incorporation into the mythology of a local people, the Yoruba. Although several African tribes attributed smallpox to "spirits" of one sort or another, formal worship of a smallpox deity in Africa apparently existed only among the Yorubas and some of their neighbors in southwest Nigeria, Dahomey (Republic of Benin), and Togo. Dahomey and the Yoruba state of Oyo (in modern Nigeria) shared many historical and cultural ties, as well as being geographically close.

When Europeans arrived in parts of West Africa near Dahomey late in the seventeenth century, Yoruba beliefs were already well established and highly organized. According to Yoruba traditions, worship of Shapona, the god of smallpox, was introduced into their country from the north (Herskovits 1938). In Yoruba land the smallpox god was also known as Obaluaye (Overlord of the Earth), or Omolu. Among the Mahis of Dahomey, he was called Sagbata. According to Le Herisse, Shapona only began to be worshipped in Dahomey during the reign of their fourth king, Agadja, early in the eighteenth century (Verger 1957).

Yoruba legend held that the supreme god delegated authority over various kingdoms of the world to his sons. To the second-born Shango, he gave control of the sky, with thunder and lightening as his tools; but to his eldest, Shapona, he gave control of the earth, to be effected by smallpox. "It was thought that the god of the earth, who nourished man by giving him maize and millet, and all other grains of the earth, when moved to punishment caused the grains men had eaten to come out on their skins" (Challenor 1971, 57–59).

Thus, smallpox was an indication of divine displeasure. But according to Herskovits, "smallpox as such is not worshipped. It is the Earth gods who are worshipped; smallpox is merely their most severe penalty for wrong doing" (1938, 2: 136). It was not a penalty to be trifled with.

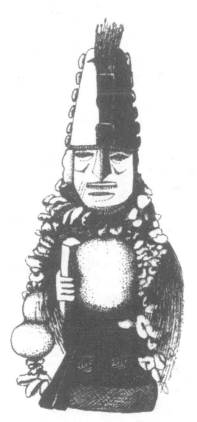

Fig. 12. Shapona, Yoruba god of smallpox. Drawing by Chris L. Smith.

According to Maclean (1965), some considered it unlucky to even mention Shapona's name.

Meek (1931) observed that since smallpox was a king, or *aku*, one did not question his right to put persons to death. The kings of Dahomey, two of whom died of smallpox, acknowledged Shapona's status by refusing to allow shrines for worship of the god to be erected within their capital. The reason, they insisted, was that "two kings cannot rule in one city" (Herskovits 1938, 2: 136).

Shapona was represented at times by laterite stones, the pitted surface of which was thought to resemble the pock-marked faces of recovered victims. Herskovits also described a seated clay figure, five feet high, with large cowrie shells embedded in the body to give a pitted appearance. Somtimes, the smallpox god was represented by a carved wooden figure of a man, adorned with cowrie shells, a monkey skull, and other meaningful objects. At other times he was represented by a broom made of bamboo palm branches smeared with camwood. Each village had its own shrine, including the major towns of Abomey and Allada. Euphorbias and cactus plants sacred to Shapona, were planted as hedges around some shrines (Herskovits 1938; Johnson 1973; Challenor 1971).

Frobenius (1926) recorded that in western Nigeria, a great festival for the god was held every September. In traditional Dahomeyan society, a smallpox epidemic was considered to be "hot earth," and "someone who dies is carried away by hot breath. During the dry season Shapona prowls about, wearing red, seeking to vent his anger. For this reason, red is a colour reserved for the god" (Quinn 1968, 157). Black and white were the other two colors of the god. Drumming was prohibited during an epidemic, we are told, "so that people may not congregate and be attacked by the smallpox god who may also come to dance" (Fadeyi 1967, V–20).

Formal worship of Shapona was controlled by specific priests, or "fetisheurs," who were in charge of the shrines. If angered, the priests were believed to be able to cause epidemics themselves. According to Dr. Bernard Challenor, the physician-advisor to the eradication programs of Togo and Dahomey in the late 1960s, most of the priests protected themselves by being inoculated, if they had not already had natural smallpox. They were also called upon to protect others by inoculation and to treat victims. While treating smallpox paitents, the fetisheurs collected and saved material from the victims, usually scabs, "for future use." Since fetisheurs traditionally "inherited" the personal belongings of persons who died of smallpox, their client's recovery was often not in their best interests. Some fetisheurs were said to have deliberately fostered small-pox epidemics by spreading infectious material from former victims, which could retain its potency for several months, among susceptible persons.

According to Lucas (1948), the British rulers of colonial Nigeria suspected the Shapona priests of spreading smallpox early in the twentieth century and therefore passed an ordinance in 1907 forbidding worship of Shapona in any form. Many priests were fined for violating this order in 1912. By 1914, the annual report to Britain's Colonial Office mentioned that "Ekiti is believed to be the last stronghold of what remains of the now almost extinct 'Shopono,' or smallpox worship, which was once the scourge of Yoruba Land" (Low 1918, 53). Half a century later, a survey of persons living in the poor areas of Nigeria's capital revealed that fully seventy percent still attributed smallpox to witchcraft and Shapona, only twenty percent recognizing the true basis of contagion (Taylor 1971).

In 1971, Challenor reported on the strong cultural resistance to vaccination still present among an estimated 4–5 million Shapona wor-shippers in southern parts of Dahomey, Togo, and western Nigeria. He noted that vaccination was sometimes strongly resisted by the villagers themselves, as well as by the fetisheurs, as a direct result of their belief in the Overlord of the Earth. "In Western Nigeria, a vaccination team was met with drawn knives when publicity posters circulated prior to the [eradication] campaign asked the population to make war on smallpox. The word for smallpox in the local language was identical to the name of the local earth god, and the population was highly incensed, feeling they were being asked to make war on one of their own deities" (Challenor 1971, 58).

Six

The Great Fire

IF THE ASIANS WHO MIGRATED across the Bering Straits to populate the Americas around 15–10,000 B.C. carried smallpox with them, and there is no evidence that they did, the disease probably did not sustain itself for long among those first immigrants. Indeed, the little evidence about early smallpox available suggests that the virus may not have appeared in eastern Asia at all until long after the ice bridge between Siberia and Alaska had disappeared, isolating the sparse bands of ancestral "Americans" from Asia altogether. Thus, the native populations of North and South America were blissfully unaware of smallpox's existence when Christopher Columbus re-established contact between the Old and New Worlds in 1492. Smallpox made its first appearance in the New World only fifteen years later.

The first outbreak struck the island of Hispanola in 1507 (Hirsch 1883, vol. 1; Do Amaral 1960; Smith 1974)and was probably imported into the colony from Spain. This initial epidemic was so disastrous, wrote the historian Hirsch, "that whole tribes were exterminated by it" (1883, 1:136). After running its course, the epidemic apparently died out. But there was much more to come. The millions of unsuspecting Indians on the American mainland, including the mighty, pre-eminent empires of the Aztecs and Incas, were about to experience one of the worst epidemic disasters of all time.

Even before the first outbreak of smallpox in Hispanola, small numbers of African slaves were being exported from Spain to Spanish estates in Santo Domingo, starting in 1503. In 1510, the Spanish king officially sanctioned use of slaves in mines on the island. According to Wilkinson (1958), by 1517, up to four thousand slaves were allowed to be imported annually. All trade with Santo Domingo, including the new trade in slaves, was supposed to be reserved for Spain, but with the increased demand, Portuguese and Genoese traders soon started bringing slaves to Santo Domingo illegally, directly from West Africa. Brau (1969) was convinced that this clandestine trade caused the next outbreak of smallpox in Hispanola.

The disease was also epidemic in Spain and Portugal, including several Spanish ports, in 1517–18, but ships from Spain usually halted at Puerto Rico or San Germán first, where any smallpox that developed during the voyage should have been discovered. However, it was only after the second epidemic ended that the authorities at Santo Domingo, not Puerto Rico, instituted the first quarantine measures in the Americas, requiring all arriving ships to be inspected. Thus this second outbreak could have originated in Spain or Africa, although the latter seems more likely, in view of where the epidemic started on the island.

The second epidemic was apparently noticed first among African slaves in the mines of Hispanola in December 1518. It then spread rapidly to the island's Amerindian population. By May 1519, up to a third of the Indians on Hispanola had died of smallpox. Meanwhile, the outbreak had spread to Cuba in 1518. Early in 1519, smallpox spread from Hispanola to Puerto Rico, where it killed over half the native population in a few months (Brau 1969; Dobyns 1963; Moll 1944).

Having reached the three main Spanish-occupied islands in the Caribbean, it was inevitable, in that age, that smallpox would spread to the densely populated mainland of Central America, where the Spanish were just beginning to discover unexpected wonders. Only a few months after smallpox arrived in Cuba, Hernando Cortez sailed from Cuba to Mexico, where he and his followers arrived at the Aztec capital, Tenochtitlán, in November 1519. The astonished Spaniards advanced over one of the broad causeways that linked the beautiful city in the middle of a large lake with the mainland of the Valley of Mexico. Recalled one of the soldiers, "We were all struck with amazement, and we exclaimed that the towers, temples and lakes seemed like the enchantment we read of in *Amadis*. Some of our soldiers kept asking themselves whether what they saw was not all a dream" (Clissold 1972, 30). The Aztec emperor, Moctezuma II, greeted Cortez and his small group of soldiers at the city gates. By this time, the governor of Cuba, who had sent Cortez to Mexico in the first place, had heard of the early successes and treasures, of Cortez's Mexican campaign. Yielding to jealous suspicions of Cortez's loyalty, the governor dispatched another expedition led by Pánfilo de Narvaez to Mexico, with orders to supercede Cortez. Only the epidemic of smallpox then raging in Cuba, said Governor Velasquez, prevented him from leading the new expedition himself (Bancroft 1883, 9: 358).

Narvaez left Cuba in early March, and landed at Cempoala, near present-day Vera Cruz, on 23 April 1520. According to D'Ardois (1961) and Smith (1974), it was an African slave in Narvaez's entourage, Francisco de Baguia, who first introduced smallpox to the American mainland. En route to Mexico, one of Narvaez's ships had also carried smallpox to Cozumel during a brief stopover at that island. Only a few months earlier, Cortez had deliberately burned his own ships at Cempoala to ensure his soldiers' undivided attention to the conquest of Mexico. The "Great Fire" that Narvaez's expedition brought ashore accidentally assured Cortez's victory.

A Spanish friar, Fray Toribio Motolinía, described the epidemic that resulted in his *History of the Indians of New Spain,* which he completed in 1541:

> at the time that Captain Pánfilo de Narvaez landed in this country, there was in one of his ships a negro stricken with smallpox, a disease which had never been seen here. At this time New Spain was extremely full of people, and when the smallpox began to attack the Indians it became so great a pestilence among them throughout the land that in most provinces more than half the population died; in others the proportion was little less. For as the Indians did not know the remedy for the disease and were very much in the habit of bathing frequently, whether well or ill, and continued to do so even when suffering from smallpox, they died in heaps, like bedbugs. Many others died of starvation, because, as they were all taken sick at once, they could not care for each other, nor was there anyone to give them bread or anything else. In many places it happened that everyone in a house died, and, as it was impossible to bury the great number of dead they pulled down the houses over them in order to check the stench that rose from the dead bodies so that their homes became their tombs. This disease was called by the Indians "the great leprosy" because the victims were so covered with pustules that they looked like lepers. Even today one can see obvious evidences of it in some individuals who escaped death, for they were left covered with pockmarks. (Foster 1950, 38)

Motolinía continued:

> it extended over all parts of their bodies. Over the forehead, head, chest. It was very destructive. Many died of it. They could no longer walk, they could do no more than lie down, stretched out on their beds. They couldn't bestir their bodies, neither to lie face down, nor on their backs, nor to turn from one side to the other. And when they did move, they cried out. In death, many [bodies] were like sticky, compacted, hard grain . . . many [of the survivors] were pockmarked . . . some were blind . . . this pestilence lasted sixty days, sixty lamentable days. (D'Ardois 1961, 1016)

Moll (1944) informs us that the Aztec word for the new disease, *hueyzahuatl,* is translated as "big pox," whereas measles, introduced later, was called by them *tepitonzahuatl,* meaning "little leprosy," or "small pox." The Aztecs' reasoning was clear, even though their nosology differed from the Europeans': "small" seemed an inappropriate adjective for the ferocious malady brought by Narvaez's slave. The Indians described the epidemic in their picture writing (plate 29).

By the summer of 1520, the disease had spread to the edge of Mexico's inland plateau. In September, it reached the towns around the lakes in the Valley of Mexico. And toward the end of the rainy season, in September or October, it invaded Tenochtitlán itself. Moctezuma, meanwhile, had been slain by his own countrymen, whereupon his aggressive brother and successor, Cuitláhuac, immediately took actions intended to expel the Spaniards from Mexico or kill them. Cortez and his soldiers were forced to abandon Tenochtitlán, with heavy losses.

When the epidemic reached Tenochtitlán in the fall of 1520, Emperor Cuitláhuac, who "had done so much to retrieve Montezuma's blunders," was one of its first victims (Helps 1904, 2: 301). He had ruled Mexico for four months. "There is no doubt that Mexico lost in [Cuitláhuac] one of the most promising sovereigns, and perhaps the only leader in face of the irresistible onslaught of foreigners" (Bancroft 1883, 9: 543–44). Cuitláhuac was succeeded by Moctezuma's twenty-five-year-old nephew.

The Aztecs lost more than their defiant emperor. When Cortez retreated to Tlascala, stronghold of his Indian allies, after his retreat from Tenochtitlán, he found the local ruler Maxixca had died of smallpox. The lord of Chalco Province also died of smallpox. In these and other instances, Cortez assumed the role of the ruler of Mexico by settling disputes about the succession and installing new chiefs in place of those killed in epidemics. No doubt other anonymous chiefs who were still fighting the Spaniards also succumbed to the virus.

It is not known for sure how many other Indians perished in this epidemic. Estimates of the total population of Mexico around this time range up to 30 million. Cartwright (1972) says nearly half of the native population of Mexico died of smallpox in less than six months. According to Magner (1942), when the terrifying conflagration ended after a few months, an estimated 2 to 3.5 million Mexican Indians had died. Crosby (1967) suggests that central Mexico's population had declined from about 25 million just before the conquest to about 16.8 million ten years later, from all causes. At a minimum, at least half of the Aztecs who caught smallpox died of it (D'Ardois 1961). Whatever the number of dead, this outbreak was a catastrophe, and of a scale far exceeding its earlier rampages on Hispanola, Puerto Rico, and Cuba.

Since most of the Spaniards had already had the disease in Spain, few of them were affected, and this differential immunity enhanced the awe in which they were held by the demoralized Indians. The importance of this timely epidemic to the Spanish side is revealed in the theurgic interpretation of one Spanish eyewitness: "When the Christians were exhausted from war, God saw fit to send the Indians smallpox, and there was a great pestilence in the city" (Crosby 1967, 329). Far from being defeated, Cortez was able to regroup and gather more Indian allies. They returned to besiege Tenochtitlán in May 1521 and captured the Aztec capital three months later. After Mexico, both smallpox and the Spaniards turned their attention south, to the land of the Mayas.

Two years after the fall of Tenochtitlán, when one of Cortez's lieutenants invaded Mayan territory, a wave of smallpox had already preceded him in 1520 or 1521. In Guatemala and Yucatán, the disease had "carried off half the Cakchiquel population, including two rulers, and greatly decreased the formerly thick population in the northern interior of the Yucatecan Peninsula" (Dobyns 1963, 495–96). According to Schram (1971), the Mayans called the rampant pestilence *nohkakil*, the "Great Fire."

The epidemic that struck Yucatán in 1520 or 1521 followed another outbreak there in 1515 or 1516, which also may have been smallpox. Diego de Landa, bishop of Yucatán, said the earlier pestilence was characterized by "great pustules that rotted the body" (Morely 1946, 99). The Indians called the earlier outbreak the "Easy Death." This epidemic might conceivably have arrived with a group of shipwrecked Spaniards, a few years before. It also might have spread north from Panama, where a similar epidemic reportedly followed the arrival of Spanish colonists there in 1514.

Spaniards in Panama had already heard rumors of another rich Indian empire further south in 1515, when Vasco Núñez de Balboa, who had discovered the Pacific Ocean just two years before, led an expedition down the Pacific coast to investigate the rumors and discovered Peru. The reigning Inca,

> Huaina Capac was in residence in his Tumipampa palaces, which were among the most beautiful in Peru, when news reached him that some strange people, of a type that was quite unknown, were cruising in a ship along the coasts of his Empire and had wanted to know what country this was. (De la Vega 1971, 339).

News of the Spaniards had reached Huayna Capac by messengers who traveled in relays along the impressive system of highways that traversed Peru's mountainous territory. The two greatest roads in this network connected the Inca capital, Cuzco, to Quito, over a thousand miles to the north (one road followed the coast and the other was cut through the mountains), and were attributed to Huayna Capac.

The Eleventh Inca valued these roads especially because they permitted him and his army to move rapidly and maintain control of his far-flung empire. But when smallpox invaded his realm, the same highways brought the enemy to Huayna Capac's doorstep before he even knew his kingdom was being attacked.

As Lastres (1954) points out, the rumors of the Inca Empire that lured Balboa south were also evidence of communication, by land and by sea, between the Indians of Peru and those living in Central America. Thus, when a devastating epidemic characterized by fever, rash, and high mortality struck the land of the Incas sometime around 1524–27, killing an estimated two hundred thousand of the empire's six million "Children of the Sun," it almost certainly was smallpox, imported from Central America. The Peruvian epidemic could easily have been a continuation of the wave that started in Mexico in 1520 and reached Guatemala by 1521, even if the unspecified pestilences that broke out in Panama in 1514 and in Yucatán in 1515 or 1516 were not smallpox.

Huayna Capac received news of the epidemic while on a campaign in the northern part of his empire, in modern Ecuador. There, at Huanca-vilca, "News came to him that a great pestilence was raging at Cuzco of which the governors Apu Hilaquito his uncle, and Auqui Tupac Inca his brother had died, also his sister Mama Cuca, and many other relations" (De Gamboa 1907, 167). The Inca returned to the Tumipampa palace near Quito and soon fell ill himself with high fever and delirium. Accord-ing to one sixteenth-century account, the emperor was "seized with a sensation of chill, which was followed by one of intense heat," after bathing in a lake near Quito (De la Vega 1971, 342). One Spanish histo-rian wrote in the early seventeenth century that Huayna Capac "was taken ill with a fever, though others say it was smallpox or measles" (De Gamboa 1907, 167). A Peruvian Indian author of the same period said the Inca died of the "pestilence of measles smallpox" (*saranpion birguelas*) (Poma de Ayala 1956, 349). According to Lastres (1954), many sixteenth-century sources also used the word *viruela*, which usually meant smallpox, to describe Huayna Capac's illness. Part of the uncertainty may have arisen because the Inca allowed no one to witness the later stages of his illness or his death.

When he realized that his illness, which progressed rapidly, would be fatal, the Son of the Sun took leave of those of his family and followers "who could reach the palace in time," and admonished them to "Dwell in peace; my father the Sun is calling me, I shall go now to rest at his side" (De la Vega 1971, 343). The Inca then

> had himself sealed with stone into his house where he was left to die unattended. After a wait of 8 days his minions went in, took out his half-decomposed body, embalmed him, dressed him in his finest armor, and carried his body on their shoulders to Cuzco where he was buried. (Schultz 1968, 506)

The emperor's courtiers thus may only have seen him during the prod-romal stages of his illness. Like many other Indians attacked by smallpox in the Americas, he may have died without ever developing a rash. Dobyns (1963) argues that the description of his illness as "measles small-pox" suggests that the disease was virulent, confluent or hemorrhagic smallpox.

The body of the conquering emperor who had doubled the size of the empire during his long reign of at least thirty years was borne back to Cuzco. The sixteenth century Peruvian commentator Garcilaso de la

Vega reported, "All along the road, crowds of people came to pay homage to his remains and to mourn the death of this beloved king" (1971, 344). Pedro Pizarro, the brother of the conqueror of Peru, stated his own belief that had "this Huayna Capac been alive when we Spaniards entered this land, it would have been impossible for us to win it, for he was much beloved by all his vassals" (Crosby 1967, 335). By Lastres's estimate, over one hundred thousand Indians died during the epidemic in Quito alone.

The emperor's general Minacnacamayta and many other officers also died in the outbreak. As unfortunate for the empire as Huayna Capac's death had been in itself, however, the suddenness of his demise and the nearly simultaneous death of his designated heir, Ninan Cuyoche, from the same disease compounded the epidemic's damage to the Inca state (Dobyns 1963). When the emperor's family had asked him to name his successor,

> His reply was that his son Ninan Cuyoche was to succeed, if the augury of the *calpa* gave signs that such succession would be auspicious, if not his son Huascar was to succeed.
>
> Orders were given to proceed with the ceremony of the *calpa*, and Cusi Tupac Yupanqui, named by the Inca to be chief steward of the Sun, came to perform it. By the first *calpa* it was found that the succession of Ninan Cuyoche would not be auspicious. Then they opened another lamb and took out the lungs, examining certain veins. The result was that the signs respecting Huascar were also inauspicious. Returning to the Inca, that he might name some one else, they found that he was dead. While the *orejones* stood in suspence about the succession, Cusi Tupac Yupanqui said: "Take care of the body, for I go to Tumipampa to give the fringe [the insignia of the emperorship] to Ninan Cuyoche." But when he arrived at Tumipampa he found that Ninan Cuyoche was also dead of the small-pox pestilence. (De Gamboa 1907, 168)

Huáscar was appointed Inca, but was later challenged by his illegitimate brother Atahualpa. These events precipitated a disastrous civil war that lasted for five years and that Dobyns believes materially aided Spanish conquest.

Details of the epidemic that killed Huayna Capac and his son are scanty, since unlike the Aztecs, the Incas had no system of writing, and the Spanish were not yet in Peru. It has been attributed by various authors to bartonellosis, typhus, measles, or smallpox. As Dr. Schultz points out, however, the rash, fever, high mortality, rapid spread, " and the intriguing fact that Huayna Capac fell ill after he had received a messenger from Cuzco, the epidemic center, also suggest that this was a disease spread by contact rather than one spread by arthropod vector," such as bartonellosis or typhus (1968, 506). The type of prodromal symptoms suggested by some accounts of the emperor's illness, and the fact that it is known to have invaded Central America a few years before this outbreak in Peru, also favor the presumption that this, too, was smallpox. The virus thus apparently spread from Hispanola to Cuba, Mexico, Yucatán, and Peru in less than twenty years.

By the time Francisco Pizarro arrived in Peru, the civil war, and the epidemic that helped cause it, were over. The Spanish conquistador finally met the Inca Atahualpa, at Caxamalca in the Andean empire's heartland, in November 1532. Prescott described the new Inca's appearance at his first meeting with the Spaniards:

> Amidst this assembly it was not difficult to distinguish the person of Atahuallpa, though his dress was simpler than that of his attendants. But he wore on his head the crimson *borla* or fringe, which, surrounding the forehead, hung down as low as the eyebrow. This was the well-known badge of Peruvian sovereignty, and had been assumed by the monarch only since the defeat of his brother Huascar . . .

The next day the Inca visited Pizarro's camp:

> Elevated high above his vassals came the Inca Atahuallpa, borne on a sedan or open litter, on which was a sort of throne made of massive gold of inestimable value. The palanquin was lined with the richly colored plumes of tropical birds, and studded with shining plates of gold and silver. The monarch's attire was much richer than on the preceding evening. Round his neck was suspended a collar of emeralds of uncommon size and brilliancy. His short hair was decorated with golden ornaments, and the imperial *borla* encircled his temples. The bearing of the Inca was sedate and dignified; and from his lofty station he looked down on the multitudes below with an air of composure, like one accustomed to command (1847, 938–39)

The same year Pizarro entered Cuzco in triumph (1533), having captured and executed Atahualpa in the interim, and again in 1535, two other epidemics of smallpox struck the Peruvian region around Quito. South America would not be free of smallpox again for nearly four and a half centuries.

That Cortez and Pizarro, each with fewer than five hundred men, were able to penetrate to the center of the well-organized, militant Aztec and Inca empires of several million Indians, seize their emperors, and subdue the inhabitants is almost unbelievable. It was made possible by a lucky coincidence of Spanish valor and weaponry, Indian superstition, and smallpox. Both groups of conquistadors enjoyed the advantages of guns, artillery, and horses, all of which were unknown to the Indians before then. The Spaniards were also exceedingly bold. During the great battle of Otumba, for example, Cortez and the remnants of his men were retreating from the Aztec capital when they were surrounded by thousands of Aztec warriors bent on their destruction: "a mighty host, filling up the whole depth of the valley, and giving to it the appearance, from the white cotton mail of the warriors, of being covered with snow," wrote Prescott (1847, 460). All seemed lost until Cortez, suddenly spotting the Aztec commander, fought his way to the Indian chief and killed him, whereupon the remaining Indians panicked and fled. Episodes such as this occurred repeatedly in Mexico and Peru.

In addition, the Indians greeted the puny bands of Spaniards with some resignation, because the Europeans seemed to fulfill old prophecies of fair-skinned beings who would assume control of the empires. In Mexico especially, the conquistadors' presumed divine status was probably confirmed when the Aztecs saw them press on relatively unscathed, while a mysterious, disfiguring, and violent epidemic reduced their own people, even their emperor, to dust. In Peru, the first epidemics erupted a few years before Pizarro arrived to conquer that country, but they weakened the Inca state by precipitating a civil war. To what extent they were associated with the coming of the Europeans in the minds of the Incas and thus served to demoralize those who escaped physical destruction can only be guessed.

Except for the removal of a few key Indian leaders, however, clearly it was the psychological impact of these coincidental epidemics on the surviving Indians, not the destruction of Aztec and Inca warriors itself, that was the key to the disease's influence in the conquest of Mexico and Peru. Whether the Spanish soldiers were outnumbered only one hundred to one rather than, say, two hundred to one, could not have made much difference in most skirmishes. Professor William McNeill (1976) concluded, and I agree, that Cortez and Pizarro would probably not have prevailed without smallpox's help.

Following their successful assaults in Mexico, Guatemala, and Peru, smallpox and the Spaniards consolidated their positions on the mainland.[1] Smallpox often accompanied, and sometimes raced ahead of, the extension of Iberian influence over South America. Soldiers, settlers, *sacerdotes*, and later slaves, all played important roles in this microbial imperialism. By mid-century the Spanish had already established municipalities at Mexico City, Quito, Lima, Buenos Aires, Asuncíon, Bogotá, La Paz, and Santiago de Chili. Although many Europeans, especially those who lived in cities, had already had smallpox by the time they reached adulthood, smallpox was not yet as rampant in Europe, particularly not in Spain and Portugal, as it became in the next two centuries. Consequently, not all Europeans who came to the New World to help found municipalities during the sixteenth century were immune, and some of them continued to import the disease.

The "Great Fire" returned to Guatemala again in 1534, 1558, and 1564. Other epidemics killed hundreds of thousands of Indians in Mexico in 1537–38, 1544–45, and 1555–56; and another two million Mexican

Indians were said to have perished during an outbreak in 1576. Cuba also suffered again during epidemic years in 1530 and 1572.

In and around the former realm of the Incas, epidemic smallpox was reported in Ecuador in 1533, 1535, 1558, 1580, 1585, and 1586–90. The latter outbreak in Ecuador supposedly originated in Colombia, where smallpox was epidemic in 1566 and where another outbreak in 1587–90 allegedly killed ninety percent of the Indians around Bogotá. In Colombia, there had been an especially long interval between the appearance and spread of the disease in the 1520s and the next reported epidemic in 1566. Not surprisingly, the epidemic of 1566 was said to have left several Colombian towns in complete desolation. A Portuguese ship imported the infection into Caravelleda, Venezuela, in 1580, where it also destroyed entire tribes of Indians.

As we saw above, fresh epidemics of smallpox struck northern Peru in 1533 and 1535. They were followed by others in 1558 and 1585. One witness to the 1585 outbreak in Peru left one of the few descriptions we have of the sixteenth-century epidemics:

> They died by scores and hundreds. Villages were depopulated. Corpses were scattered over the fields or piled up in the houses or huts. All branches of industrial activity were paralyzed. The fields were uncultivated; the herds were untended; and the workshops and the mines were without laborers. It was only with difficulty that the ships could be manned. The price of food rose to such an extent that many persons found it beyond their reach. They escaped the foul disease, but only to be wasted by famine. (Moses 1914, 1:385)

Spanish soldiers introduced smallpox into Chile for the first time in 1554, around the time that the local Araucanian Indians killed the Spanish explorer and colonizer Pedro de Valdivia. This outbreak continued into the next year, and one writer described a district of about twelve thousand persons, "of which number not more than one hundred escaped with life" (Molina 1809, 2:159). Seven years later, when the new Spanish governor of Chile arrived to take up his appointment on 5 June, the ship that brought him from Peru also brought several persons suffering from smallpox, which then spread rapidly, "especially among the Indians" (Moses 1914, 1:359). According to Elliot (1911), in the next recorded Chilean epidemic, in 1591, about three hundred Spaniards, some of whom may have been born in the New World, died of the disease, and the Araucanian Indians again "suffered terribly." Elliot (1911) also records that this outbreak was so severe it temporarily halted a war in progress between the Spanish and the Indians.[2]

A year after Spanish soldiers introduced the virus into Chile, French Huguenots carried the infection to Brazil while establishing a small settlement at the site of Rio de Janeiro in 1555. According to Moll, this epidemic "attacked the Indians and made them flee the coast" (1944, 512). Five years later, African slaves may have also introduced smallpox into Brazil. A more severe epidemic originating in Portugal in 1562 started at Itaparica Island and ravaged Bahia, killing at least thirty thousand Indians within three months.

Less than a year after the epidemic on Itaparica Island, a ship from Portugal introduced smallpox into Ilhéus in January 1563, and this epidemic also spread to Bahia, killing between one-fourth and two-thirds of those who had escaped the preceding epidemic. From Bahia, the contagion spread along the coast to Pernambuco, and deep into the Indian populations of the forested interior, where it was followed by famine. It killed a hundred thousand persons in Chito Province alone. Jesuit settlements of Indians around Bahia and Olinda were destroyed or abandoned. A letter from a Portuguese resident of Bahia, dated 12 May 1563, stated:

> This was a form of smallpox or pox so loathsome and evil-smelling that none could stand the great stench that emerged from them. For this reason many died untended, consumed by the worms that grew in the wounds of the pox and were engendered in their bodies in such abundance and of such great size that they caused horror and shock to any who saw them. (Hemming 1978, 142)

Another author was probably referring to the epidemic of 1563 when he concluded that "historically, the most important occurrence during the French occupation [1555–65] was the outbreak of a deadly epidemic of smallpox which wiped out more than half the natives of the State of Bahia" (Crow 1946, 241–42). As we have seen, however, smallpox apparently had been imported into coastal Brazil at least four times over that decade: once from France, once from Africa, and twice from Portugal.

When another epidemic struck other groups of Indians in Jesuit-controlled settlements in Espírito Santo in 1565, it was described as "a pitiful spectacle. The houses served equally as hospitals for the sick and cemeteries for the dead" (Hemming 1978, 144). Rio de Janeiro, founded by the Portuguese in 1567, experienced its first outbreak of smallpox the very next year. Smallpox proclaimed its ascendency, erupting in epidemics over the entire South American continent in 1588.

As wave upon wave of savage smallpox epidemics continued to decimate native populations throughout Latin America, depopulation became as important to the continent's subsequent history as the disease's earlier supporting role in the conquest of Mexico and Peru. G. Fernández Oveido, who witnessed smallpox's impact on Hispanola first hand, said the Indians of that island, who numbered as many as three hundred thousand to one million when Columbus arrived, were down to five hundred in 1541. He attributed their decline to "so many diseases, especially pestilential smallpox" (Simpson 1954, 680). Thirty years after the Peruvian conquest, the descendents of the Incas had been reduced at least by half, and possibly by three-quarters. In 1568, only about three million of Mexico's former 15–30 million remained.

In Brazil especially, Jesuit missionaries unwittingly made the Indians even more vulnerable to smallpox by herding them into *aldeias*, or settlements. The resettlement program commenced immediately before the early epidemics struck coastal Brazil in the 1560s. According to John Hemming, who recently chronicled the conquest of the Brazilian Indians, their reaction to these epidemics, which they associated with the Europeans, was to "fear the missionaries and respect them more" (1978, 141). As their converts died almost as fast as they were baptized, the Jesuits responded by rounding up even more Indians from the interior. Some of the Jesuits, observed Hemming, "may have believed that it was better for Indians to be baptized but dead than heathen but alive and free" (ibid., 145).

SEVENTEENTH CENTURY

Some of the sixteenth-century epidemics on the Brazilian coast were carried inland by terrified Indians trying to escape the infection. Indians living deep in the interior of Brazil lost their relative isolation altogether in the seventeenth century, when Jesuit missionaries penetrated the upper regions of the Amazon and began to herd them into missions. Whatever benefits of religion, civilization, or freedom from slavery the Indians gained were achieved at a horrendous price, as smallpox helped strip the continent's interior of its native inhabitants.

Around the middle of the century, Jesuits established ten missions in "Mainas," a region stretching 1,500 miles along the banks of the Marañón, Huallaga, and Ucayali rivers in Peru, and along the Amazon as far as Manaus in Brazil. Thirty years later, some one hundred thousand Indians were gathered around these missions. They might as well have been in a slaughter house. The first smallpox epidemic in 1660 killed forty-four thousand Indians, nearly half the mission population in Phelan's estimate (1967). A second epidemic of smallpox nine years later carried off another twenty thousand victims and continued to claim victims among other Indians in the forest. The missions were finally abandoned under the impact of epidemics, Indian revolts, and Portuguese slave raids.

Mexico's Indian population reached its nadir of about 1.6 million persons in 1620. Thereafter, it began to recover, although as D'Ardois has documented epidemic smallpox continued to plague Moctezuma's heirs at seventeen- to eighteen-year intervals.

As we shall see in chapter 7, smallpox had an equally devastating effect on the North American Indian population, though it started there a century later. Moreover, although there is no lack of evidence that the Spanish often abused and punished Indian slaves brutally, there appears to have been a fundamental difference in the way smallpox's decimation of the indigenous population was regarded by predominantly Protestant colonizers in North America and their Catholic counterparts to the south. Portuguese and Spanish immigrants generally deplored the disease's impact on the Indians and actively tried, albeit ineffectively, to minimize it (there were economic as well as humanitarian considerations at work here). In North America, in contrast, although there were some who sympathized with the Indians' plight, most early European immigrants viewed smallpox as God's beneficent way of removing an obstacle to their settlement, and some deliberately spread it to the Indians.

Smallpox's impact on the economies of seventeenth-century Latin American colonies was considerable and derived largely from its destruction of the Indians. In 1700, for example, the Crown was asked to grant a Portuguese settler permission to obtain 120 fresh Indian slaves for a sugar mill after his previous slaves were wiped out by smallpox, and in 1703, another Brazilian town was authorized to bring in a whole tribe in order "to make good the loses of its native laborers from smallpox" (Hemming 1978, 370, 419). Because of the acute shortage of labor caused by another epidemic, in a letter dated 3 March 1644, a local Portuguese official recommended importing Indians from Pará "to repopulate the villages wiped out by smallpox" (Kieman 1973, 58).

As Amerindian populations declined, the difficulty of finding Indian replacements intensified the demand for African slaves to work on plantations and in the mines. African slaves also suffered severely in New World epidemics, but many had been exposed to smallpox in Africa, by design or by accident, and as a group they were usually less susceptible than the Indians. As the slave trade was stepped up, however, so was the risk of imported smallpox.

The danger posed by newly imported, infected slaves was widely recognized. In 1603 slave ships introduced smallpox into Buenos Aires, which suffered six other major epidemics before the century was out. The viceroy of Peru ordered all new slaves to be quarantined and inspected for smallpox in 1630. When smallpox was reintroduced into Venezuela in 1693, a local official was prosecuted for falsely certifying the good health of a shipload of slaves (Moll 1944, 86). As we saw in chapter 5, toward the end of the 1680s, Bahia almost stopped sending slave ships to Angola, because of an epidemic of smallpox in the African colony. By this time, slave ships were also exporting smallpox from the West Indies to North America.

In Brazil, the first large epidemic of the seventeenth century struck the coastal city of Maranhão in 1621. According to Hemming (1978) most of the predominantly Indian victims did not survive more than three days after becoming ill. Other epidemics raked the whole coast in 1631, 1642, 1662–63, and 1665–66. The epidemic in 1642 killed an estimated three thousand free and slave Indians in Maranhão alone. This epidemic, wrote Hemming, "raged so violently among the Indians that entire aldeias were almost totally extinguished. The survivors retreated into the forest, since they no longer dared to remain in their homes" (ibid., 293). Maranhão was also hit hard by the epidemic of 1662–63. In the words of one local Jesuit,

> Maranhão was burning with a plague of smallpox. The missionary fathers often dug graves with their own hands to bury the dead, for there were aldeias where there were not two Indians left on foot. Parents abandoned their children and fled into the forests in order not to be struck by that pestilential evil. (Ibid., 338)

At one interior village near the town of Cametá, the same priest came upon a group of Indians who had fled into the forest:

> They were so covered in pox and putridity that they caused horror to their own families. When they saw that a Father wanted to confess them they told me not to approach, for the rotten smell they were giving off was intolerable. I rather feared that I would not hear them well, but it was God's pleasure that I heard them better than the others; and the rotten smell seemed to me like the smell of white bread when it is removed from the oven. To confess them I was forced to put my mouth close to their ears, which were full of nauseating matter from the pox, with which they were entirely covered. (Ibid., 339)

During the next epidemic, in 1665–66, mortality was especially high among African slaves:

> This was a fatal year to Brazil. The small pox broke out in Pernambuco and spread along the coast to Rio de Janeiro. The mortality was dreadful; families of forty or fifty persons sickened at once, so that there was not in the whole establishment one who had strength enough to assist the rest, go for medical assistance, or seek such remedies as were at hand. . . . The disease became less fatal as it proceeded southward; but its ravages were dreadful. Many *Engehhos* in the Reconcave lost all their Negroes, and wealthy proprietors were thus at once reduced to irremediable poverty. So great was the mortality that hands were wanting for agriculture; many years of famine followed; and Rocha Pitta, writing about half a century afterwards, declares that the effects of the visitation were still felt. (Southey 1817, 2: 554–55)

Bahia's economy also suffered a severe blow in 1680–84, when a more localized epidemic coincided with a three-year-long drought. Russell-Wood (1968) reports that this outbreak reduced the number of slaves of the Reconcavo (bay area) at Bahia so severely that sugar production was reduced drastically. Elsewhere, in the Spanish territories, there were similar problems.

Chile and Guatemala each recorded three epidemics of smallpox in the seventeenth century. In Chile, some fifty thousand deaths were attributed to smallpox in 1619–20 alone. During the Chilean epidemic of 1654, Jesuit missionaries baptized an unusually large number of Araucanians, because of the desperation smallpox caused among the Indians. In Ecuador, smallpox was epidemic seven times during the century, killing over sixty thousand persons in 1680 (Moll 1944; Dobyns 1963). Even so, the historian J. L. Phelan believed Indian populations in Ecuador's highlands suffered less than those in Mexico and Peru.

Laval (1967–68) and Penna (1885) describe other epidemics that affected the Spanish military garrison in Chile in 1660 and in Peru a few years later. One of the few military engagements disrupted by smallpox in this period and region took place in 1597, when French soldiers and their Indian allies attacked a Portuguese fort on the Paraiba River. When the Portuguese counterattacked, their column of about a thousand men lost ten to twelve of its members daily during an epidemic of smallpox. The same outbreak affected the French's Indian allies even more, however, and prevented several French offensives (Hemming 1978, 169).

EIGHTEENTH CENTURY

Almost two hundred years exactly after it removed the last independent Peruvian Inca, smallpox killed the youthful king of Spain, who claimed the thrones of Huayna Capac and his fellow New World sovereign, Cuitláhuac. The Spanish king's painful death from smallpox three years after inoculation was introduced into Europe didn't hasten the adoption of inoculation in Spain's American colonies anymore than in Spain itself. With no traditional knowledge of effective empirical countermeasures, since the disease had only appeared among them a few generations earlier, the rapidly dwindling indigenous populations of South America were entirely dependent on European and African immigrants for specific ways to combat smallpox. As it turned out, inoculation was introduced into Portuguese Brazil over thirty-five years before it was practiced in one of the Spanish colonies.

The fact that Brazilian slaves were mostly imported from southern Africa, especially Angola, during the sixteenth to eighteenth centuries, whereas Yoruba-speaking slaves from West Africa were imported in large quantities only after 1770, may account in part for why inoculation became known in Brazil as late as it did. Although the Yoruba almost certainly practiced inoculation by this time, inoculation, and apparently smallpox, were relatively recent arrivals in southern Africa. Even North Americans, whose slaves were largely from West Africa, where inoculation had been widely known for generations, and possibly for centuries, only learned of inoculation from one of those slaves in 1706.

Before Roman Catholic missionaries introduced inoculation into Brazil in 1728, early Brazilian settlers who caught smallpox are said to have favored "powdered horse excrement" as a cure (Crow 1946). Like other Europeans, the Portuguese were only beginning to understand basic facts about the disease, how it spread, and how it should be treated. In the meantime, various antiquated therapies were still employed, according to the beliefs of the therapist. The use of powdered horse excrement was based on the belief that smallpox resulted from evil spirits in the body and required a repulsive medicine such as this to be taken orally in order to drive them out.

Other seventeenth-century epidemics in Brazil were fought the only way physicians of the period and well-intentioned, medically-minded missionaries knew how: by bleeding. Thus, a deadly epidemic of hemorrhagic smallpox that struck Jesuit missions in Brazil in 1695 was doubly sanguinary. In the words of one of the Jesuits:

> As soon as I heard that this epidemic was raging in other reductions, I wanted to let the blood of mine as fast as possible, from children of ten up to old people, so that if the disease attacked it would find the rotten blood eliminated. . . . It was something to see the streets reddened with quantities of spilled blood—a horrible, cruel spectacle that brought tears to the eyes and sighs to the heart. (Hemming 1978, 468)

Elsewhere in Latin America, religious ceremonies undertaken to mitigate epidemics of smallpox may have helped spread the disease. B. W. Diffie noted that "the system of combatting smallpox and other diseases by holding religious processions guaranteed that everybody in the community would be exposed" (1945, 448). A diphtheria epidemic in Cuzco, Peru, in 1614, for example, "called forth a great burst of Catholic ritual activity aimed at propitiating saintly intercessors so as to end the threat" (Dobyns 1963, 509). Laval reports there were repeated religious processions during the epidemic of smallpox in Santiago, Chile, in 1660. In such circumstances, there was little to lose by trying an unproven, but reportedly effective way of preventing smallpox.

In 1728 a Carmelite missionary who had read European newspapers describing the recent successful introduction of inoculation into Europe resorted to the same practice in desperation as smallpox raged among Indians in his mission at Pará (Belém), near the mouth of the Amazon. Fifteen or twenty years later, the same missionary described his exploit to a Frenchman who was exploring the Amazon and told the explorer how another missionary had later also successfully inoculated Indians on the Río Negro, about eight hundred miles upstream. The French explorer was Charles Marie de la Condamine, and this encounter in the Amazon helped stimulate him to become the foremost advocate of inoculation in France. (Miller 1957, 209). Jesuits introduced inoculation into Bahia in 1743.

While it was more effective than blood-letting, and if undertaken with proper precautions, it was perhaps only slightly more risky to the public during epidemics than large religious processions, inoculation didn't end Brazil's problem. In eighteenth-century Bahia, the threat was so acute that "some land owners refused to leave their plantations in the Reconcavo to come to the city from fear of catching smallpox. At the same time, "any criminal sent from the interior to the gaol in Bahia could regard his imprisonment a death sentence because of this disease" (Russell-Wood 1968, 290). During an epidemic in 1750, a local governor reported "one could calculate the total loss at 40,000 persons around Belém alone" (Hemming 1978, 446). Indians in Amazon mission settlements suffered severe smallpox epidemics during the eight years 1743–50, and again in 1762 (Lersch 1896; Boxer 1962). Only about one-fifth of ninety thousand Indians in the settlements survived the latter outbreak. There were other major epidemics of smallpox in Brazil in 1707, 1725, 1753, and 1793–1800.[3]

New World Spaniards had a longer wait for specific countermeasures, which did not reach their colonies until the second half of the century. Even so, inoculation was practiced in several of the Spanish colonies before it was used in Madrid. Inoculation was introduced for the first time into Chile in 1765, Venezuela in 1769, Argentina in 1777, Peru in 1778, Mexico in 1779, and Guatemala in 1780. It was not adopted in Spain until 1771. Only in 1785 did the Spanish Crown officially recommend isolation of victims to help alleviate the scourge of smallpox in the colonies.

Smallpox thus was almost uncontrolled in the Spanish colonies, except for quarantine, during most of the eighteenth century. Buenos Aires led the continent's major cities with the greatest number of smallpox epidemics reported during this century. It had nine, in 1700, 1705, 1733, 1734, 1738, 1744, 1770, 1778, and 1792–93. Quito, Ecuador, had seven. The entire Plata region was affected in 1716, and two years later, an epidemic killed more than seventeen thousand persons at Córdoba, Argentina. The disease claimed another seventeen thousand lives, mainly Indians, in the Río de la Plata area the year after the Córdoba epidemic.[4] Epidemics engulfed all of Argentina in 1778–79.

Chile was struck by an epidemic of smallpox and an earthquake in 1730, followed by four other major epidemics later in the century. In 1765, the year inoculation was introduced into Chile, smallpox killed over five thousand persons at Santiago alone. During the outbreak of 1788–89, Concepción lost one fourth of its six thousand inhabitants to the disease.

Smallpox was pandemic again throughout South America in 1764–65, and also in Mexico, as we shall see.

Imported slaves continued to be a dangerous source of smallpox on the South American mainland and in the Caribbean. A shipment of infected slaves caused a fresh epidemic in French Guiana in 1766. The importation of infected Africans to the Caribbean brought much suffering to the inhabitants of the islands themselves, as well as to North American ports that received transshipped slaves from the West Indies. The population of most of the islands was small enough that epidemics died out after a while—until another ship brought the virus back again. Cuba had five epidemics in this century. On the island of Hispanola, smallpox was epidemic in Haiti in 1738, and returned for an encore with measles in 1740–41. Ten years later, Haitian authorities refused to allow a ship with smallpox aboard to dock without undergoing quarantine (Moll 1944).

At mid-century, an epidemic of smallpox interrupted Trinidad's economic recovery from a disastrous failure of its cocoa crop, one year before the English invaded the island. Local Indians bore the brunt of that epidemic. On Barbados, smallpox contributed to the excess of three hundred more deaths than births in 1759, and with yellow fever, reduced that island's slave population from 68,548 to 57,434 during the decade ending in 1783. Another epidemic of smallpox on Barbados in 1751 counted George Washington, who was there helping his convalescent brother recover from tuberculosis, among its survivors.

Even without inoculation, which as we saw, was only introduced into Mexico in 1779, Mexico's population recovered from its low point after the early seventeenth century, so that by the beginning of the eighteenth, there were about four million Mexicans. However, Peru's population continued to decline, until there were only about six hundred thousand to one million Indians remaining at the end of the eighteenth century. Smallpox epidemics in 1756, 1762, and 1764 contributed to the Peruvian decline. Outbreaks of smallpox are mentioned in Baja California for the first time in 1709, and elsewhere in Mexican California in 1737 and 1747, but Mexico apparently escaped any major epidemics during the century's first half.

Mexicans recalled what they'd been spared in the first half of the century when three widespread epidemics of smallpox struck the country again during the second half. The first killed some ten thousand people in Mexico City in 1762. The next epidemic in 1779 was more terrible than the first, causing an estimated eighteen thousand deaths. In December 1779, the viceroy wrote King Carlos III, saying: "There is nothing but corpses seen in the streets and throughout the city one hears only outcries and laments" (Cooper 1965, 63; D'Ardois 1961, 1018). It was during this latter outbreak that inoculation was introduced into Mexico. Outbreaks in

Baja California during 1780–82 "carried off thousands of natives" (North 1908, 51; Meigs 1935, 135).

The third epidemic, which struck Mexico City in 1797, was better documented than any of its predecessors in Latin America, a distinction it fully deserved. The following summary of that outbreak is largely based on S. F. Cook's 1939 account. The epidemic was popularly thought to have derived from smallpox imported into northern Guatemala or Acapulco by a ship from Peru in April 1796. Two of the patients on board were daughters of the regent of the Royal Audiencia, one Don Ambrosio Cerda. Smallpox was already endemic and increasingly prevalent in Mexico as long as six years before the contaminated ship sailed from Peru, however, and Cook concluded that the shipborne smallpox was irrelevant to the epidemic in question. During one of the smaller outbreaks in 1793, the Mexican viceroy's lawyer wisely advised him to count the number of known cases before deciding whether an epidemic was present (Cooper 1965, 89).

The series of outbreaks in question began late in 1795 in southwestern Mexico, spread along the main line of communications to Oaxaca in December 1796, to Mexico City in July and August 1797, and then spread radially from the capital, ending in 1798. Eighty-two thousand cases and nearly eleven thousand deaths from this epidemic were counted in Mexico City, Orizaba, and Puebla alone. Overall, Cook estimated, between 100,000 and 150,000 Mexicans were infected, of whom 14,000 to 25,000 died. Even so, local officials insisted that the outbreak in 1797 was less severe than the 1779 epidemic.

The epidemic in 1797 might have been even worse, had not some 60–70,000 inoculations been performed during the outbreak (Stearn & Stearn 1943). However, the inoculations could also have made the epidemic worse, depending on how the inoculees were cared for. The mortality rate among about 3,300 inoculated persons was 3.5 percent, compared to 18.5 percent in about 58,000 naturally acquired cases of smallpox. Three out of every four patients were less than twenty years old.

Mexican officials made vigorous attempts to contain the outbreaks, in addition to encouraging inoculation. The reader is referred to Robin Price's recent analysis (1982) of this epidemic and the valiant administrative measures taken against it. Patients were isolated in makeshift hospitals, although this was resisted in most instances by parents who were loathe to part with their children. Infected villages and towns were placed under strict quarantine, at great inconvenience to the inhabitants. The only legal exception to the strict quarantine of Oaxaca was to allow the silver from the mines in that area to be shipped to Mexico City and the colonial treasury. In the end, the deliberate interruption of traffic along the main highways between Oaxaca and Mexico City merely delayed the virus's march on the capital.

Although primary responsibility for control of outbreaks remained with local officials, all officials, clergy, and physicians were expected to report even a single case of smallpox directly to the central government, which lent any necessary assistance. Priests were particularly fruitful sources of information. Cook reported an example from Mexico City in which a curate realized during a funeral for a child in August 1797 that "the family was covering the face of the corpse and putting gloves on the hands, in order to avoid the discovery that the death was from smallpox" (1939a, 960).

At the height of the epidemic in Mexico City, the archbishop of Mexico, Alonzo Núñez de Haro y Peralta, who presided over the Junta Principal de Caridad, the main charity organization in the city, appointed a priest to each district board of charity and appealed for alms from the rich, promising "to return any unused balance adjusted to the original rate of contribution" after the epidemic ended. In a circular letter dated 31 October 1797, the archbishop temporarily empowered priests not otherwise so authorized to hear confessions of smallpox victims for the duration of the epidemic (De Haro y Peralta 1797).

This was Mexico's last outbreak during the prevaccination era.

Nineteenth Century

The nineteenth century brought three events that drastically reduced the death rate from smallpox in Latin America. The first was the introduction of vaccination. The second was abolition of the slave trade. And finally, *V. minor* appeared and spread as a kind of natural immunization against the more virulent variety of smallpox.[5]

Latin America's main concern in the nineteenth century, however, was the colonies' successful struggles for independence from their European mother countries. Haiti led the way, declaring itself independent of France in 1804. Within eight years rebellions began in Chile, Mexico, Paraguay, Uraguay, Venezuela, Bolivia, and Central America. Brazil proclaimed its independence from Portugal in 1822. Two years later, Spanish rule on the continent was ended at the Battle of Ayacucho, fought in a suitably spectacular Andean setting 9,000 feet (3,000 meters) above sea level, "on the road between Lima and Cuzco" (Pendle 1969, 108). Before these wars for political independence began, however, there was time for one last magnanimous gesture by the king of Spain, intended to aid his New World subjects in their struggle against smallpox.

Smallpox was epidemic in Buenos Aires, Chile, Uraguay, Peru, Guiana and Cuba as the century began. According to the medical historian A. A. Moll (1944), it was the description of the devastation caused by smallpox in Lima in 1802 that moved King Carlos IV to his "truly royal gesture." The king had also been primed for his action four years earlier, when smallpox attacked his daughter, Princess Maria Luisa, only a few months after Jenner announced his discovery of vaccination. Alarmed by his daughter's illness (she recovered), Carlos had his sons inoculated, and also promoted inoculation among his subjects. Spain, which had taken up the practice of inoculation only half a century after it became known in Europe, adopted Jennerian vaccination much more quickly. Thus, in 1803, the king issued a royal order for his Expedición Filantrópica de la Vacuna, or the Balmis-Salvany Expedition, as it came to be called after its leaders:

> Royal Order of September 1, 1803. The King, desiring to ameliorate the havoc wrought by the frequent smallpox epidemics in his dominions of the Indies and in order to furnish his royal subjects the protection they deserve and for the good of the State, and of the people and the immense number who suffer more because they are poor as well as others who expect the royal bounty, it was resolved, after hearing the opinion of the Council and of the men of science that the vaccine should be sent to North and South America, and if it were possible, to the Philippine Islands also, at royal expense, employing vaccination which has been proven in Spain and in almost the rest of Europe as a preventive against smallpox. (Bantug 1953, 107)

Michael Smith (1974) provides an excellent account of the background and course of this expedition. Carlos's motives were not only humanitarian. There was also "the good of the State" to consider. Before the Balmis-Salvany Expedition left Spain, a report by one of the king's physicians declared smallpox to be the "first and principal cause of the depopulation of America." The governor of the Council of the Indies noted further that the depopulation meant less tribute, commerce, mining, and farming in the colonies, and that the economic benefits of such a mission would justify paying for it from the royal treasury.

Thus the Spanish monarch decided to provide Jenner's vaccine to all his colonies around the world. He commissioned his Surgeon Extraordinary, Don Francisco Xavier Balmis, to lead a maritime expedition that would visit each of the colonies in turn, bringing cowpox virus. The vaccine was maintained during the voyages by sequentially vaccinating, arm to arm, susceptible children brought along specifically for that purpose. In addition to Balmis and twenty-two young orphans, the expedition included four physicians, two stewards, and three nurses.

Sailing from the Spanish port of Corunna on 20 November 1803, the tiny fleet of three ships made its first landing in the new world at Puerto Rico, on 9 February 1804, after a stopover in the Canary Islands. At their next stop, Venezuela, the expedition divided into two groups. Balmis led one group to Cuba, then Yucatán. After crossing Mexico and collecting twenty-six new children, he continued to the Philippines and two Chinese ports before returning to Spain in 1806, whereupon he "had the honour of kissing his Majesty's hand" at San Ildefonso on 7 September ("Diffusion of Vaccination," 1896, 1269). The second group, commanded by the expedition's deputy director José Salvany, was shipwrecked in the mouth of Colombia's Magdalena River. After they were rescued, they proceeded to Cartagena, crossed the isthmus of Panama, and vaccinated "no fewer than 50,000 persons along the Peruvian coast" (ibid.) After a stop in Buenos Aires, this group called at Chile in January 1808 before it also returned to Spain via the Philippines.

In return for their services the orphan boys were educated at the king's expense. Smith (1974) says that when the first group arrived at Mexico City, their tutor had a hard time discouraging the swear words they had learned from the Spanish sailors. The Balmis-Salvany Expedition allegedly discovered natural sources of cowpox in the Mexican valley of Atlixco and in the Venezuelan province of Caracas.

For all its fanfare, the Balmis-Salvany Expedition was preceded by numerous other attempts, some of which were successful, to introduce vaccine and vaccination into Spanish and Portuguese America. Indeed, Moll states that "in Brazil the vaccine had been brought by Mendes-Ribeioro [to Rio] as early as 1798, . . . and again in Bolivia in 1804, and in Rio and Sao Paulo in 1805" (1944, 235, 542). Vaccine was also introduced into Guatemala in 1800, and into Cuba, Puerto Rico, Mexico, Costa Rica, Peru, Uruguay, Argentina, and Chile between 1802 and 1807. The vaccine introduced into Montevideo, Uruguay, in 1805 was from vaccinated slaves aboard a slave ship en route from Lisbon to Bahia.

Other attempts to introduce cowpox vaccine into Latin America failed. Haiti, which took advantage of yellow fever to defeat Napoleon's soldiers, still had not secured an effective supply of smallpox vaccine before 1816, as is clear from King Henri Christophe's letter to James Moore, director of London's National Vaccine Institute (Saunders 1982, 365–66):

Palace of San Souci
5, February, 1816

The King to James Moore
Director, National Vaccine Inst.

Mr. Prince Sanders presented to me the work, bearing my direction, on the subject of the smallpox; I accepted it with pleasure and I feel infinite obligation for your generous attention and the great interest you take in the preservation of the Haitians. . . . my intention is to give all possible latitude to the happy results of that immortal discovery which I have not hitherto been able to put into practice, on account of the difficulty I experienced in my application to Jamaica, St. Thomas and the United States relative to this object.

Henry

Haiti vaccinated its army against smallpox in 1825.

Smallpox continued to plague the Latin American colonies, and later the young republics, throughout the nineteenth century, although with decreasing intensity. In Mexico, smallpox dampened independence celebrations by staging an epidemic in 1813–14, which was followed by five other epidemics later in the century. One of the later outbreaks, in 1839–40, coincided with the great pandemic then raging among Indians in the United States and Canada.

Smallpox was unusually prevalent in Argentina in 1818, 1829, 1836–37, 1843, 1847, and 1890. Buenos Aires had thirteen epidemics in this century, two of the later ones (in 1872 and 1890) causing about eight thousand, four hundred and two thousand, two hundred deaths, respectively. In Bolivia, an epidemic killed ten percent of the residents of Sucre in 1888–89. In Uruguay, the disease was epidemic seven times. Chile, which had eight epidemics in this century, buried twenty-two thousand smallpox victims between 1840 and 1876, and another twenty-seven thousand between 1890 and 1898.

Densely populated port cities were favored sites for epidemics in nineteenth-century Brazil. Rio de Janeiro suffered eleven major outbreaks, while Pará had seven. As the century ended, smallpox was epidemic in Rio in 1895 (1, 865 deaths reported), in Pernambuco in 1896 (2,119 deaths), Bahia in 1897 (1,676 deaths), and Rio again in 1899 (1, 395 deaths). Much later, a resident of Rio recalled that when he first came to that city in 1887, it

> was periodically devastated by smallpox and yellow fever. In the center of the downtown area, where the coffee businesses were located, the toll was great. . . . There was no isolation of the victims; the patient was treated at home. It was said that yellow fever hit the foreigners in particular and smallpox struck the Negroes. (Freyre 1970, 342–43)

At Fortaleza on the northeast Brazilian coast, a massive epidemic erupted in 1878 among refugees who converged on the city after fleeing a severe drought in the surrounding region of Ceará. Refugees had swollen the town's population to about 125,000 before smallpox broke out and killed 56,791 victims in a few months, half of them in November and December. One witness described the grisly scene in December:

> If the pestilence was hidden in the city, it was visible everywhere about the camps. Half-recovered patients sat apart, but scarcely heeded;

in almost every hut the sick were lying, horrible with the foul disease. Many dead were waiting for the body carriers; many more would be waiting at the morning round. Yet here, among the sick and dying and dead, there was the same indifference to danger that I noticed in the city. The peasants were talking and laughing with each other; three or four were gathered about a mat, gambling for biscuits; everywhere the ghastly patients and ghastlier corpses were passed unnoticed; they were too common to be the objects of curiosity. (Smith 1880, 422–23)

Another witness to the same epidemic wrote that

S. verified 808 deaths in one day.... The cemeteries have long since been filled. Graves åre supposed to hold twelve bodies; but so great was the demand for space that often twenty-five were put into the same hole; there is no burial service, and the diggers faint while digging, from fearful stench. ("Smallpox in Brazil," 1879, 156).

One of the victims was the wife of the provincial president. She died of hemorrhagic smallpox at the end of December.

Other notable epidemics struck the islands of St. Thomas in 1843 (infecting at least one sixth of the population), Antigua in 1862 (where the disease had been absent for more than fifty years but emancipated slaves neglected vaccinations), Jamaica in 1851 (the virus was imported by a group of liberated Africans), and Hispanola in 1882 (more than three thousand persons died in Port au Prince).

Twelve years after the previous outbreak in Jamaica, smallpox again broke out in Kingston and adjacent St. Andrew's Parish early in 1863. Unlike its well-known, ferocious antecedents in Latin America, however, this was "a peculiar epidemic." According to one physician, who treated 115 patients, none of his patients died:

In some of the cases I saw, the eruption was apparently that of simple [chickenpox], while in others, from mere inspection of the eruption, a medical man unacquainted with the character of the prevailing epidemic would unhesitatingly state that they were instances of genuine variola. (Anderson 1866, 414).

This was "the first unequivocal description" or world premiere, of *V. minor* (Dixon 1962, 203). Where it came from, and where if anywhere, it had been while *V. major* was attacking people for so long, no one knows. Some authors have speculated that it spread to Jamaica from southern Africa. Earlier, less complete descriptions of "mild smallpox" could have resulted from confusion with chickenpox, or confusion with modified smallpox in persons with waning vaccinal immunity. Over the next several decades, *V. minor* essentially replaced *V. major* in much of Latin America.

V. minor unfortunately didn't spread to Trinidad before a mail steamer brought virulent smallpox to that island on 4 August 1871. The disease had already killed one passenger during the fourteen-day voyage from England. Smallpox was prevalent in England that year as part of the European pandemic started by the Franco-Prussian War. By the time the outbreak on Trinidad ended in 1872, the island's medical officer of Health had resigned in frustration and disgust, and over twelve and a half thousand cases of smallpox were reported, of whom 2,449 died. During the epidemic, one of Trinidad's residents wrote to the *Medical Times and Gazette* of London:

> Business is at a standstill; the only thing thought about or talked about is the epidemic. The worst of it is that no one can get away; all the steamers refuse to take passengers, and there are, as yet, but very few sailing vessels for Europe. ("Epidemic of Smallpox in Trinidad," 1872, 1: 264)

The economic impact of outbreaks such as the one in Trinidad was further illustrated when a traveler imported smallpox from Canada to Barbados in 1902, causing a year-long outbreak with 1,466 cases and 118 deaths. The epidemic caused Barbados to be quarantined by its neighbors, reduced government revenues by nearly 22,000 pounds, increased government expenditures by almost 18,000 pounds and resulted in a total loss of trade estimated at 6,000 pounds (Starkey 1939). Thus, smallpox could still paralyze countries of the region, which was still surprisingly vulnerable to unpredictable epidemics, but not for much longer.

Slavery and the slave trade were abolished in stages during the nineteenth century, beginning with abolition of the trade by Britain and the United States in 1807, and ending with the abolition of slavery itself in the United States in the 1860s, and in Cuba and Brazil in the 1880s. This removed one of the most important sources of imported smallpox. It obviously did not end the threat altogether, since the disease was endemic in many countries. Moreover, Spain was still one of the most highly endemic countries in Europe, and other types of trade and traffic with Spain continued after the attainment of political independence. Spanish troops introduced smallpox into Colombia in 1815, causing the first large outbreak in that country in several years. In Cuba, which experienced thirteen epidemics of smallpox during the nineteenth century, the epidemic of 1887-88 was also started by the arrival of troops from Spain. One nineteenth-century author believed the Spanish used smallpox at least passively in their struggle with the Cubans (Woodson 1898).

Beginning in 1897, Puerto Rico showed what a determined effort to make maximum use of Jenner's vaccine could do. Smallpox was epidemic in Puerto Rico five times between 1804 and 1885, and over three thousand cases were reported on the island in 1896. Soon after the United States occupied Puerto Rico in 1898, about eighty percent of the island's one million inhabitants were vaccinated in a mass campaign. Vaccine for the crash program was produced locally by using calves borrowed from local cattlemen. Another epidemic in December 1898, and the threat of quarantine by New York City and other U.S. ports, greatly stimulated the later stages of the campaign. By October 1899, smallpox had been eradicated from Puerto Rico (Wadhams 1889–90; Hyde 1901).

TWENTIETH CENTURY

Although health authorities in Puerto Rico had to use borrowed calves to make enough vaccine for their successful eradication campaign, several Latin American nations had already established institutes to produce smallpox vaccine in sufficient quantities for national use. Availability of locally produced vaccine was more important then than later in the twentieth century, when addition of glycerine and freeze-drying techniques made shipment of potent vaccine from one county to another easier. Vaccine institutes were established in Brazil in 1846, in Peru in 1896, in Venezuela in 1898, in Argentina and Bolivia in 1903, in Guatemala and El Salvador in 1904, and in Honduras in 1911.

Mexico, Chile, and Brazil were the Latin American countries most severely affected by smallpox during the first decade of the twentieth century.[6] In Brazil, smallpox was epidemic in Belém in 1904–5, Recife (3,800 deaths in 1905), and Rio (3600 deaths in 1904). When the Brazilian government passed a bill for compulsory vaccination in 1904, "an anti-vaccination agitation was started against the measure, and this culminated in open revolt with riots in the streets necessitating the use of a military force to establish order" (Low 1918, 85–87). Epidemic smallpox returned to cause another 1,800 deaths in Recife, and 6,500 deaths in Rio three and four years after the compulsory vaccination bill was enacted. From Rio, the 1908 outbreak spread "along the Central Railway Line" to Sao Paulo and Santos. An epidemic also struck Bahia again in 1908–10.

In Chile, smallpox killed over 3,500 people in Santiago (pop. 350,000) in 1905, and spread to the country's second-largest city, Valparaiso (pop. 180,000), where it caused more than 5,600 deaths the same year. Both cities shut down their schools because of the outbreak. In Valparaiso, municipal authorities removed from the streets at least thirty-five corpses of persons "who had died from smallpox and had been abandoned in panic by their relatives" (ibid., 81). The disease spread by ship from Valparaiso to five other Chilean ports. As in Brazil the year before, the epidemic moved the Chilean government to pass a law making vaccination compulsory.

Like Chile and Brazil, other governments had begun to pass and implement compulsory vaccination laws, often as a direct response to severe local epidemics. Such laws, which usually required all infants to have primary vaccination, and often required revaccination in early childhood, were put forth in Uruguay as early as 1850, in Costa Rica (1884), Argentina (1904), Guatemala (1905), Venezuela (1909), again in Uruguay (1911), Bolivia (1912), Dominican Republic and Haiti (1921), and in Mexico, in a renewed effort, in 1925. The value of these legislative efforts was seriously limited, however, in Latin America as elsewhere at that time, by the fact that they were rarely enforced, and because the vaccines used then were sometimes unreliable.

In its own way, *V. minor* was also helping to reduce deaths from smallpox by "immunizing" susceptible persons in epidemics of its own, in which relatively few of the infected persons died. This mild variety of smallpox had spread over North America starting in 1896, and was already widely prevalent in the Caribbean, where outbreaks had recently been reported in Trinidad, Puerto Rico, British Guiana and Barbados.

In 1910, *V. minor* was described in Brazil for the first time, where it was thought to have been introduced at Bahia before spreading to southern states, including Sao Paulo and Paraná. During the outbreak in Paraná in 1910, some five to six thousand persons were infected, of whom less than 2.3 percent died. As *V. minor* spread throughout Brazil, it came to be known locally as *alastrim*, a word reportedly derived from "a Portuguese verb, *alastrar*, which conveys the idea of something which melts and spreads" (Greenwood 1935, 242). Twenty years after alastrim's first appearance in Brazil, the low proportion of deaths (under two percent) among the many cases of smallpox still occurring gave proof that alastrim had virtually replaced *V. major* in that country. Virulent smallpox made its final appearance in Rio de Janeiro in an epidemic which killed two thousand, two hundred persons in 1926.

V. minor ushered in the 1920s with epidemics in Jamaica, Cuba, and Haiti. From Haiti, it spread to the Dominican Republic, and returning sugar cane workers carried it home to Anguilla from the Dominican Republic in August, 1921. Parsons (1930) argues, however, that since about ten percent of the more than three thousand victims treated in Port au Prince's General Hospital in 1920–21 died, however, *V. major* must also have been present in Haiti. *V. minor* was also epidemic in Venezuela in 1922–23. Virulent smallpox was still widely prevalent in Argentina, where it claimed nearly ten thousand lives in 1922, and in Chile, where eleven thousand died in 1921–23.

In Mexico, which had a population of about fifteen million in 1910, smallpox killed an average of over ten thousand persons annually in the 1920s—the highest amount of smallpox in proportion to its population of any country in the world at that time. Thus, when *V. minor* appeared in the populous, but poorly vaccinated country in 1932, it may have been a blessing in disguise. Unlike in Brazil and the United States however, it did not displace *V. major*.

Cuba, which had reported over seven thousand cases of smallpox in 1921, rapidly reversed its situation and eradicated the disease from the island by the end of 1923. Chile reported its last large outbreak of smallpox the same year. Bolivia, Brazil, Colombia, Mexico, and Peru, meanwhile, continued to report large numbers of cases of smallpox for twenty more years.

The last colossal outbreaks of *V. major* in Latin America occurred in Peru, where the disease killed nearly ten thousand persons in 1941–43, and in Mexico, where over eight thousand persons perished in 1942–43. Epidemics were also recorded in Colombia in 1943 and 1947, and Bolivia in 1944–46. Brazil reported a nationwide outbreak of alastrim in 1944–45.

By the end of World War II, the disease had been eradicated from all of the Caribbean Islands, the Guianas, Central America, Panama, and Chile. Mexico, which by now had drastically reduced its levels of smallpox, reported only eleven hundred cases in 1947, a year when much smaller Ecuador reported three thousand cases, and Colombia reported nearly four thousand cases. In Venezuela, an outbreak of over six thousand cases in 1947–48 resulted in a national eradication campaign (Halbrohr 1973).

Following a decision by the Pan American Health Organization in 1950 to begin an effort to eradicate smallpox in the Western Hemisphere, Venezuela, Mexico, Peru, and Bolivia each succeeded in doing just that before the end of that decade. Bolivia, which had had the highest amount of the disease proportionate to its population in the Americas in 1957, saw its last case in 1959. Uruguay freed itself in 1962, Ecuador in 1964, and Colombia and Paraguay in 1966. That left only Brazil, where smallpox was still highly endemic, and Argentina, where smallpox was imported repeatedly from Brazil. According to Rodrigues (1975), fifty-six thousand of the sixty-one thousand cases of smallpox reported in South America in the 1960s were from Brazil.

Brazil began a special campaign to systematically vaccinate its ninety million citizens in 1966. After a strenuous, five-year-long effort, in which over seventy-five million Brazilians were vaccinated, smallpox was eliminated from Brazil in April 1971. Latin America's final outbreak of smallpox occurred in a poor, densely populated area of Guanabara State outside Rio de Janeiro (WHO 1971). Argentina had had its last epidemic of smallpox, which was imported from Brazil, in 1970.

OMOLU/OBALUAYE: GOD OF SMALLPOX
IN THE NEW WORLD

As slaves in northeast Brazil sought to maintain the beliefs of their homeland, some of the traditional gods of the Yoruba-speaking people were reborn in the New World as hybrid Roman Catholic saints. Shapona, the Yoruba god of smallpox, was among those that survived the voyage from West Africa to Bahia. Worshipped as the god of smallpox and other pestilences in the New World, Shapona came to be called most frequently

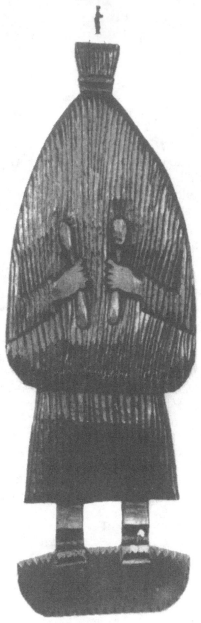

Fig. 13. Omolu/Obaluaye, god of smallpox in the New World. Courtesy Dr. D. A. Henderson.

by another of his names from West Africa, Obaluaye ("King of the Earth"), or simply Omolu. The same diety was sometimes called Obaluaye at Ile Ife in Nigeria, and Ayinon or Sagbata ('Master of the Earth") among the Mahis of neighboring Dahomey (Davidson 1961; Pierson 1967; Verger 1954).

Verger says that in northeast Brazil, Obaluaye was syncretized with the Christian saints Roche, Sebastian, Lazarus, and Benoit. (Elsewhere in the Roman Catholic world, St. Sebastian and St. Roche were patron saints of syphilitics, although St. Roche was invoked for various contagious diseases.) H. C. Dent (1886) observed a procession with images of Christ and St. Sebastian in a Catholic service to ward off smallpox at Brumado, Brazil, in 1883. Another observer recalled that worshippers of Obaluaye at Recife danced with their hands crossed behind their backs, possibly alluding to the usual depiction of St. Sebastian's martyrdom (Verger 1957, 255).

Interestingly, Obaluaye is not mentioned as having been syncretized with St. Nicaise, the patron saint of smallpox in Europe. St. Nicaise may have been called upon in Mexico, where early missionaries reportedly "found a day set aside for prayer to the Aztec god of syphilis, and consecrated it instead to the saint who granted relief from smallpox" (Clark 1955, 327).

At appropriate ceremonies, Obaluaye was typically represented by a male dancer in a costume of straw, who, according to Pierre Verger, danced doubled over, as if in pain, while imitating the suffering, trembling, and itching of a patient with fever—all to special music and chants. In his hand the dancer carried the symbol of the smallpox god, a *shashara*: a thick rod made of palm stems decorated with cowrie shells. The smallpox god's followers were identified by the red and black or white and black necklaces they wore (Verger 1954, 1957).

African cultural practices also persisted in some other areas of Latin America besides northeast Brazil. Omolu may have been worshipped in Haiti, a known stronghold of Dahomeyan cultural influence, but I have seen no reference to such practice. In Cuba, Obaluaye (= Baba luaye) was identified with St. Lazarus and symbolized by a crutch or by a broom or bundle of palm stems decorated with cowrie shells (Verger 1957). In the United States, the same "Baba Luaye" was the subject of a highly popular recording by Cuban-American entertainer Desi Arnez in the early 1950s (Dr. Robert Thompson, personal communication, 1981).

Seven

A Destroying Angel

As LATE AS 1600, smallpox was still unheard of among the one-half to two million Indians living in the vast area north of Mexico. By this time, Spanish settlers and the smallpox they had brought with them had been established in South America for nearly a century. But the disease had not yet appeared in the north, even though several European expeditions explored parts of North America in the sixteenth century, and fishermen from French ports made annual voyages to rich fishing areas off the northeast coast during the latter part of that period. About the same time that Britain, France, and Holland finally began establishing the first permanent European settlements in North America early in the seventeenth century, smallpox descended on the unsuspecting native North Americans.

Around 1617–19, a devastating epidemic wiped out nine-tenths of the Indian population along the Massachusetts coast. The cause of this epidemic, which almost certainly was a foreign disease introduced by Europeans, is disputed, but it appears to have been smallpox's debut in America north of Mexico. The physician Herbert U. Williams (1909) reviewed contemporary descriptions of this outbreak and concluded that it was probably caused by bubonic plague, but might have been due to smallpox. Both diseases had recently been epidemic in England. Williams based his conclusion largely on the fact that several European witnesses referred to this outbreak as "plague," or "the plague." However, observers could well have been misled by the outbreak's unusual virulence in the Indians if it was caused by smallpox. Even in the nineteenth century, it was observed that

> [smallpox] kills a greater part of them [North American Indians] before any eruption appears. . . . It generally takes the confluent turn of the most malignant kind (when the patient does not die before the eruption) which in 95 out of 100 is fatal. (Stearn & Stearn 1943, 610–11)

One witness to the epidemic of 1617–19, Captain Thomas Dermeer, reported having seen "sores" on some Indians who had escaped death, and described "spots" on others before they died (Williams 1909, 348). Another opinion is that "neither malaria, nor yellow fever, nor the plague, but smallpox was the blessing in disguise that gave our emigrant ancestors an opportunity to found the State" (Woodward 1932, 1182). As the latter statement suggests, this epidemic fortuitously cleared a place for the first pilgrims. Seven years earlier, "the Narragansetts alone were said to be able to muster some 3,000 warriors," whereas Miles Standish and his companions found only "a few straggling inhabitants, burial places, empty wigwams, and some skeletons" when they arrived at Plymouth in 1620 (ibid.).

By its calamitous impact on the remainder of the indigenous population, smallpox also helped the settlers maintain their precarious position. Another epidemic of smallpox struck the Indians near Plymouth Colony in 1633. Increase Mather (d. 1723), one of Boston's leading Puritan clergy and an early president of Harvard College, later related this outbreak to a dispute between the colonists and the local Indians, leaving no doubt that as far as Mather was concerned, God was on the settlers' side:

> About the same time the Indians began to be quarrelsome touching the Bounds of the land which they had sold to the English; but God ended the controversy by sending the small-pox amongst the Indians at Saugust, who were before that time exceeding numerous. Whole towns of them were swept away, in some of them not so much as one Soul escaping the Destruction. (Simpson 1954, 680)

The epidemic also killed twenty settlers from the *Mayflower*, including the only physician at Plymouth Colony.

Once it had made its premiere appearances on the coast, the virus soon began to move inland. The Indians' complete susceptibility made spread inevitable. A year after the outbreak at Plymouth Colony, smallpox spread from Dutch traders to Indians in the valley of the Connecticut River, "one of the easier routes to the St. Lawrence." This was the beginning of an enormous epidemic, which reverberated in a series of outbreaks among Indians in the Great Lakes–St. Lawrence River region over the next seven years. Jesuits also reported smallpox outbreaks among the Indians in eastern Canada in 1634. (Duffy 1951, 328).

Among the Huron Indians north of Lake Ontario in 1636, it was reported that "terror was universal. The contagion increased as autumn advanced; and when winter came . . . its ravages were appalling. The season of the Huron festivity was turned to a season of mourning" (ibid.). The epidemic among the Hurons lasted until 1640 and reduced their numbers by half. Since they blamed the Jesuits for this disaster, "only the need to maintain trade relations with the French prevented the Hurons from granting all the missionaries the martyrdom they each coveted" (Eccles 1973, 45). Eight years later, the weakened Hurons were nearly destroyed in an attack by their traditional enemies, the Iroquois. By 1650, wrote the medical historian J. J. Heagerty, "the Hurons as a tribe had ceased to exist" (1928, 1: 26).

The powerful Iroquois were also attacked themselves. The Stearns (1945) record that in 1649, smallpox broke out in the ranks of a joint English-Iroquois war party, and forced them to turn back from their intended assault on the French at Montreal. Fourteen years later, the disease again caused consternation among the tribe: "The small-pox . . . has wrought sad havoc in their villages and has carried off many men, besides great numbers of women and children; and as a result their villages are nearly deserted, and their fields are only half-tilled" (Duffy 1951, 329). The governor of Canada described yet another outbreak among the Iroquois in 1679: "The small pox desolates them to such a degree, that they think no longer of meeting nor of wars, but only of bewailing the dead, of whom there is already an immense number" (ibid., 71).

Jesuits conducted a flurry of baptisms among the dying Indians in Canada, but surviving Indians, including the Hurons, believed the baptisms were causing the deaths that rapidly followed. The Indians may have been partly correct, since missionaries going from cabin to cabin baptizing and with crucifixes to be kissed, as well as funeral ceremonies for Christian Indians, probably did help spread the infection (Stearn & Stearn 1945; Eccles 1973).

A group of Canadian Indians gave their opinion of the extraordinary new phenomenon that the whites called "smallpox" at a meeting with Jesuit missionaries around this time:

> This disease has not been engendered here; it comes from without; never have we seen demons so cruel. The other maladies lasted two or three moons; this has been persecuting us more than a year. Ours are content with one or two in a family; this, in many, has left no more than that number and in many none at all. (Heagerty 1928, 1: 58)

It is sobering to note that some colonists actively and deliberately fostered smallpox's spread among native North Americans in order to break the Indians' resistance and facilitate European settlement. In *The Effect of Smallpox on the Destiny of the Amerindian*, the Stearns report that "history records numerous instances of the French, the Spanish, the English and later on the American, using smallpox as an ignoble means to an end" (1945, 13–14). One such incident, described by Heagerty, involved a white trader who avenged the loss of his equipment in an Indian raid by inviting leaders of the tribe to smoke a peace pipe. The trader presented the Indians with a keg of rum wrapped in a flag which had been contaminated with smallpox virus, and told the Indians not to unwrap the keg until after they returned to their village. Many died in the outbreak that followed. Increase Mather's unconcealed gratitude for the disease's catastrophic impact on the Indians and the similar reactions of many other settlers in the North American colonies during the seventeenth and eighteenth centuries stood in curious contrast to the attitude of most Spanish and Portuguese colonists in Latin America.

Regardless of whether they were infected deliberately or accidentally, the Indians suffered terribly in part because of other factors peculiar to them. Their universal susceptibility to the disease, crowded housing, and their migratory habits all helped spread the infection. In this virgin population, smallpox often assumed one of its deadly hemorrhagic or confluent forms, but even those with less severe manifestations were apt to be killed by their indigenous "treatment": sweating in a hot house followed by a plunge in cold water. Even at the end of the nineteenth century, fatality rates averaged thirty-five percent among infected Indians, and rates of ninety percent or more were not rare (Searn & Stearn 1945).

Some Indians were said to believe that "smallpox has eyes, and sees who is afraid of it" and thought it best to pretend one was not afraid, staying as close to the victims as possible, with predictable results (Corlett 1935, 107). More commonly, however, when the disease entered a village, converting victims into hideous monsters before killing, blinding, or scarring them, terror-stricken neighbors and relatives fled, taking the seeds of infection with them. Some of the encounters with this terrible unknown disease, for which there was no effective remedy, were so stressful that uninfected Indians became mentally ill or committed suicide.

For all the havoc it brought to the Indians, smallpox was far from being an unmixed blessing for European settlers, a lesson they first learned at Plymouth Colony in 1633. While the disease was not as rampant among Europeans in North America as it was among the Indians or among Europeans in Europe, it was still a serious hazard, particularly in the port cities along the eastern seaboard. Usually it arrived by ship with settlers from Europe, or with slaves from the West Indies or Africa. This pattern of importation was evident from the earliest days of the colonies.

When John Winthrop brought nine hundred settlers from England to found several towns, including Boston, around Massachusetts Bay in 1630, smallpox sailed with them. It killed one child during the voyage, but the epidemic apparently ended before the ships landed. Just the year before, the Reverend Francis Higginson had lost his young daughter to smallpox while sailing from England "to prepare the way for Governor Winthrop and his party" (Cone 1978). The year after Winthrop's voyage, another ship from England lost fourteen persons to the virus while crossing the Atlantic. Half a century later, William Penn arrived to found the city of Philadelphia minus thirty members of his company, who died of smallpox during the voyage (Duffy 1953; Tandy 1923).[1]

Boston suffered major epidemics of smallpox in 1636, 1659, 1666, 1677–78, 1689–90 and 1697–98. English ships were responsible for the outbreak in 1677–78. Whereas a total of forty Bostonians had died in the previous outbreak, this epidemic claimed thirty lives in one day, 30 September 1677. The next epidemic was imported from Barbados with infected slaves. The final epidemic in the seventeenth century killed a thousand of the town's seven or eight thousand residents (Winslow 1974; Woodward 1932).

The epidemics not only killed people, they also disrupted the fledgling cities in other ways. In 1636, the General Court of the Massachusetts Bay Colony convened in Cambridge, then in Roxbury, to escape an outbreak of smallpox in Boston, where it usually met. Two years later, the entire Massachusetts Bay Colony declared a fast in an attempt to halt an outbreak of "spotted fever" (probably typhus) and smallpox. In 1659, the general court held its sessions outside Boston again, this time in Charlestown, to avoid another outbreak in the city. In June 1680, a New York City diarist noted that military exercises had been suspended in that city for the past year because of smallpox. Sixteen years later, an epidemic in Jamestown, Virginia caused that colony's assembly to recess (ibid.; Duffy 1953, 1968). When the outbreak in Jamestown was spread further south by Indians, it caused a series of epidemics in South Carolina, including an outbreak that killed between two and three hundred residents of Charleston (Waring 1964).

We should underscore here certain important differences between seventeenth-century Europe and North America. In relatively densely populated Europe, the disease was increasing in severity, but by and large, it was already endemic in the larger cities, where it mysteriously erupted in epidemics from time to time. As we have seen, some Europeans blamed the "epidemic constitution" of the atmosphere for these periodic surges in contagion. To many European colonists in the small port cities along the eastern coast of North America, however, it was clear that epidemics resulted from ill persons arriving on board ships, from which the disease spread. In these small North American ports, the infection died out between epidemics, as the population was not yet large enough to maintain the infection endemically. Thus, despite their strong religious beliefs about pestilence-as-divine-punishment and the need for appropriate religious countermeasures during an outbreak and the persisting beliefs of some that the disease derived from unsanitary neighborhoods, European settlers in North America, particularly in Boston, took effective, practical steps to protect themselves against smallpox early on by quarantining arriving ships.

According to Blake (1959), by 1647, vessels arriving in Boston from the West Indies with infected passengers or crew were quarantined in the harbor. Heaton (1945) records that New York City instituted its first quarantine measures, against a ship that arrived from St. Nevis with smallpox-infected slaves, in 1690. Other specific communal countermeasures started as early as 1639, when the hospital Hotel-Dieu was established in Quebec City, originally to care for persons with smallpox. Gibb's account (1855) tells us that during another epidemic eleven years later, Quebec also had to establish a special burial ground for smallpox victims.

The earliest evidence of local quarantine and isolation, as opposed to maritime quarantine, is found in an order issued at East Hampton, Long Island, in 1662, which sought to prevent spread of smallpox from local Indians to the town's population. A similar order was issued by the selectmen of Salem, on Massachusetts Bay, in 1678. The colony of Virginia also undertook one of the earliest attempts to legislate mandatory isolation of smallpox victims at home in 1667, after a sailor imported the virus from Bermuda into one of the southern colonies for the first time. The sailor had been quarantined in a cabin in the woods. In his delirium, however, he escaped to an Indian village, causing a widespread epidemic in which Indians "died by the hundred" (Tandy 1923; Duffy 1953; Wilkinson 1958).

Ten years after Virginia reacted to its first outbreak of smallpox, Boston's terrible outbreak of 1677–78 provoked a different sort of reaction. The first minister of Boston's Old South Church, Reverend Thomas Thacher, published a broadside entitled *A Brief rule to guide the Common-People of New-England How to order themselves and theirs in the Small Pocks, or Measles*. Based on a recent work by the English physician Thomas Sydenham, Thacher's broadside "explained the nature of smallpox, gave directions for its control, described its course, offered simple sensible rules of treatment, presented a theory of its cause, gave its symptoms, and outlined early, doubtful, hopeful and fatal signs" (Bloch 1973). This was the first medical pamphlet published in America.

The risk of smallpox infection was still much less in seventeenth-century North America than in densely populated English cities, where most surviving European adults were immune to the disease. Because of North America's sparsely settled population, many mature young colonials had never had smallpox. In North America, the disease appeared periodically in epidemics, sometimes after intervals of thirty years or more. As a result many vulnerable North American students never returned home from studies in England because of smallpox. Would-be ministers of the Church of England in the colonies, who could not be ordained in America, had understandable reservations about traveling to England during this period. As the seventeenth century progressed, the increasingly obvious danger of smallpox in England became "a decided stimulus to the development of colleges in the colonies" (Duffy 1953, 109). Thus, when a Frenchman visited William and Mary College in Virginia in 1702, a school founded by Queen Mary II in 1693, one year before she died of smallpox,

> he learned that wealthy parents who formerly had sent their sons to England now preferred the intellectual crudities of a colonial education

to the perils of the English smallpox. The Rev. Hugh Jones, in 1724,
observed that more Virginians would have been given an English education "were they not afraid of the Small-Pox, which most commonly
proves fatal to them." (Boorstin 1958, 220)

Thus, by the end of the seventeenth century, smallpox had taken a
substantial toll of European settlers in North America despite their control measures and wary avoidance of England. The New World epidemics
were all the more notable since they killed adults as well as children. But
the disease took an even heavier toll of Indians in the eastern third of the
continent. Epidemics were reported among Indians as far west as the
Illinois, the Quapaw (Arkansas), and the Biloxi (Mississippi), and smallpox was well along the way toward decimating the native population of
eastern North America just as it had the Amerindian tribes in Latin
America during the sixteenth century. Apart from the hundred-year
delay, the only factor in the North American Indians' favor was that they
were not as densely settled as the Aztecs, Incas, and Mayas had been.

As the English colonies expanded to cover most of the eastern seaboard of North America, France established a sparse presence to the
north and west, from the mouth of the St. Lawrence River to the mouth of
the Mississippi. A clash between rival French and British colonists in the
1690s set the stage for one of smallpox's most influential interventions in
North American history.

King William's War, which pitted the British and French and their
Indian allies against each other, helped spread smallpox throughout New
England and Canada in 1690, and many who survived the fighting died of
the disease. During the war, the English planned a two-pronged attack on
Quebec, capital of New France. Unfortunately for them, the British and
Mohegan emissaries who were sent to arrange part of the joint assault
with the Iroquois bore scars of recent smallpox, and the Iroquois accused
them of bringing the infection with them. The Iroquois did become, or
already were, infected, and after about three hundred died, the others
refused to join the expedition. The English thus had to abandon this part
of their campaign, which had called for two thousand troops and one
thousand, five hundred Indians to march on Quebec from the south
(Duffy 1951; Heagerty 1928).

Meanwhile, Sir William Phipps led a fleet of thirty-four ships with two
thousand men out of smallpox-ridden Boston in August and reached
Quebec two months later. It is not clear whether Phipps ever attempted to
land after he arrived at Quebec. Eccles (1973) argues that since the British
plan for an overland force had collapsed, the French were able to rein-
force their defenses at Quebec City against Phipps's maritime attack.
Moreover, many of Phipps's soldiers had also caught smallpox. Fronte-
nac, the French commander, hardly needed his cannon. Many of Phipps's
men died of the disease "both during the advance and the retreat, while

many more perished on shore" after the fleet returned to Boston (Wood-ward 1932, 1183). Referring to these unsuccessful expeditions, a Jesuit remarked that "smallpox stopped the first completely, and also scattered the second" (Duffy 1953, 73).

EIGHTEENTH CENTURY

European settlers and African slaves in the port cities along the Atlantic coast and St. Lawrence River continued to suffer periodic epidemics of smallpox throughout the eighteenth century. The disruption was even worse than in seventeenth century. As urban populations increased, so did the size and intensity of the outbreaks.

Quebec, Boston, and New York City were each affected in 1702. A terrible epidemic in Quebec City in 1702–3 killed between two and three thousand persons, or nearly one-fourth of that city's inhabitants. Accord-ing to Heagerty, "The nursing sisters of the Hotel-Dieu fell ill in such great numbers that there were not enough left to attend the sick." In the town at large, "the mortality was so great that the priests could scarcely bury the dead and assist the dying" (Heagerty 1928, 1: 68). The epidemic had been imported into Quebec City by a Huron Indian from Albany, New York. Boston's outbreak began in the summer of 1702, lasted until the following spring, and was accompanied by an outbreak of scarlet fever. At the epidemic's midpoint, Cotton Mather—Increase Mather's son—wrote in his diary: "More than four score people were in this black month of December, carried from this Town to their long Home" (Wins-low 1974, 27). That year, the Massachusetts Bay Colony passed an act that specifically authorized selectmen of local towns to provide for isolation and quarantine (Tandy 1923). Previously, selectmen of some of the towns had acted under much vaguer authority delegated to them by the Gov-ernor and Company of Massachusetts Bay. In New York City, the assem-bly and the supreme court adjourned to Long Island in September 1702 because of smallpox in Manhattan (Heaton 1945).

The same three cities were attacked again in another wave of epidemics between 1729 and 1732. The outbreak in Boston was intro-duced by a ship from Ireland late in 1728. It infected approximately four thousand of Boston's thirteen thousand inhabitants, killed about five hundred of them, and caused the colony's general court to convene in Cambridge (Woodward 1932).

A year later, smallpox was imported into New York City with slaves from Jamaica. During this epidemic, New York's assembly had to defer meeting for more than eleven months after it was observed that their meetings had become "very thin, and more likely to grow thinner than fuller, by Reason that the Small-pox are very rief in the City of New York, a Distemper which at least 9 of the Members never had" (Heaton 1945, 23). About half of the city's population was infected, and nearly seven percent of the eight to ten thousand New Yorkers died within three months during this outbreak of 1730–31. The city was still paralyzed in August 1731 when a correspondent for Boston's *Weekly News-letter* reported from New York:

> Here is little or no Business, and less Money, the Markets begin to grow very thin; the Small-Pox raging very violently in Town, which in a great measure hinders the country People from supplying this Place with Provisions. (Duffy 1953, 78–79)

Over seventeen hundred Quebecers died when a similar epidemic peaked there in 1732–33, and it was noted that "there were counted at one time two thousand cases in the general hospitals in Quebec" (Heagerty 1928, 1: 72).

Early in 1731, the disease was also widespread in New Jersey and Pennsylvania. Because of the danger of smallpox, authorities in Burlington City, Pennsylvania, published an order in the *Gazette* cancelling a fair that had been scheduled for 16 April. The notice warned "All Persons are hereby to take Notice accordingly, as they will answer for their Contempt at their Perils" (Labaree 1961, 1: 215).

Few colonials needed to be reminded of their "Perils" when smallpox was around. Rather than risk getting infected, and perhaps thinking also of the panicky disruption that accompanied epidemic sieges even if one did somehow manage to escape the unpredictable contagion, many people left town at the first sign of the disease. Nearly two thousand Bostonians fled their city when smallpox broke out there in early January 1752. The epidemic started on Christmas Eve 1751, when residents of Chelsea, a community on the bay just north of Boston, went to the aid of a ship from London that was wrecked in the Bay. Some of the ship's passengers had smallpox, which proceeded to kill a fifth of Chelsea's population. After the disease spread to Boston, an eye-witness wrote that "half of the houses and shops are shut up and the people retired to the country" (Duffy 1953, 58).

At mid-century, smallpox disrupted assemblies in Maryland (1747), Virginia (1748), and New York (1752). The president of Kings College fled New York City with his family because of another smallpox epidemic in 1756 (ibid., 88).

When the disease returned to Boston in 1764, "the townspeople remembered the previous outbreak only too well, and the news of smallpox in town precipitated a mass exodus" (ibid., 64). Ten of the first twelve victims in this outbreak died, a statistic that must have gotten the attention of even the most complacent susceptible Bostonian. The General Court of the Massachusetts Bay Colony joined the exodus that year too, and retreated to Cambridge, where they held their session in Harvard Hall. Keeping themselves warm with the fireplaces there, the elderly lawmen accidently set the building on fire. It burned to the ground, and with it "the best collection of scientific apparatus and the finest library in the American colonies" (Simpson 1954, 681).

Philadelphia, founded a half century after Boston, quickly became notorious for its deadly epidemics of smallpox. Benjamin Franklin wrote to his sister on 19 June 1731 about one such outbreak:

> We have had the small pox here lately, which raged violently while it lasted. . . . In one family in my neighborhood there appeared a great mortality. Mr. George Claypole, (a descendent of Oliver Cromwell) had, by industry, acquired a great estate, and being in excellent business (a merchant) would probably have doubled it had he lived. . . . He died first, suddenly; within a short time died his best negro; then one of his children; then a negro woman; then two children more, buried at the same time; then two more: so that I saw two double buryings come out of the house in one week. None were left in the family, but the mother and one child. (Labaree 1961, 1: 200–201)

Even some Bostonians hesitated to travel to Philadelphia because of smallpox. In another letter to his sister dated 20 September 1750, Franklin wrote that "Mr. Cooper [Reverend Samuel Cooper of Brattle Square Church, Boston] is not yet arrived. I shall be glad to see him; but as he has not yet had the small pox, I suppose he will not come so far, for it is spreading here" (ibid., 4: 64). A month later Franklin wrote to Samuel Jackson:

> Since your Way to us is at present block'd up by the Spreading of the Small Pox among us, which (if you do not incline to inoculate) may be a perpetual Bar to your settling here, as we have it every 4 or 5 years, we must endeavor to make ourselves Amends, by obtaining as much of your Advice as we can at a Distance. (Ibid.)

The virus was at large in Philadelphia again in 1773, when the Bills of Mortality registered over three hundred deaths from Smallpox. Thus, when delegates from the colonies agreed to meet in Philadelphia for the First Continental Congress in September 1774, the city's physicians "voluntarily agreed to stop inoculating for a given period," since "several of the Northern and Southern delegates [were] understood not to have had that disorder" (Duffy 1953, 41). Even so, Major Erastus Wolcott and Mr. Richard Law resigned from Connecticut's delegation to the congress and had to be replaced. Neither man had had smallpox or been inoculated, and after consulting with their physicians, they decided the risk of going to Philadelphia, or being inoculated before leaving, was too great (*Connecticut Courant*, 2 August 1774).

The eighteenth-century epidemics were not limited to the colonists, nor to the cities, any more than those in the previous century had been. Indians all over New France suffered from smallpox in 1708. In the winter of 1711–12, whites, blacks, and Indians at Charleston, South Carolina, were affected by an outbreak of "smallpox, pestilential fevers, pleurisies and fluxes" (Duffy 1953, 75). When the disease was introduced into Charleston again with a cargo of slaves from West Africa in 1738, it infected over two thousand of the town's less than five thousand inhabitants before spreading to the nearby Cherokee Indian nation (population included an estimated 6,000 warriors) where it annihilated half of the population in a year's time. Charleston's general assembly met at Ashley Ferry that September, and passed a bill that specified measures to be taken against smallpox, including quarantine of victims at home (Waring 1964).

Twenty-one years later, smallpox spread from the Cherokees to Charleston, when soldiers returned from an expedition against the Indians in the late fall of 1759 after Governor Lyttleton of South Carolina concluded the Treaty of Fort St. George. The disease was rampant among Indians in Georgia and South Carolina that year, having first been noted in August. It erupted in the governor's camp almost as soon as he had concluded his treaty. According to one contemporary historian,

> As few of [Governor Lyttleton's] little army had ever gone through that distemper, and as the surgeons were totally unprovided for such an accident, his men were struck with terror, and in great haste returned to the settlements, cautiously, avoiding all intercourse one with another, and suffering much from hunger and fatigue by the way. (Duffy 1953, 93)

One of the "settlements" to which Governor Lyttleton's soldiers fled was Charleston, where the disease was epidemic by January 1760. By April, about three-fourths of Charleston's eight thousand inhabitants had had smallpox, and one out of every eleven citizens had died of it. In March that year, a newspaper correspondent wrote that

> what few escape the Indians, no sooner arrive in Town, than they are seized with Small-Pox, which generally carries them off; and, from the Numbers, already dead, you may judge the Fatality of the Disease. Of the white Inhabitants 95; Acadians 115; Negroes 500, were dead two days ago, by the Sexton's Account. (Ibid., 94–95)

Smallpox visited the Cherokees again in 1783, and this time the disease "broke their last resistance" (Stearn & Stearn 1945, 49).

Indian movements coincident to various wars and skirmishes sometimes helped spread the disease, frustrating many Indian attacks on behalf of, or against, the colonists. Early in 1717, an Iroquois war band was turned around by smallpox in their ranks (ibid., 37). Two decades later, when a war party of 330 Monsoni, Cree, and Assiniboin Indians in western Manitoba set out to avenge the massacre of a French priest and some of his compatriots by a group of Sioux Indians, smallpox "paralyzed their movements and ended their quest for vengeance" (Heagerty 1928, 1: 37). At mid-century, the disease rendered the Miami Indians south of Lake Michigan unfit to support the French in one of their battles with the English, and in the 1780s, Indians who were planning a massacre of local white settlers in the old "Northwest" (Ohio, Illinois, Michigan) were themselves decimated by smallpox (Duffy 1953, 86; Stearn & Stearn 1945, 47).

Long after it was over, Canadian Indians remembered 1755 as the "Year of the Great Smallpox Epidemic," the worst in their history. The epidemic started among the French settlers before spreading to the Indians. The governor of Quebec wrote that "smallpox prevails in the cities and rural districts, few houses are exempt from it" (Heagerty 1928, 1: 74). Among the Indians, the epidemic lasted until 1757 and interrupted many anti-English skirmishes in the French and Indian War.

The French and Indian War, which resulted in the British capture of Quebec in 1759, and with it, Canada, led to a general upsurge in smallpox among Indians and settlers. Aided by the war, smallpox spread west from Quebec past Montreal to Niagara. At Albany, New York, "it was found necessary to garrison the town with British troops and discharge all the [terrified] colonial soldiers except one regiment raised in New York" (Duffy 1953, 88). Although Britain's First Regiment of Foot was inoculated before embarking for Canada in 1756, smallpox appeared among British soldiers during the siege of Louisburg in 1758 (Ward 1960; Howell 1933).

Montcalm, trying to hold Canada for France, at one time had over two thousand of his men ill with smallpox. At Fort William Henry between Albany and Lake Champlain, an 8,000-man French-Indian force commanded by Montcalm overran the English defendents, but Montcalm was unable to prevent his Indian allies from looting the place and massacring the inhabitants. The Indians soon regretted their impulsive behavior. The massacre had interrupted an epidemic of smallpox at the fort. A few months later Montcalm wrote

> A number of the upper country Indians, who came last year to the expedition against Fort William Henry, died of the smallpox on their way home. The English had it. This is a real loss to us and will cost the King considerable in consequence of the expenses it will occasion at the posts to treat them, cover the dead and console the widows. (Heagerty 1928, 1: 41)

Soldiers returning from the campaign at Quebec in September 1760 were responsible for outbreaks in many New England communities. In New York City, the French and Indian War was blamed for smallpox's appearance in the city almost every year for ten years, beginning in 1756 (Duffy 1953, 1968).

As in the previous century, fleeing Indians also helped spread the disease. The Stearns record that Senecas panicked by an outbreak in northern New York province in 1731–32 carried the infection to Massachusetts, New Hampshire, and spread it among the other five nations of the Iroquois. The next year Governor William Cosby of New York sent the Iroquois his condolences, regretting the "great mortality among you by the small pox" (Duffy 1953, 81). Indians in Ohio, Illinois, and Michigan were also hard hit again around this time.

Some of the eighteenth-century epidemics among the Indians were actively fostered or initiated by vengeful or frightened whites. Probably the most notorious instance of smallpox being deliberately recommended as a weapon against North American Indians occurred when Sir Jeffery Amherst, commander-in-chief of British forces in North America, became concerned about a coalition of Indian tribes led by the Ottawa chief Pontiac that was harassing the western frontiers of Pennsylvania, Maryland, and Virginia. Pontiac and his followers captured several forts in defiance of the whites, who were pushing westward. Among other countermeasures, Amherst suggested in a letter written to Colonel Henry Bouquet in 1763: "Could it not be contrived to send the smallpox among these disaffected tribes of Indians? We must on this occasion use every strategem in our power to reduce them." That July, Bouquet replied: "I will try to inoculate the ——— with some blankets that may fall in their hands, and take care not to get the disease myself" (Duffy 1951, 340). The result of this conspiracy is unknown.

Twenty years later, smallpox spread to the Sioux Indians of the Plains after they attacked white families who were suffering from it (Heagerty 1928, 1: 46). With the Sioux, the disease then crossed the Rocky Mountains. By 1785, smallpox was reported among Indians in Alaska and in California (at San Gabriel Mission), having appeared in southern Alaska for the first time around 1775. Catholic missionaries in the area now known as New Mexico recorded local epidemics of smallpox as early as 1719, 1733, 1738, 1747 and 1749.

Meanwhile, the colonists continued efforts begun in the seventeenth century to prevent the introduction of smallpox into port cities on the East Coast, quarantining ships and isolating patients. Boston established a quarantine hospital on Spectacle Island in Boston Harbor in 1717. The Massachusetts Bay Colony passed "An Act to Prevent Persons from Concealing the Small Pox" in 1731, which required heads of households to report any smallpox to the local selectmen and display a red flag on the affected home to warn others. South Carolina enacted a similar law in 1738. In both Massachusetts and South Carolina the penalty for breaking these laws was fifty pounds. (Tandy 1923). New York City passed its first Quarantine Act, and established a quarantine station at Bedloe's Island, which was later to be the site of the Statue of Liberty, in 1755. By then, the colonists were also beginning to fight smallpox with a third method, inoculation, as were their contemporaries in Europe. Though it soon proved to be the most effective weapon of all until the end of the eighteenth century, its introduction during a severe epidemic in Boston in 1721 provoked a violent controversy.

One Saturday in mid-April 1721, two British ships fresh from the West Indies sailed past the quarantine station on Spectacle Island and docked at Boston's Long Wharf. On board the *Seahorse*, two blacks were ill with smallpox and several other crewmen were incubating the infection. The first two men were confined to houses near the shore, but the disease still began to spread. On 26 May, Cotton Mather wrote in his diary, "The grevious calamity of the smallpox has now entered the town" (Winslow 1974, 45). Thus Boston's two main defenses against smallpox, isolation and quarantine, as well as supplementary sanitary measures undertaken in haste, failed to prevent smallpox from attacking the city once again. It had been eighteen years since Boston's last epidemic, and much of the population was susceptible.

By June, Harvard University declared that its commencement that year would be private, in order to avoid the risk of spreading smallpox among the large numbers of persons from Boston and other towns who otherwise would have attended. Dr. William Douglass was soon lamenting that smallpox had "rendered this large and populous town of Boston . . . a mere Hospital" (Rudolph & Musher 1965, 695). In July, complaints about the funeral bells for smallpox victims were so numerous that they "led to an order that only one bell might be tolled at a time and that only at designated hours" (Winslow 1974, 55). Across the river in Charlestown, "so many were ill that by Christmas the selectmen ordered that the sexton do not on any account whatsoever, without an order from them, toll above three bells in one day for the burial of any person, lest it be a discouragement to those that were ill with the smallpox" (Woodward 1932, 1184). Ola E. Winslow described the impact on Boston in *A Destroying Angel* (1974, 54):

> As July ended and August began, the severity of this epidemic increased with terror in proportion as the disease mounted to its usual peak in the months of September, October, and November. Whole families were laid low at the same time. More and more deaths were reported by the day. Funeral bells tolled all day long. Many shops were closed and business was almost at a complete standstill. Streets were deserted except for groups of mourners on their way to a funeral at one of the meeting-houses or waiting at the entrance to hold a service. At night the "dead cart" rumbled over the cobbled streets.

The 1721 outbreak was Boston's worst epidemic of smallpox in the eighteenth century. According to Blake's 1952 and 1959 estimates, whereas the average death rate from smallpox in Boston between 1720 and 1775 was about 37 per 1,000 population, a rate that doubled in the epidemics of 1702, 1730, and 1752, the death rate from smallpox in 1721 was 103 per 1,000. Three-fourths of all the deaths in Boston that year were due to smallpox. One of those who died in the epidemic was a Boston member of the Massachusetts General Assembly, which had adjourned to Cambridge because of the outbreak. Despite its grave impact, however, the outbreak of 1721 is remembered less for the monumental havoc it wrought than for the fact that it was the occasion when smallpox inoculation was introduced into the New World.

Reverend Cotton Mather (plate 30), a graduate of Harvard, was pastor of North Church when the *Seahorse* sailed into Boston. He had a longstanding interest in science and studied medicine briefly before entering the ministry. Cotton Mather and his father, Increase, who also was a Puritan minister and served as Harvard's sixth president, were well known in Boston, having actively fanned public opinion during the Salem witch trials of 1692. The younger Mather had published a book on witchcraft entitled *The Wonders of the Invisible World* three years before the trials. On 26 May 1721, as the epidemic took hold of Boston, Cotton Mather noted in his diary that "the practice of conveying Small-pox by Inoculation has never been used in America, nor in our Nation, But how many Lives might be saved by it, if it were practiced. I will procure a Consult of our Physicians, and lay the matter before them" (Bernstein 1951, 231–32).

Mather had been thinking about inoculation for a long time. In 1714, Dr. William Douglass lent him a copy of the *Philosophical Transactions of the Royal Society of London*, containing Dr. Timoni's account of inoculation in Constantinople. According to J. J. Barrett (1942), Douglass, the only Doctor of Medicine in Massachusetts, had recently arrived after training in Edinburgh, Paris, and Leyden with "letters of introduction to the more important men of [Boston], among them Cotton Mather." Barrett characterized the young Scot as "obstinate, a hard and unrelenting fighter and an excellent hater," as became clear from later events.

Mather also read Dr. Pylarini's paper on inoculation, which appeared in the 1716 *Transactions*. He wrote to Dr. John Woodward of the Royal Society that year relating the papers in the *Transactions* to a routine inquiry he'd had ten years earlier with a slave who had been presented to him by his parishoners:

> I am willing to confirm you, in a favourable Opinion, of Dr. *Timonius's* Communication: And therefore, I do assure you, that many months before I mett with any Intimations of treating ye *Small-Pox*, with ye Method of Inoculation, any where in *Europe*; I had from a Servant of my own, an Account of its being practised in *Africa*. Enquiring of my Negroman *Onesimus*, who is a pretty Intelligent Fellow, Whether he ever had ye

Small-Pox; he answered, both, *Yes*, and, *No*; and then told me, that he had undergone an *Operation*, which had given him something of ye *Small-Pox*, & would forever Praeserve him from it; adding, That it was often used among ye *Guramantese*, & whoever had ye Courage to use it, was forever free from ye fear of the Contagion. He described ye Operation to me, and shew'd me in his Arm ye Scar, which it had left upon him; and his Description of it, made it the same, that afterwards I found it related unto you by your *Timonius*.

This cannot but expire, in a Wonder, and in a request, unto my Dr. *Woodward*. How does it come to pass, that no more is done to bring this operation, into experiment & into Fashion—in *England*? When there are so many Thousands of People, that would give Thousands of Pounds, to have ye Danger and Horror of this frightful Disease well over with ym. I Beseech you, syr, to move it, and save more Lives than Dr. *Sydenham*. For my own part, if I should live to see ye *Small-Pox* again enter into our City, I would immediately procure a Consult of our Physicians, to Introduce a Practice, which may be of so very happy a Tendency. But could we hear, that you have done it before us, how much would That embolden us! (Leikind 1940, 374)

When he issued his appeal to Boston's physicians on 6 June, urging them to adopt inoculation as a desperate means of stopping the terrible epidemic then in progress, Mather apparently did not know that Charles Maitland had inoculated Lady Montague's daughter in London the same month the *Seahorse* docked in Boston. Boston's ten physicians would probably have hesitated before attempting such a drastic unknown step no matter who suggested it, but the fact that it was proposed by Mather virtually guaranteed a controversy. Only forty-one-year-old Zabdiel Boylston, a physician born in Muddy River (Brookline), Massachusetts, and trained by Dr. John Cutler of Boston, agreed to try the new method. Boylston himself had already had smallpox as a child. He was one of the one or two physicians in and around Boston who "enjoyed the courtesy title of Doctor," having learned his craft by apprenticeship without the benefit of university training or formal medical degree (Miller 1953, 345).

On 26 June 1721, Boylston used a "sharp toothpick and quill" to inoculate his only son Thomas (age six), and two Negro slaves with pus from a smallpox patient. The operation took place at or near the First Parish Church, which still stands in Brookline. All three developed favorable mild infections, which made them immune (Moore 1971; "MD Remembers," 1971, 97).

Physicians, ministers, and citizens were outraged and horrified that Boylston had deliberately infected someone with smallpox. They raised a storm of abuse against Boylston and Cotton Mather. Dr. William Douglass was in the forefront of the opposition, publishing several articles condemning inoculation in the *New England Courant*. (The *Courant* was a Boston newspaper published by James Franklin, whose younger brother

Benjamin was then serving an apprenticeship at the paper.) Recalling these events, Mather wrote:

> I never saw the Devil so *let loose* upon any occasion. A Lying Spirit was gone forth at such a rate, that there was no believing anything one heard. If the inoculated patients were a little *sickish*, or had a *Vomit* given them, it was immediately reported, that they were at the *point of Death*, or *actually* dead, . . . But never any Patient had so many *Pustules* of the *Small-pox*, as there were *Lies* now daily told, and spread among our deluded People. (Miller 1957, 100–101)

Boylston allegedly had to hide in his own home for two weeks, at one point, "while parties entered by day and by night in search of him" (Woodward 1932, 1185). Others threatened to hang him. One unfortunate gentleman, mistaken for Dr. Boylston while visiting a neighbor, came outside to find his saddle tarred. In November, a homemade grenade was thrown into Cotton Mather's house but failed to explode. An attached note read, "Cotton Mather, you dog. Damn you! I'll inoculate you with this with a pox to you" (Barrett 1942, 179).

In addition to the public controversy, Cotton Mather faced an agonizing personal dilemma as well. His son Samuel came home from Harvard in June 1721 frightened because his roommate had died of smallpox, and he had not yet had it. By 1 August, father and son were still wrestling with the problem. On that date Cotton Mather wrote in his diary:

> Full of Distress about *Sammy*; He begs to have his life saved, by receiving the *Small-pox*, in the way of *Inoculation*, . . . and if he should after all dy by receiving it in the common Way, how can I answer it? On the other Side, our People, who have Satan remarkably filling their Hearts and their Tongues, will go on with infinite Prejudices against me and my Ministry, if I suffer this Operation upon the child. (Cone 1974, 756)

Samuel was inoculated in August, and was the only one of Cotton Mather's sixteen children who survived him.[2]

Arguments similar to those described in the European controversy were raised in Boston, but with some significant differences. The chief antagonists were Cotton Mather and William Douglass. Part of Douglass's special anger derived from the fact that they were his copies of the *Transactions* that Mather, a minister, had borrowed "and select[ed] therefrom communications upon a medical subject and recommended them to the consideration of the physicians of Boston without consulting with the owner of the books in question" (Fitz 1911, 318). But Mather's presuming to assert leadership on this question involved more than a clash of two different, strong personalities. The controversy also was a struggle over the larger issue of institutional "prestige and authority," that is, the extent to which the Puritan ministers should continue to dominate virtually all aspects of the community's secular and religious life. As John Blake noted, "Douglass' attitude toward the clergy brought him allies who opposed them chiefly for political reasons" (1952, 504). Interwoven with the important issue of leadership of the community, which the historian Perry Miller (1953) believed was fundamental in this controversy, were equally difficult medical and religious questions.

Mather, who with his ally the Reverend Benjamin Colman of the Brattle Street Church espoused the animalcular theory, was more than superficially conversant with the latest European medical thought. By way of explaining the mild disease that followed inoculation and provided protection against subsequent infection, Mather wrote somewhat colorfully:

> The Miasms of the Small-Pox, being admitted in the Way of Inoculation, their approaches were made only by the Out-Works of the Citadel, and at a considerable Distance from it. The Enemy, 'tis true, gets in so far as to make some Spoil; even so much as to satisfy him, and leave no prey in the Body of the Patient, for him ever afterwards to seize upon; but the vital Powers are kept so clear from his Assaults, that they can manage the Combat bravely; and . . . oblige him [the Invader] to march out the same Way he came in, and are sure of never being troubled with him anymore. (Beall 1954, 116–17)

We saw in chapter 1 how close Benjamin Colman came in 1722 to a modern understanding of how the virus invaded and spread in humans and why inoculated smallpox was milder than smallpox acquired naturally "by our Breath." Colman also understood the principle of contagion, theorizing at one point during the controversy that religious men such as himself might be spreading the infection by their frequent visits to sickrooms of victims.

For his part, Douglass was firmly convinced that smallpox was contagious, and spread from person to person, not as a result of seasonal or climatic factors. In a letter written in 1722, he "pointed out that the smallpox [in the Boston area] in 1721 affected only two or three adjacent towns, 'which demonstrates that no constitution of air can produce the small Pox without some real communication of Infection from a small Pox Illness' " (Blake 1959, 39). While it is tempting in retrospect to perceive Douglass as an unenlightened conservative physician, it must be noted that in 1721 he honestly believed inoculation to be "a dubious and dangerous Practice." Moreover, "what Mather and Boylston were attempting was a rash, headstrong, and irregular procedure which, for all they knew or could know, was as likely to spread contagion as to check it; and for authorization they (or at any rate Cotton Mather) relied primarily upon their sanctimoniousness" (Miller 1953, 350).

The two immediate medical questions in Boston, as in London, were whether inoculation worked and whether it posed a threat of spreading the disease to others in the community. It soon became clear that while some persons died of inoculation, most inoculees survived the operation, which made them immune to smallpox, although it could not be known right away that their immunity was virtually lifelong. The risk of dying from inoculated smallpox was substantially less than the risk of dying from naturally acquired smallpox (see below). The real bone of contention, however, was the potential risk to the public. It was one thing to infect oneself deliberately, but quite another to infect one's neighbor as a result. Boylston,

> though aware that the inoculated had pustules "capable of Infecting and producing the *Small Pox* in the ordinary way on others," made no attempt to isolate his patients. Rather, they sat up in their rooms, with the disease upon them, entertaining their friends, and Douglass noted that inoculated persons with sores still running were going about their business in public. (Blake 1959, 67)

Thus, in this crucial respect, the needs and desires of the individual to protect himself and his family conflicted with those of his neighbor, and of the community at large. In Puritan Boston, that conflict took on enormous religious significance.

For all his scientific sophistication, to Cotton Mather, as to most other Puritan New Englanders in the early eighteenth century, sickness, including smallpox, was considered to be one of the ways God punished sinners. If, despite quarantine and other protective measures, certain individuals came down with smallpox, it was because they had fallen from God's grace. Some of the colonists opposed inoculation, therefore, because of a vague fear of interfering with the will of Divine Providence. Others opposed it because of more specific concern that "the Almighty was more than apt to be so angered by the presumption of inoculation as to make it fatal" (Miller 1953, 348). (A sentiment shared by many modern Indians in respect to the Hindu goddess of smallpox, Shitala mata.) But the most difficult religious opposition arose from the peculiarly New England Puritan conception of a covenant between the community as a whole and God. Smallpox and other epidemic pestilences were afflictions "pronounced upon the sins of the community" (ibid., 349). If inoculation spread smallpox in the community, those responsible committed a "supreme violation" of that covenant. Despite the tortuous theology their stand implied, most of the Boston clergy supported inoculation in 1721, apparently because they believed it was "safe" and protected people from dying of smallpox. At least one authoritative historian believed that in helping to establish inoculation as an effective preventive measure against smallpox, the ministers and inoculators "overturned—without quite knowing what they were doing—the corporate doctrine [of the covenant]" (ibid., 363). Thus no longer could the people be told convincingly that their suffering resulted from their sins, or that repentance was the only road to salvation.

When the dust finally settled in Boston the following spring, Boylston had openly defied an order from the selectmen of Boston by inoculating 244 persons. In Cambridge and Roxbury, two other doctors had inoculated 36 others. Only 6 of Boylston's patients died (2.4 percent). Of the 5,980 Bostonians (total population about 11,000) who caught smallpox naturally in the outbreak, 844 died (14 percent). Most of the other five thousand-odd inhabitants had either fled the city during the epidemic or were already immune from a prior attack. After the outbreak ended, Boylston promised the selectmen he would stop inoculating, in order not to prolong occurrence of the disease in the city (Barrett 1942; Winslow 1974; Cone 1976).

Two years after the outbreak ended, Boylston visited London at the invitation of Dr. Hans Sloane, who was president of the Royal Society and one of the main figures responsible for introducing inoculation into England the same year it was introduced into Boston. Boylston was elected a member of the society in 1726, when he also published *An Historical Account of the Small-pox Inoculated in New England* in London. He returned to Boston after two years and practiced medicine until he was over seventy years old. Ironically, when smallpox returned to Boston in 1730, Dr. William Douglass was among the first to advocate inoculation, although he remained estranged from Dr. Boylston. By 1755, Douglass could write, "I am at a loss for the reasons, why inoculation is not much used in our mother country, Great-Britain" (Boorstin 1958, pp. 225–26). That same year, Douglass published the second volume of his authoritative *A Summary, Historical and Political, of the First Planting, Progressive Improvements and Present State of the British Settlements in North America.* Cotton Mather went on to complete *The Angel of Bethesda*, a book he had begun in 1720, and which Beall (1954) describes as the "first general treatise on medicine prepared in the English Colonies."

North Americans could have learned about inoculation long before it was introduced into Europe. It is intriguing that the operation, already so widely known in West Africa, was only "discovered" in America nearly a hundred years after the first African slaves were brought to the colonies. Writing from New York to support Douglass's early opposition to the practice in New England, Cadwallader Colden sought to explain why:

> It is not to be wondered at, since we seldom converse with our Negroes, especially with those who are not born among us: and tho I learned this but lately when the smallpox was among us last spring, by some discourse being accidently overheard among the Negroes themselves, I have had the same Negroes above 20 years about my house, without knowing it before this time. (Miller 1957, 54)

After Boston, inoculation was introduced into Philadelphia in 1730, New York in 1731, and Charleston in 1738, during epidemics in those cities, but without the searing controversy that marked its debut in Boston. In Charleston, a British surgeon on a warship in the town's harbor suggested inoculation to the local physicians during the outbreak in 1738. All the practitioners declined except one, John Kilpatrick. He inoculated eight hundred persons, of whom only eight died. Like Boylston, Kilpatrick later sailed to London where he also published a treatise on his experiences, *An Essay on Inoculation*, in 1743. His account helped stimulate renewed interest in the practice in England (ibid., 135).

Six years after inoculation was introduced into Philadelphia, Benjamin Franklin lost his four-year-old-son Francis to smallpox during another epidemic, and he "regretted to the end of his life, . . . that he had not had the boy inoculated" (Labaree 1961, 1: 154). At the time of the boy's death it was rumored that he had died from inoculation, since his father's sentiments in favor of the practice were already known. The distraught father, concerned at the effect such a rumor might have on other parents considering inoculation of their children, published a letter in the *Pennsylvania Gazette* of 30 December 1736, to "hereby sincerely declare, that [Francis] was not inoculated, but receiv'd the Distemper in the common Way of Infection" (ibid.). Twenty-two years later, the newly elected president of Princeton College, Jonathan Edwards, "one of the greatest thinkers produced in America during the eighteenth century" did die as a result of smallpox inoculation in New Jersey (Cohen 1949, 351).

Franklin, Boston-born "son of the Enlightenment," was editor of the *Pennsylvania Gazette* during inoculation's introduction into Philadelphia, a position he used skillfully to promote the new method. In thus reversing the position in which he had found himself in Boston in 1721, as an apprentice at his older brother's anti-inoculationist newspaper, Franklin symbolizes the different civic responses to smallpox in the two rival colonial communities. According to Blake (1959) Boston and Philadelphia were roughly comparable, in size, frequency of exposure to imported disease, and medical thought. Boston and the rest of the Massachusetts Bay Colony, however, had been settled mainly by Puritans, and evolved a relatively democratic community, the institutions of which were responsive to the political will of the general populace, who dreaded smallpox. Boston's comparatively conservative, locally trained medical leaders and its disciplined citizenry instituted a strict policy of quarantine, isolation, and later "exclusion of travelers and of traders from neighboring communities" when smallpox appeared, beginning in the seventeenth century (Wolman 1978, 344).

Quaker-founded Philadelphia had a much more heterogeneous population, which feared smallpox no less than Bostonians, but in Philadelphia, "the wealthy few exercized effective political control to their own, at times short-sighted, advantage" (Blake 1959, 110). "Although a lazaretto and quarantine laws for the inspection of incoming ships existed in Philadelphia," wrote Roslyn Wolman—a "reception center" for ill passengers on incoming ships was established on Province Island in 1733—"no attempt was made to isolate cases of smallpox occurring among residents of the city, or to debar travelers from neighboring communities" (1978, 344). Quarantine was inimical to Philadelphia's mercantilist interests. Pennsylvania apparently provided no local authority for isolation until after the Revolutionary War.

When inoculation became available, it was embraced by many of Philadelphia's medical leaders, a large number of whom had trained in Europe and "tended to be more worldly and more responsive to new concepts" (ibid.). It was also favored without restriction by Philadelphia's wealthy city fathers, who could afford to have their families inoculated. By 1761, thanks in part to Franklin's propagandizing, Philadelphia "became a center of inoculation and attracted patients from all the English colonies in the Americas, including the West Indies" (ibid., 342).

For those who could afford it, inoculation and the recommended one or two weeks of preparation and isolation became social occasions, to be shared with close friends. An invitation to one such "smallpox party" survives in a letter from Joseph Barrell of Boston dated 8 July 1776:

> Mr. Storer has invited Mrs. Martin to take the small-pox at his house: if Mrs. Wentworth desires to get rid of her fears in the same way we will accommodate her in the best way we can. I've several friends that I've invited, and none of them will be more welcome than Mrs. W. (Drake 1971, 389)

Martha Washington turned down an invitation to be inoculated at the home of John Hancock, who wrote General Washington that "Mrs. Hancock would esteem it to have Mrs. Washington take the smallpox in her house" (Furman 1973, 16). Martha elected instead to be inoculated in New York, and convalesced in Philadelphia, while en route from Cambridge, Massachusetts, to her own home in Virginia. Abigail Adams "took her four children to the home of an Aunt in Boston, and was inoculated while her husband was at the Continental Congress in Philadelphia" (ibid.).

Because of the recognized risk of spreading smallpox, some colonies forbade inoculation at first. In 1747, for example, Governor Clinton of New York issued a proclamation "strictly prohibiting and forbidding all and every other person within this Province to inoculate for the small pox any person or persons within the City and County of New York, on pain of being prosecuted to the utmost rigor of the law" (Blanton 1931, 61). Ambivalent attitudes toward inoculation persisted until Jenner discovered vaccination, whereby protection could be obtained without the risk of spreading the disease. In addition to New York, the practice of inoculation was restricted or legally barred altogether in Connecticut, Virginia, and Maryland during the remaining colonial period. In Boston, the conflict over inoculation was eventually reconciled by legislation that forbade the operation in the town itself in interepidemic periods and permitted it during epidemics only when more than twenty families were known to have the infection (1731–32). Gradually, inoculation hospitals were established outside the city, and finally in Boston itself (1764). In 1764–65, Massachusetts assemblymen authorized local selectmen to install guards at any house where someone had the disease to control persons going in or out. The colony of South Carolina enacted similar legislation in 1738, banning inoculation in, or within two miles of, the city limits of Charleston (Blake 1953; Tandy 1923).

After demonstrating the efficacy of the practice and finding a reasonable way to accommodate differing personal and public interests, the third challenge to inoculationists was to help ensure inoculation of the poor. The operation was not readily available to the poorer classes earlier in the eighteenth century, in either North American cities or in England, and poor whites, slaves, and Indians continued to die of smallpox in large numbers. Inoculated patients required a period of preparation and isolation, which cost time and money. The charge for inoculation was at least three pounds in colonial Philadelphia, and eight dollars at Dr. William Aspinwall's inoculation hospital in Brookline, Massachusetts, when it opened in 1788 (Wolman 1978; Blake 1959). Partly because of the cost, Benjamin Franklin began advocating inoculation at home in 1759. The first arrangements for the poor in North America were made at Boston during an epidemic in 1764. Philadelphians established a Society for Inoculation of the Poor in 1774. In Boston, particularly, the poor had generally opposed establishment of inoculation hospitals up to the 1760s, because of their own vulnerability, while wealthier segments of the population had favored them.

Inoculation was practiced more widely in the seaboard cities as the eighteenth century progressed, and it gradually mitigated smallpox's impact among more prosperous groups.[3] About four hundred Bostonians were inoculated during the city's epidemic in 1730, over two thousand were inoculated in 1752, and nearly five thousand in 1764. The outbreak of 1752 was particularly well documented. Two thousand of Boston's 15,684 residents fled to the country; 5,545 of the remainder caught smallpox, of whom 539 died; 2,124 were inoculated, with 30 deaths; and 5,998 persons had already had smallpox when the outbreak began. Only one hundred and seventy-four susceptible persons who stayed in the city escaped infection. When the virus broke out in Boston again in 1792, "practically the whole town was inoculated within a few days" (Woodward 1932, 1188). Whereas 842 Bostonians died of naturally acquired smallpox in 1721, only 69 such deaths were recorded in a population twice as large in 1792.

By adding widespread inoculation under careful control, particularly inoculation of the poor, to its earlier strict policies of quarantine and isolation, Boston and other towns in Massachusetts developed effective systems for controlling smallpox before the vaccination era. In Boston, the average annual death rate from smallpox fell from about 300 per 100,000 population before 1764 to about 100 per 100,000 in the 1790s. Whereas Boston suffered six major epidemics between 1702 and 1776, Philadelphia suffered ten between 1712 and 1773. In the last of these outbreaks, over 300 Philadelphians died of smallpox out of a population of about 35,000 in 1773, while only 57 of Boston's 17,000 inhabitants died of smallpox in 1776. Philadelphia's relative neglect of quarantine and isolation, and uncontrolled inoculation in the city undoubtedly accounted for a large part, if not all, of the difference. In the late eighteenth century, it should be noted, most larger British cities were closer to Philadelphia in respect to inoculation than to Boston.

Notwithstanding increasingly better control of the disease, smallpox continued to be an important, and sometimes deciding factor as political events moved toward the American colonies' declaration of independence from Britain. The revolutionary fervor was matched by an associated rise in the prevalence of smallpox. In and around Boston, reported Blake, "the chief public health problem during and immediately after the Revolution was smallpox" (1959, 126). One result of this increased risk was that inoculation became even more popular in Boston after the war. In Norfolk, Virginia, controversy over inoculation combined with the community's division over loyalty to Britain—proinoculators were generally "Loyalists"; anti-inoculators, "Patriots"—to cause riots in 1768 and 1769 by mobs seeking to prevent inoculation (Henderson 1965). Once or twice, in the military action during the American Revolution, "Major Variola" outmaneuvered the generals.

In Boston, where the British maintained their North American headquarters, authorities transferred the quarantine station for incoming ships to Rainsford Island, further out in the harbor, in 1773. On 7 December of that year, the brigantine *Beaver* arrived from London, and was forced to anchor off Rainsford Island because of smallpox on board. After being cleaned and smoked, the *Beaver* was released on 15 December and joined two other ships at Griffins Wharf—barely in time to be included in the Boston Tea Party the next night (Fryatt 1972).

Although quarantine successfully excluded smallpox from the Tea Party, the disease was already present in Boston and other towns of eastern Massachusetts, where it persisted into 1775. Three days after open fighting began in April 1775, "Capt. Brown of Watertown was admonished to make sure that the soldiers guarding the prisoners taken at Lexington and Concord had had smallpox in order to prevent the spreading of that disease" (Cash 1973, 39). After all, if smallpox could be used against the Indians, mightn't it also be used to advantage against the Continental army, many of whom were also vulnerable? George Washington thought so.

After the Battle of Bunker Hill in June 1775, General Washington and the Continental army lay in wait around beleagured, British-occupied Boston for nine months, refusing to attack. Refugees streaming into Boston from the countryside had apparently carried smallpox into the city, since Boston was having another epidemic. Some of General Howe's British troops were susceptible, although most had had the infection, either naturally or by inoculation. But Washington's army was more susceptible than Howe's, since unlike the British, many of the colonials had not had the disease when they were children. Washington, whose own pockmarked face attested to his having crossed La Condamine's "river," knew about smallpox first hand, having survived an attack in 1751 while visiting Barbados. Now he was afraid his uninoculated army might get infected. From Cambridge he wrote to Congress on 21 July:

> I have been particularly attentive to the least symptom of the smallpox: and hitherto we have been so fortunate as to have every person removed, so soon as noting, to prevent any communication, but I am apprehensive it may gain in the camps. We shall continue the utmost vigilence against this most dangerous enemy. (Stark 1977, 429)

Washington suspected that the British were deliberately planting smallpox victims among the refugees they permitted to leave Boston during the siege, in an attempt to infect the Continental army. Moreover, it was said that General Howe had decided to inoculate his army in Boston "as a surety against any attempt of [Washington] to attack" (Thursfield 1940, 314). Washington had all refugees from Boston thoroughly inspected and smoked to guard against contamination. On 11 December 1775, he wrote again to Congress:

> The information I received that the Enemy intended spreading Smallpox among us I could not suppose them capable of. I now must give some credit to it as it made its appearance on several of those who last came out of Boston. Every necessary precaution has been taken to prevent its being communicated to the Army, and the General Court will take care that it does not spread throughout the country. (Gibson 1937, 89)

When Howe finally sent word that the British were preparing to leave Boston, Washington issued a general order declaring the city off limits to his own men: "As the enemy has with malicious assiduity spread the smallpox through the Town, no officer or soldier may go into Boston when the enemy evacuates the Town." When the British did leave on 17 March, Washington ordered "one thousand men *who had had the smallpox*" to take possession of the city (Thursfield 1940, 314). Two days later, he was forced to send in most of his men to secure the badly needed supplies left by the British against the civilians who were pouring back into Boston. As the historian Thursfield summed up, "It appears certain that the long deadlock of nine months, from June 1775 to March 1776 was due in great degree to the existence of smallpox in Boston and to Washington's fear of it for.his army" (ibid.). But when John Adams complained in 1776 "This Distemper is the King of Terrors to America this year" he was thinking not of Boston, but of Quebec (Blanton 1931, 63).

Even as Washington was deadlocked at Boston, smallpox was moving to center stage in Quebec, again, for an encore as Defender of Canada. The colonials had decided to attack eastern Canada to prevent the British from using it as a base against them, and perhaps expected to win a large new territory as well. Quebec was unprepared for such an attack, and Guy Carleton, the overconfident British governor of Quebec, had dispatched most of his troops to Boston in 1774 to help shore up General Gage's forces. This had left him "fewer than six hundred regulars for the defense of the province" (Eccles 1973, 235).

In the fall of 1775, General Montgomery led two thousand men from Crown Point up the western side of Lake Champlain and captured Montreal in September. General Arnold led another eleven hundred troops out of Boston overland along the Kennebec River and across to the Chaudière River, which they followed to the St. Lawrence, at Quebec City. Meanwhile, Governor Carleton retreated from Montreal to lead the defense of Quebec. Montgomery and part of his forces joined Arnold for a combined assault on the Canadian capital. If the colonials had taken Quebec City, the province would have been theirs.

The first attack, in a snowstorm on 31 December 1775, was repulsed. Arnold was wounded and Montgomery was killed. The colonials began a siege of the fortress city. Major-General John Thomas, a native of Kingston, Massachusetts, arrived at Quebec to assume command of the colonial force on 1 May 1776. But by that time, nearly half of the colonial troops were ill with smallpox. When British reinforcements began arriving later in May, the colonials abandoned the siege, and fled. One of the participants, Charles Cushing, wrote, "The line of retreat extended near thirty miles distance and a great part of them sick with the Smallpox. . . . I am creditably informed no less than thirty Captains died of it" (Gibson 1937, 96). And later: "We have now been at Crown Point for eight days and since then have buried great numbers, some days not less than fifteen or twenty; but few have died except of the smallpox" (Thursfield 1940, 314). Sullivan, the new commanding officer, reported to Washington in June or July: "The raging of the smallpox deprives us of whole regiments in the course of a few days. Of the remaining regiments, from 50 to 60 in each are taken down in a day" (ibid.). On 10 June, Colonel Trumbull wrote: "I did not look into a tent or hut in which I did not see either a dead or dying man" (Gibson 1937, 229).

According to Bardell, "Montgomery's troops had taken smallpox to Montreal; they also brought it to the soldiers besieging Quebec City" (1976, 527). Others believed the British took advantage of the northern army's long absence from home to intentionally introduce the infection into the colonial ranks by sending young infected women out of Quebec City. (Dann 1980). Boston also was experiencing epidemic smallpox when General Arnold departed. General Thomas, who was himself a physician, could not help clarify the source of the disastrous outbreak. He died of smallpox on 2 June at Fort Chambly, where his grave may still be seen (plate 31). When Thomas arrived at Quebec to find smallpox among the troops and desperate soldiers inoculating themselves, he had "deemed it necessary, for the safety of the army, to prohibit the practice of inoculation . . . not excepting himself" (*Military Journal*, 1862, 45).

Thursfield (1940, 314–15) quotes John Adams:

> Our misfortunes in Canada are enough to melt the heart of stone. The smallpox is ten times more terrible than the British, Canadians and Indians together. This was the cause of our precipitate retreat from Quebec.

and another observer:

> Our Northern army has left Canada and retreated to Ticonderoga and Crown Point. The smallpox has made great havoc among them. . . . In short the Army has melted away in a little time as if the Destroying Angel had been sent on purpose to demolish them.

He concludes that "with such evidence it is hardly an exaggeration to say that smallpox was the main cause of the preservation of Canada to the British Empire."

The bitter lessons at Quebec and Boston heightened General Washington's concern should his army have to fight in the South, where the disease was more prevalent than in the northern colonies. Smallpox already was a widely recognized hazard of military duty during the first two years of the War of Independence. Fear of smallpox reduced the flow of new recruits substantially and was a serious cause of desertion. It was George and Martha Washington's awareness of the risk she was taking in visiting his camps that led her to be inoculated. Some soldiers inoculated themselves clandestinely before and after the army forbade it.

The commander of Fort Ticonderoga reflected popular sentiment about the risks of inoculating soldiers, when a doctor prepared to inoculate militia arriving in August 1776. The practitioner could hardly have chosen a more sensitive time or place. General Gates wrote, "Such a slave to private gain who would sacrifice the Army for the sake of obtaining a few dollars for himself, deserved to be immediately brought to condign punishment. Were he within my reach it would not be many minutes before he would feel the weight of my resentment. . . . As fine an army as ever marched into Canada has this year been entirely ruined by the smallpox" (Bernstein 1951, 242).

As smallpox continued to harass the Continental army during his campaigns in New York and New Jersey, Washington finally wrote to Dr. William Shippen, Jr., the medical director of the army, from Morristown in January 1777, insisting that the army be inoculated:

> Finding the smallpox to be spreading much, and fearing no precaution can prevent it from running through the whole of our Army, I have determined that the troops shall be inoculated. . . . I would fain hope . . . that in a short space of time we shall have an Army not subject to this the greatest of all calamities that can befall it when taken in the natural way. (Thursfield 1940, 316)

On 12 February 1777, the Medical Committee of the Continental Congress, chaired by Dr. Benjamin Rush of Philadelphia, passed a resolution authorizing the army's inoculation. Washington issued the orders immediately, and instructed Shippen to also inoculate new recruits "as fast as they arrive" (Stark 1977, 430). This was apparently the first instance of compulsory inoculation on a large scale. To Governor Trumbull of Connecticut, who inquired about Washington's bold decision, the general wrote, "Inoculation at Philadelphia and in this neighborhood has been attended by amazing success" (ibid., 431). In April 1777, Washington chided his fellow Virginian, Governor Patrick Henry, whose colony still banned inoculation:

> I am induced to believe that the apprehensions of the Smallpox and its calamitous consequences have greatly retarded enlistments. But may not those objections be easily done away with by introducing inoculation into the State? . . . You will pardon my observation on the Smallpox because I know it is more destructive to an Army in the natural way than the sword. (Bardell 1976, 528)

Inoculation of the Continental army didn't end smallpox's role in the Revolution completely. According to Waring (1964) captured members of the local militia began to develop the disease while imprisoned on British ships in Charleston harbor in 1780 and successfully petitioned the British to let them inoculate themselves. As late as the Yorktown campaign in 1781, a group of British soldiers were able to discourage some of the Virginia militia from pursuing them by leaving a Negro ill with smallpox lying on the roadside. That same year, the marquis de Lafayette wrote Thomas Jefferson that "by the utmost care to avoid infected grounds we have hitherto got clear of the small pox" (Blanton, 1931, 64). In late April 1781, two wounded American brothers in a British military prison at Camden, New Jersey became ill with severe smallpox. Two days later, Robert Jackson was dead and his brother Andrew was delirious. Fourteen-year-old Andrew Jackson recovered and would become the nation's seventh president.

Thursfield summarized the influential part played by smallpox during the Revolutionary War:

> I do not, of course ignore the many other factors which enabled the American colonists to secure their independence: the military genius of Washington; the desperate plight of England with an Irish rebellion of formidable proportions on her hands in addition to a war with France and Spain: the strong feeling on the part of many Englishmen in favour of the American claims; nor least of all the magnificent spirit of American patriotism: but I think it is fair to claim that an intelligent and properly controlled application of the only method then known of defeating the ravages of smallpox, which in the years 1775–76 threatened to ruin the American cause, was a factor of considerable importance in the eventual outcome of the War of Independence. (1940, 317)

Less than twenty years after Washington inoculated his army, Edward Jenner discovered vaccination in England.

Soon after Jenner published his *Inquiry into the Causes and Effects of Variola Vaccinae* in London in 1798, he sent a copy of the treatise and a sample of cowpox "vaccine" to his friend and former classmate, Reverend John Clinch, M.D., in Trinity, Newfoundland.[4] Clinch vaccinated his own children, and several hundred other local persons, but did not pursue it further. Fortunately for the rest of North America, Benjamin Waterhouse did. We shall briefly consider the exploits of this memorable man.

Benjamin Waterhouse

Waterhouse was born 4 March 1754 at Newport, Rhode Island, the son of a tanner and cabinetmaker. Raised as a Quaker, he was sixteen years old when he began his medical education in an apprenticeship to Dr. John Halliburton of Newport. This phase of his medical education lasted until March 1775, when Waterhouse sailed to England on the last ship which the British permitted to leave Boston.

In London, Waterhouse lived and studied at the home of his mother's cousin, Dr. John Fothergill, then one of England's foremost physicians, who was also a Quaker. Waterhouse's boyhood friend and classmate, Gilbert Stuart, later joined him in London, where they lived for about two years in a house run by Fothergill's niece. Stuart studied painting while Waterhouse studied medicine. Some time during this period, Fothergill commissioned the young artist to paint a portrait of the young medical student (plate 32).

Waterhouse also studied medicine at Edinburgh before receiving his M.D. degree from Leyden University in 1780. The twenty-six-year-old physician then spent an extra year in Europe traveling and studying history and law. Partly as a result of his relationship to Dr. Fothergill, Waterhouse met such persons as Joseph Priestly, John Adams, John Quincy Adams, and Benjamin Franklin before leaving Europe, but according to Trent (1946b), he did not meet Edward Jenner, who was already practicing medicine in Gloucestershire. Fothergill's home was also the site of a preliminary meeting between the famous inoculator Dr. Thomas Dimsdale and the Russian ambassador to England in 1768, before Dimsdale agreed to inoculate Catherine the Great later that year. I do not know whether Waterhouse met Dimsdale, but he must have heard of the empress's fabulous remuneration of Dimsdale—which may have influenced his controversial attitude about his own "reward" for introducing vaccination into the United States.

Waterhouse returned to set up practice at Newport in 1781 as one of the most thoroughly educated physicians in North America. The very next year, he was named the first professor of medicine ("Theory and Practice of Physic") at the new medical school (Harvard) in Cambridge, Massachusetts. He was one of a faculty of three.

Over the next eighteen years, Waterhouse taught natural history, botany, and minerology, as well as medicine. He established a botanical garden in Cambridge, donated a valuable mineral collection to the university, and served as curator of Harvard's minerology museum. He also maintained a small medical practice. For his medical appointment at Harvard he received fifteen dollars annually for a season of fifty lectures. After eleven years of service, his stipend was raised to four hundred dollars per year.

Waterhouse kept in touch with his many European friends, and early in 1799 one of them, Dr. John Lettsom of England, sent him a copy of Jenner's recently published paper on cowpox vaccination. Knowing well the continued importance of smallpox in the United States, Waterhouse was excited by Jenner's description of experiments demonstrating that a benign cowpox inoculation conferred immunity to the dreaded disease. Waterhouse immediately published an account of Jenner's findings in the *Colombian Sentinel* of March 1799, in an article entitled "Something Curious in the Medical Line." A few weeks later, he presented the news from England at a meeting of the American Academy of Arts and Sciences, presided over by the president of the academy, who was also the president of the United States, John Adams. Waterhouse later received a supply of vaccine from another English friend, Dr. John Haygarth.

On 8 July 1800, Waterhouse vaccinated his five-year-old son, Daniel, and, later, six other members of his household. These were the first vaccinations performed in the United States. Waterhouse then asked Dr. William Aspinwall, who ran the smallpox inoculation hospital at Sewell's Point in Brookline, to inoculate the vaccinated child with smallpox virus to test his immunity. Having thus proved his son's immunity, Waterhouse declared: "one fact in such cases, is worth a thousand arguments" (Hawes 1974, 38). Later that year, he published an account of these vaccinations in a work entitled *A Prospect of Exterminating the Smallpox; Being the History of the Variolae Vaccine, or Kine-pox, Commonly Called the Cowpox; As It Appeared in England: With an Account of a Series of Inoculations Performed for the Kine-pox, in Massachusetts.*

Waterhouse had been married for twelve years to Elizabeth Oliver, who bore him six children. (He later married again, but had no children by his second wife.) Perhaps for that reason and because his means were small, he tried to maintain a monopoly on smallpox vaccine in the early fall of 1800. Letters to and from Waterhouse and other New England physicians mention Waterhouse's willingness to supply vaccine in return for one-fourth of the profits from its use, or for a flat fee of $150 (Blake 1957, 23). Citing earlier tragedies in Europe in which persons inoculated with inactive material later contracted smallpox, Waterhouse said his main concern in temporarily restricting the vaccine was that incompetent practitioners might use poorly selected or fraudulent vaccine, and thus give the new practice a bad reputation before it had a chance to start (Block 1974).

In early October just such a disaster struck the community of Marblehead, outside Boston. A physician inoculated his daughter with material from the arm of a sailor allegedly vaccinated in London several days before. After fifteen days, the daughter developed a rash, and her father inoculated several other persons with material taken from her arm. It was later realized that the girl's rash and the sailor's pustule were smallpox, not cowpox. Sixty-eight persons died in the epidemic that resulted from the mistake (Blake 1957).

A few months later, Waterhouse and the president and vice-president of the Massachusetts Medical Society were appointed by the society to conduct an inquiry into the Marblehead disaster. Because of a mix-up in communications, Waterhouse found himself facing the irate residents of Marblehead alone on the appointed day. Under the circumstances, he acquitted himself well, as far as the residents of Marblehead were concerned, but the incident magnified Waterhouse's mistrust of the Boston medical establishment (Martin 1881).

By mid-October, several other practitioners had received vaccine from Europe and the possibility of maintaining a monopoly disappeared. At about this time, Waterhouse began to receive requests for vaccine from physicians in the southern states. He wrote to President Thomas Jefferson asking his aid in introducing the practice into that part of the country. Jefferson responded immediately and enthusiastically in a letter written on Christmas Day 1800:

> Sir. I received last night, and have read with great satisfaction, your pamphlet on the subject of the kine-pock, and pray you to accept my thanks for the communication of it.
>
> I had before attended to your publications on the subject in the newspapers, and took much interest in the result of the experiments you were making. Every friend of humanity must look with pleasure on this discovery, by which one evil more is withdrawn from the condition of man. (Furman 1973, 23–25)

After Waterhouse's first two shipments of vaccine to Jefferson in Washington in the summer of 1801 failed to produce successful "takes," Jefferson designed a special vessel to protect the vaccine from hot weather, suggesting that the next consignment be put "into a phial of the smallest size, well corked & immersed in a larger one filled with water & well corked. It would be effectively preserved against the air, and I doubt whether the water would permit so great a degree of heat to penetrate to the inner phial" (ibid., 30–31). In the meantime, Waterhouse's third shipment of vaccine to Jefferson on 24 July was successful.

As a result of the Waterhouse-Jefferson collaboration, vaccination was introduced into Washington by Dr. Edward Gantt, into Philadelphia by Dr. John Coxe, and into Monticello by Dr. Wardlaw. Drs. John Crawford and James Smith began to vaccinate in Baltimore in 1801, and Drs. Valentine Seaman and David Hosack in New York the same year. In December 1801, Jefferson initiated vaccination among American Indians for the first time by sending for an embassy of tribesmen already in Washington, explaining the new preventive, and arranging for Dr. Gantt to vaccinate them. He then gave them a supply of vaccine and instructions in how to use it (Furman 1973; Garrison 1914).

When Waterhouse received a fresh supply of vaccine directly from Jenner and a personally inscribed silver case early in 1801, he supplied vaccine free of charge to practitioners throughout New England.

Over the next few years, Waterhouse devoted his energies to promoting vaccination. In 1802, he prevailed upon the Boston Board of Health to conduct a public experiment on Noddles Island. In this, the first controlled medical test on humans in the United States, nineteen vaccinated and two unvaccinated children were inoculated with smallpox virus. At its successful conclusion, Waterhouse remarked: "this decisive experiment has fixed forever the practice of the new inoculation in Massachusetts" (Blake 1957, 46–47). In his efforts to promote vaccination among the general public, Waterhouse elaborated on a theme earlier used by La Condamine. Writing in the *Columbian Sentinel*, the "Jenner of

America" likened natural smallpox to swimming across a dangerous stream; inoculation was like crossing the stream in a leaky boat; but vaccination was like crossing the stream on a new and safe bridge (Welch 1885).

Waterhouse maintained a cordial correspondence with Jenner, and in a letter to Dr. Lettsom in 1802, he wrote, "Dr. Jenner has been to me what the sun is to the moon" (Fitz 1942, 261). In contrast to his friendship with Jenner, however, Waterhouse's relationship with most of his Boston colleagues continued to worsen. In 1806, he published a broadside attack on the Massachusetts Medical Society in retaliation for continued sniping about his alleged personal profit making during the first months of smallpox vaccination in the United States. Block (1974) reports that two years later, the Massachusetts Medical Society published the report of its Committee on Vaccination and that the report did not once mention Waterhouse's name. In 1809, Waterhouse was forced to resign his lectureship in natural history and his position as curator of the minerology collection at Harvard. In 1812, after nearly thirty years' service, he was dismissed from his Harvard professorship when he was only fifty-eight, after associates on the faculty declared themselves unwilling to work with him. Nine years before, Harvard had been the first university to award Edward Jenner an honorary degree.

As a young boy growing up in Cambridge, Oliver Wendell Holmes knew the elderly, retired Waterhouse and had vivid memories of "his powdered hair, . . . his gold-headed cane, his magisterial air and diction" (Struik 1948, 157). It was indeed Waterhouse's "magisterial air," and the unfortunate way he chose to promote vaccination in the summer of 1800 that embroiled him in bitter, unseemly controversies for the rest of his life. He was contentious, and arrogantly proud, first denying, but later admitting that he had attempted to secure a monopoly on vaccination for a few months after it was introduced. He insisted, however, that his major concern was not personal profit, which he felt he deserved for risking his professional reputation on the new technique, but rather to make sure vaccination was performed at first by persons he thought he could trust to perform it properly. Waterhouse's mistake was not just that he attempted to profit unduly, however briefly, from introducing vaccination. In England the Suttons profited handsomely by selling their "secret" improved method of inoculation in the 1760s, Delacoste had hoped to obtain a patent for inoculation in France in 1723, and there were doubtless others who gained personally in similar ways from inoculation or vaccination (Razzell 1977a; Miller 1957). But Waterhouse attempted to maintain his early monopoly on vaccination while denying it and loftily maintaining that his intentions were entirely philanthropic. The fact that he was appointed as Harvard's first professor of medicine at such a young age, that he was from outside Massachusetts and was a Quaker, that he was exceptionally well educated and later quite famous all made him a tempting target. He also found himself at odds politically with some of his detractors, who regarded him with suspicion and hostility.

After appointing Waterhouse physician of the Marine Hospital in Charlestown in 1807, President Jefferson expressed his own opinion of Waterhouse in a letter to Benjamin Rush:

> Dr. Waterhouse has been appointed to the Marine hospital of Boston as you wished. It was just tho small return for his merit in introducing the Vaccination earlier than we should have had it. His appointment makes some noise, there and here being unacceptable to some; but I believe that schismatic divisions in the medical fraternity ar (*sic*) at the bottom of it. My usage is to make the best appointment my information and judgment will enable me to do, and then . . . abide, unmoved, the peltings of the storm. (Trent 1946a, 362)

Waterhouse died at home in Cambridge on 2 October 1846 and is buried in Mount Auburn Cemetery, not far away. His home still stands at 7 Waterhouse Street. His widow raised a poignant monument over his grave, on which is inscribed a detailed summary of his life and accomplishments, "in testimony of his private worth and of his merit as a public benefactor." In the last entry in his diary, dated eighteen months before he died, Waterhouse wrote:

> All the seed which I myself have thrown broad-cast has not all rotted in the ground. Some of my feeble efforts must have prospered, even at this late hour of my day. Some very useful things would probably never have existed or been postponed to a late and chilling distance of time, but for my exertions. I cut the claws and wings of smallpox, and in the venerable Dr. Sawyer's opinion uprooted if not destroyed several contagious disorders. . . . I am not, I hope, a boaster, but I have done my part. (Ibid., 367).

NINETEENTH CENTURY

Thanks to Waterhouse's "exertions" and those of many others, from the first part of the nineteenth century vaccination was widely employed and prevented many cases of smallpox among white North Americans. Steps were taken early to provide enough vaccine of good quality to satisfy the demand. James Smith established the first vaccine institute in the United States at Baltimore in 1802. Eleven years later the United States Congress established a National Vaccine Agency under his direction, as part of the Act to Encourage Vaccination (promoted by former president Jefferson). The Vaccine Agency was closed, however, and the Act to Encourage Vaccination repealed, in 1822, after Dr. Smith mistakenly mailed smallpox virus instead of cowpox to a vaccinator in Tarboro, North Carolina. Dr. Smith's error caused at least ten deaths (Long 1955, 498–99). Ironically, one of the provisions of the act required the United States Post Office to carry mail weighing up to one half ounce and pertaining only to vaccine or vaccination, free of charge.

Vaccine quality was greatly improved only after the practice of propagating the vaccine virus in cows, rather than arm to arm in people, was introduced into North America in the 1860s in a herd near Boston around the time of the Civil War. According to an article in a local newspaper, natural cowpox had been found in American cattle by three country physicians in southern New England in 1801 (Blake 1957). But a more reliable account maintains that "the first and only authenticated case of spontaneous cow-pox in America was discovered by Dr. Alexander," on a farm near Marietta, Pennsylvania, near the end of the century. Dr. Alexander used that source to found his Lancaster County Vaccine Farms, the forerunner of Wyeth Laboratories, in 1882 ("H. M. Alexander," 1894, 597–98). Even propagation in cattle did not always guarantee safe, effective vaccine, however. According to Herrick (1888), during an outbreak in San Francisco as late as 1887–88, the Board of Health was notified of the establishment of an opportunistic "vaccination farm" at nearby San Rafael. When tested, the farm's "vaccine" produced no successful vaccinations in 351 attempts.

Speaking of nonnative North Americans, Waterhouse once remarked that the most democratic people on earth "have voluntarily submitted to more restrictions and abridgements of liberty to secure themselves against that terrific scourge [smallpox] than any absolute monarch could have enforced" (Blake 1959, 109). The potential conflict between inoculated individuals and their communities' desire to be protected from smallpox did not obtain of course with vaccination. Instead, nineteenth- and early twentieth-century legislators struggled with another recurring dilemma: that of balancing the need for vaccination laws and other legal measures to protect communities from smallpox against indignant demands for personal freedom of choice. The result was a potpourri of laws, alternately progressive and regressive, which seemingly depended on how well legislators recalled past or current epidemics and which varied from state to state. Massachusetts, for example, repealed a law in 1838 that required patients who had smallpox to be isolated in special hospitals. Largely as a result of that change, 1,491 persons died of smallpox in Boston between 1839 and 1861, whereas only 52 persons had died of the disease between 1811 and 1838. Smallpox was epidemic in Boston in 1855, the year the state legislature passed the first mandatory school vaccination law in the United States. Massachusetts' example was soon followed by New York. When epidemic smallpox broke out again in Boston in 1859, killing 318 persons, forty percent of the victims were children less than five years old—the age they had to be vaccinated for school (Ware 1861; Duffy 1978).

Despite less than perfect vaccines and inconsistent legislative measures, widespread vaccination continued to reduce smallpox among white North Americans, although the larger cities still recorded epidemics. In the first half of the nineteenth century alone, Philadelphia had eight epidemics of smallpox, Boston had six, and Baltimore had three. In 1824, the year of a severe epidemic in New York City, smallpox was also introduced into Quebec aboard two ships from Ireland (Heagerty 1928, 1:87).

White Americans who lived in rural areas were also still subject to periodic outbreaks. Dr. J. Barnes described an interesting epidemic in Port Gibson, Mississippi, in the late spring of 1838 that illustrates the potentially lethal disaster of one mistaken diagnosis. After a graphic description of the clinical symptoms and death of the first patient, a man with hemorrhagic smallpox whom he misdiagnosed as having typhus, Barnes candidly admitted that he was none the wiser a few weeks later when he was called to "visit a family residing about two miles distant from the late residence of [his] deceased patient":

> After the usual interchange of civilities, the head of the family, a shrewd and intelligent planter, asked me what was the disease of which his neighbor had died. I replied that I regarded it as a case which most physicians, in all probability, would call malignant typhus; but what perplexed me, in the consideration of the case, was its occurrence at that season of the year, and in that vicinity.
>
> He then requested me to accompany him into an adjoining apartment, to see his daughter, who, he said, was suffering from disease. Upon entering the room, I had before me a young lady about fourteen years of age, presenting all the appearances of a well marked case of distinct small pox in its pustular state, especially of those pocks situated on the face, neck and breast. I remarked to the father that I had seen a large number of cases of small pox, and that his daughter's affection was unquestionably a genuine case of that disease. He then remarked, that there were in the neighborhood more perhaps than twenty cases of the same disease as that with which his daughter was afflicted, and that the persons affected had all visited the house of my deceased patient, either during the period of his illness, or at the time of the funeral. (1848, 535–37)

As in Europe, vaccine-induced complacency soon led to relative neglect of vaccination, and the need for revaccination was not yet appreciated, so that beginning in the 1830s, the disease became increasingly prevalent again. Resurgent epidemics among non-Indians were still appreciably less severe than in the prevaccination era, but they were dreaded, deadly events nonetheless. Epidemics struck Chicago, Quebec, and killed nearly a thousand New Yorkers in 1853–54. During the New York City outbreak, a mother who didn't trust the vaccine's ability to prevent the disease deliberately exposed her four children to smallpox, "in order that they might have the disease at once, and thus relieve her from the anxiety." Three of them died (Hutchinson 1854, 354).

In the meantime, as terrible as the recrudescent epidemics among whites were, smallpox's greatest impact by far in North America during the first half of the nineteenth century was among the Indians. Two massive, devastating pandemics, in 1801–2 and 1836–40, delivered the coup de grace to many tribes of indigenous Americans.

The first ravaged Indian communities throughout the Plains states and Louisiana, from the Gulf of Mexico to the Dakotas. Along the Missouri and Columbia rivers, the Omaha, once the most numerous and powerful tribe of the prairies, lost "about two thirds of their number" (Stearn & Stearn 1945, 74). Their reknowned chief, Blackbird, also died in this epidemic. It is said he asked to be buried "astride his favorite horse on the summit of a promontory overlooking the valley of the Missouri, 'that he might overlook his ancient domain, and behold the barks of the white men as they came up the river to trade with his people' " (Heagerty 1928, 1: 48).

Meriwether Lewis and William Clark reported evidence of the recent epidemic among the Omaha after President Jefferson engaged them to explore the huge Louisiana Territory he had just purchased from France in 1803. Noting the ages of pock-marked Indians in another area, they concluded that smallpox must have been prevalent there thirty years before their arrival (ibid.). Jefferson took advantage of this opportunity to try to promote vaccination among the Indians. He directed the two explorers to "carry with you some matter of the kinepox (cowpox), inform those of them with whom you may be of its efficiency as a preservative from the smallpox; and instruct & encourage them in the use of it" (Furman 1973, 37–38). Four months later, Lewis wrote back to request fresh vaccine, saying the original material they had been provided had "lost its virtue."

Edward Jenner also was moved by the plight of the American Indians and sent the Abenaquis a book explaining vaccination, inscribed, "For Chief of the Five Nations, From Dr. Jenner, London, 11th August, 1807." In November the Indians replied:

> Brother, Our Father has delivered to us the book you sent to instruct us how to use the discovery which the Great Spirit made to you, whereby the small-pox, that fatal enemy of our tribe, may be driven from the earth. We have deposited your book in the hands of a man of skill whom our Great Father employs to attend us when sick or wounded. We shall not fail to teach our children to speak the name of Jenner and to thank the Great Spirit for the bestowing upon him so much wisdom and so much benevolence. We send with this a belt and string of Wampum in

token of our acceptance of your precious gift, and we beseech the Great Spirit to take care of you in this world, and in the land of spirits. (Heagerty 1928, 1: 49)

The United States Congress took its first step towards securing public support for vaccination of the Indians by appropriating $12,000 for that purpose in 1832, two years after President Andrew Jackson began a massive resettlement of Indians from the eastern part of the country to the West. The act stated

That it shall be the duty of several Indian Agents and subagents under the direction of the Secretary of War to take such measures as he shall deem most efficient to convene the Indian tribes in their respective towns, or in such other places and numbers and at such seasons as shall be most convenient to the Indian population, for the purpose of arresting the progress of smallpox among the several tribes by vaccination. (Stearn & Stearn 1943, 607)

The artist George Catlin, whose painting of the Plains Indians exposed him to their plight, discovered that in spite of the Indians' great suffering, some were still wary of vaccination: "They see white men urging the operation so earnestly they decide that it must be some new mode or trick of the pale face by which they hope to gain some new advantage over them" (ibid., 608–9). Catlin reported in the early 1830s that the Omaha, Oto, and Missouri Indians had been so decimated by smallpox that the few remaining members merged with the Pawnee tribe.

The second pandemic appears to have been even worse than the first, although it may only have been better documented. For five years, 1836–40, a savage pandemic raged among the Indian population over the entire North American continent west of the Mississippi River, from Texas to Alaska, St. Louis to California. The Stearns estimate that one to three hundred thousand or more Indians perished in this conflagration. Among its many devastating effects, this pandemic was responsible for the extinction of the "People of the Pheasants," the amiable Mandan.

The Mandan, whose population numbered about 1,500 to 2,000, having been halved by the previous pandemic, were reputed to be the "most interesting, friendly, and gentlemanly of the Western Indians" (Barnes 1848, 541). In June 1837 a steamboat belonging to the American Fur Company brought smallpox from St. Louis, up the Missouri River past Chief Blackbird's burial spot, to the Mandan in North Dakota. Three months later, there were only 27 Mandan left. Among the dead were Catlin's friend, Chief Ma-to-toh-pa, "The Four Bears," whom the artist had immortalized (plate 33). Although Catlin (1841), who did not personally witness his friend's death, said that Ma-to-toh-pa starved himself to death after watching his wives and children die of smallpox, the Mandan leader is said by Chardon to have died of the disease himself on 30 July 1837. According to the latter source, in his dying speech Ma-to-toh-pa told his tribesmen,

> I do not fear *Death* my friends, You Know it, but to *die* with my face rotten, that even the Wolves will shrink with horror at seeing Me, and say to themselves, that is the 4 Bears the Friend of the Whites. (Devoto 1947, 283).

From the Mandan, smallpox spread to the Assiniboin, Crow, Dakota, and others; from the Dakota to the Pawnee; from them to the Osage, Kiowa, Choctaw, Apache, Comanche, into New Mexico and from there to the eastern United States via traders from Santa Fe. The Choctaw chief Mo-sho-la-tub-bee, "He who puts out and kills," had also been portrayed by Catlin and also died of smallpox. In the Kiowa calendar, the winter of 1839–40 became known as the "Smallpox Winter" (Stearn & Stearn 1945; Catlin 1841).

Catlin also witnessed smallpox's effects among the Sioux and Winnebago on the Upper Mississippi River:

> Every other man amongst them was slain by it: and O-wapa-shaw, the greatest man of the Sioux, with half his band, died under corners of fences, in little groups, to which kindred ties held them in ghastly death, with their bodies swollen, and covered with pustules, their eyes blinded, hideously howling their death song in utter despair. (Barnes 1848, 538)

A giant warrior of the Winnebago tribe, Wah-chee-hahs-ka, "The man who puts all out of doors," commonly called the "boxer," died of smallpox the summer after Catlin painted him (Catlin 1841).

An unsigned letter from New Orleans, dated 6 June 1838, summarized the impact of this epidemic among the Indians

> We have, from the trading posts on the western frontier of the Missouri, the most frightful accounts of the ravages of the small pox among the Indians. The destroying angel has visited the unfortunate sons of the wilderness with terrors never before known, and has converted the extensive hunting grounds, as well as the peaceful settlements, of those tribes, into desolate and boundless cemeteries. The number of the victims within a few months is estimated at 30,000, and the pestilence is still spreading. The warlike spirit which but lately animated the several Indian tribes, and but a few months ago gave reason to apprehend the breaking-out of a sanguinary war, is broken. The mighty warriors are now the prey of the greedy wolves of the prairie, and the few survivors, in mute despair, throw themselves on the pity of the Whites, who, however, can do but little to help them. The vast preparations for the protection of the western frontier are superfluous. . . . Every thought of war was dispelled, and the few that are left are as humble as famished dogs. No

language can picture the scene of desolation which the country presents. In whatever direction we go, we see nothing but melancholy wrecks of human life. The tents are still standing on every hill, but no rising smoke announces the presence of human beings, and no sounds but the croaking of the raven and the howling of the wolf interrupt the fearful silence. (Stearn & Stearn 1945, 89-90)

In November 1835, the wave of epidemic smallpox spread to Russian America (Alaska) from British Columbia, killing over 100 of the 161 Indians who were infected at Novo-Arkhangelsk. Between July 1837 and January 1838, the disease killed 736 Kadiak Aleuts, or about one-third of the largest group of Aleutian Islanders. The second-largest group, the Unalashka Aleuts, were spared a similar fate only because authorities of the Russian-American (fur-trading) Company vaccinated them just in time. Only five Unalashka Aleuts died of smallpox. By the time the epidemic was over in 1839, it had reduced the total Aleut population from 6,991 to 4,007 (Sarafian 1977).

Cook attributed the apparent absence of severe smallpox epidemics in Mexican and Spanish California between 1770 and 1830 to "the extreme isolation of the region, the active preventive efforts on the part of a paternalistic government, and the introduction of vaccination at a relatively early phase of the country's development" (1939b, 154). California's luck ran out in 1828 when a large epidemic started in the northern part of the territory and spread south to San Diego, "killing large numbers of both Mexicans and Indians" (Stearn & Stearn 1943, 606). The Russians sent a shipment of vaccine to San Diego and Monterey to help fight the epidemic the following year. In 1833, California's San Joaquin Valley suffered a very terribly destructive epidemic.

Four years later, during the great pandemic, a small group of calvarymen sent from their base at Sonoma, California, to collect supplies at Fort Ross on the coast, introduced smallpox into Sonoma, whence it spread among the Indians all over north central California, and among some of the white settlers around San Francisco Bay, finally dying out in 1839. One report estimated the deaths at "200 whites, 3,000 Mestizos and 100,000 wild Indians." Other estimates of deaths simply said upwards of sixty thousand or three-fifths of the Indian population. Laundry from crewmen of a vessel who had been infected in San Blas, was carried ashore at Monterey and started another severe epidemic in May 1844 (Cook 1939b).

"Such," says Cook, "was the situation when the Americans came [to California]: three epidemics in twenty years, the Indians decimated, the whites either vaccinated or endowed with natural immunity, the disease thoroughly established in all parts of the territory and waiting only for a new mass immigration to continue its deadly ravages" (ibid., 190). The incentive for such a migration came when gold was discovered in the Sacramento Valley in 1848, the same year Mexico ceded California to the United States.

Further north, a gold rush in British Columbia attracted eight or ten thousand men from California in 1862. They brought smallpox, which spread to the local Indian population and "perceptibly thinned their ranks" (Heagerty 1928, 1: 53). Six years earlier, another steamer with traders carried smallpox to Indians in the Upper Missouri River area around Fort William. One group of Indians, who had been reduced from about one thousand two hundred lodges (six to eight Indians per lodge) to four hundred lodges in the epidemic of 1836, were down to two hundred lodges after the epidemic in 1856.

The second pandemic of the nineteenth century permanently altered the balance among tribes in the Missouri region, allowing other tribes to assume prominence and power in the vacuum created by smallpox's decimation of the Mandan, Blackfoot, Assiniboin, and Pawnee. The shift occurred on the eve of the United States' annexation of Texas (1845), the Oregon territory (1846), and a large part of northern Mexico, including California (1848) (DeVoto 1947; Hauptman 1979).

The cumulative effect of the two pandemics on the Indians during the first half of the nineteenth century, and of increasingly vigorous federal efforts to vaccinate and isolate the survivors, was to sharply limit the occurrence of major epidemics of smallpox among the remaining Indian population during the latter half of the century. According to the Stearns, by the end of the century, smallpox was generally less of a problem among the Indians—who by then were better vaccinated, less contentious, and much fewer in number—than among their white and black neighbors, many of whom resisted vaccination. The story of smallpox in late nineteenth-century North America, therefore, is mainly the story of three widespread epidemics among the non-Indian population in 1865–66, 1871–75, and 1881–83.

The upsurge in the mid–1860s exposed the United States' inadequate vaccination and its inadequate supply of safe, effective vaccine. Like similar outbreaks stimulated by the French and Indian War and the Revolutionary War, the latest wave of epidemics was caused by disruptions associated with the Civil War. Deficiencies in vaccination and of vaccine were more acute in the Southern states than in the North, but smallpox was not a significant factor in the outcome of the war, although it almost was.

The United States Army had been ordered vaccinated a half century before, on the eve of the War of 1812. Properly administered, Jenner's cowpox vaccine made the immunization of troops far less risky than in General Washington's day, since "after vaccination, the men could continue with their duties as before, but after inoculation they were confined to their beds for some days" (Ward 1960, 198). In spite of the army regulation requiring vaccination, however, when the Civil War began in the early 1860s, "regiments were raised by the various States and rushed to the front," according to one authority, "without a thought of smallpox or vaccination" (Smart 1888, 626).

In the United States Union army, black troops, who numbered 61,132 and suffered a total of 6,716 cases and 2,341 deaths, were affected proportionately more than white troops, who totaled 431,237, and experienced 12,236 cases and 4,717 deaths from smallpox. Soldiers posted in the vicinity of cities, were more likely to be infected than those in the field, and men recently returned from furlough or general hospital were at highest risk (ibid., 624, 627). Long (1962) records that some of General Grant's men suffered from smallpox, measles, and malaria during the siege of Vicksburg in April 1863. According to Smart (1888), captured Union soldiers carried smallpox as far south as the Confederate prison in Andersonville, Georgia.

Smallpox was widely present in the South even before the war. South Carolina, the first state to secede, had to move its secession convention from Columbia to Charleston in December 1860 because of an outbreak of smallpox in the capital. In Virginia, infected Confederate soldiers carried the disease to hospitals in Charlottesville, Lynchburg, and Richmond. The medical director of general hospitals in Virginia stated that the Confederate Army of Northern Virginia became infected "while in Maryland during the campaign which culminated in the battle of Antietam, September 17, 1862" (Smart 1888, 628). One physician reported that the Confederate soldiers were "panic stricken" by the spread of smallpox. Confederate prisoners of war introduced the disease into Union prison depots in Illinois, Indiana, Ohio, New York, Delaware, and Maryland. Over two thousand cases of smallpox, with 618 deaths, were recorded among Confederate prisoners at Camp Douglas, Illinois, alone between February 1862 and June 1865. The contagion at Camp Douglas was one source of an epidemic in nearby Chicago that lasted for five years (ibid.; Rauch 1894).

In the Southern states especially, owing to the debilitated condition of many of the troops and bad vaccine, attempted vaccination was sometimes almost as dangerous as smallpox. The Confederate inspector general reported that "as many as 5,000 men were unfit for duty because of disability arising from vaccination" during the battle of Chancellorsville in May 1863 (Smart 1888, 638). The severity of many of the reactions to attempted vaccination of Confederate soldiers may be judged from the typical history of one such patient admitted to a hospital in Richmond, Virginia:

P. Davidson, K, 10th Ga; age 17 and in good health, was vaccinated from the arm of another man Feb. 15, 1863, by Ass't Surgeon Wright. His arm became very sore and in a week was useless, continuing so until he entered this hospital, May 12. There were four elevated reddened scars about an inch apart on the right arm; the axillary glands were enlarged; he had diarrhoea and his general health was bad; he had no syphilitic taint. He was given one grain of opium, five of idodide of potassium and one drachm of syrup of sarsaparilla three times daily. By July 8 his diarrhoea had subsided, but as he was exceedingly debilitated iron and quinine were given. He was returned to duty August 6. (Ibid., 639)

In addition to causing severe reactions, and often failing to protect against smallpox, the spurious vaccinations were widely suspected of spreading syphilis. Although the latter allegation was generally not confirmed by physicians, some soldiers were reluctant to be vaccinated. All in all, vaccinal reactions were so widespread and severe in the South, that for a while even after the war, some Southerners and their physicians "manifested a fear of resorting to this protective measure" (ibid., 638).

In Northern cities, smallpox vaccine "was supplied in the form of crusts by the medical dispensaries"; the stock derived "wholly from infants." A small fraction of the vaccine was provided by Dr. Ephraim Cutter of Woburn, Massachusetts, who was already raising crusts "from the calf by vaccinating with humanized virus" (ibid., 634). In the South, civilian physicians were also implored to supply the Confederate army with scabs from healthy vaccinated children. One Southern physician, Dr. Bolton of Richmond, Virginia, propagated vaccine virus for use by the Confederate army on the arms of slave children on plantations. Still, vaccine was sometimes in such short supply that during an epidemic of smallpox in Macon, Georgia, in 1864, the superintendent of Vaccination resorted to inoculation with *Variola* virus (ibid., 645,646).

In Washington, D.C., some of the epidemiologic consequences of the war were manifest early. The "usually quiet" capital "swarmed with newly-enlisted men" (Warner, 189). Epidemics of measles, mumps, and smallpox broke out in the first summer of the war. When the federal government ran short of smallpox vaccine that fall, the Sanitary Commission, a nonfederal body, "provided for vaccination of over twenty thousand men" (Leech 1941, 215). Smallpox broke out in Washington again during the winter of 1861–62. By then, a smallpox hospital had been opened in May 1861 on First Street, between C and D Streets, N.E., but there was no systematic isolation of victims. After August that year, smallpox patients were hospitalized at Kolorama Hospital on Twenty-first Street, N.W., which at that time was on the periphery of the city. But when the epidemic reached black families crowded into rooms on "Duff Green's Row" in 1862, the ill persons were left in place while everyone else was moved to a special camp. By 1863, "scarcely a neighborhood" in Washington was "wholly free of smallpox" (Green 1962, 253–54).

Towards the end of 1863, the smallpox epidemic in Washington intensified. On 20 September, President Abraham Lincoln wrote to his wife, who had traveled to New York with their youngest son, Tad: "I neither see nor hear anything of sickness here now; though there may be much without my knowing it" (Randall 1955, 167–68). Four months later, the president sent a quite different telegram to his older son Robert, who was attending college in Cambridge, Massachusetts: "There is a good deal of small-pox here, your friends must judge for themselves whether they ought to come or not" (Nicolay & Hay 1905, 9: 286). During the Christmas holidays that winter, it is reported that "delirious Negroes stumbled through the streets, and died on doorsteps and in police stations" (Leech 1941, 283). The *Chicago Tribune* reported on 8 January that there was "great terror" in Washington because of smallpox. The Congress became alarmed when a United States Senator, Republican Lemuel L. Bowden of Virginia, a graduate of William and Mary College, died of smallpox in Washington on 2 January 1864. By then, the infection had also spread to the White House.

En route back to Washington by train on the evening of 19 November 1863, President Lincoln was hardly in a condition to ponder the memorable address he had just given at Gettysburg, Pennsylvania, that afternoon. According to one witness who was a guest of the president, Lincoln "was suffering from a severe headache and lying down in the drawing room with his head bathed in cold water " (Shutes 1933, 84–85). Another witness, who saw the president during his speech at Gettysburg, recalled much later:

> I was very much struck, many times as I had heard him, by the appearance of Mr. Lincoln when he arose and stood before the audience. It seems to me that I had never seen any other human being who was so stately, and, I may say, majestic, and yet benignant. His features had a sad, mournful, almost haggard, and still hopeful expression. (Carr 1909, 67)

When he arrived at the White House around one that night, the president went to bed complaining of "pain in head and back, fever and general malaise." Two days later, a rash appeared (See chronology below for sources).

Dr. Stone, the president's family doctor, diagnosed the illness first as a cold, later as "bilous fever," and then after the rash appeared, as scarlatina. The correct diagnosis of smallpox apparently was made only sometime later, after a Baltimore physician, Dr. van Bibber, was called in as a consultant to Dr. Stone. Since the president's rash was "small and widely

CALENDAR OF EVENTS IN RELATION TO PRESIDENT LINCOLN'S SMALLPOX

November 1863

5	Rides to Georgetown Heights accompanied by John Hay. (Miers 1960)
8	Walks or rides to photographer Gardner's studio with Noah Brooks. (Sandburg 1939)
9	Presidential party attends performance at Ford's Theatre. (Miers 1960)
12	Attends wedding of Kate Chase to Governor Sprague in Washington.
18	Departs Washington by train at noon for Gettysburg. Tad Lincoln in bed with "scarlet fever." Arrives Gettysburg at 5 P.M. (Marx 1960)
19	Delivers Gettysburg Address at 2 P.M: "sad, mournful, almost haggard." Departs by train to Washington at 7 P.M: "weary, talked little"; "severe headache and lying down." (Carr 1909; Sandburg 1939; Shutes 1933)
20	Arrives in Washington from Gettysburg 1 A.M. Goes to bed complaining of "pain in head and back, fever and general malaise." (Marx 1960)
23	Exhibits "blisters small and widely scattered." (Ibid.)
25	Retires to bed early feeling unwell. (Miers 1960)
26	Thanksgiving Day. Confined to sick room. John Hay (asst. private secretary) writes Nicolay: "The President is sick in bed. Bilious." (Sandburg 1939)
27	Prohibited by physician from receiving visitors. Cabinet meeting cancelled. Sends note to Secretary of State in unsteady handwriting: "I am improving but I cannot meet the Cabinet to-day." Tad Lincoln "much better." (Basler 1971–72; Meirs 1960)
28–29	Peeling and itching of skin, but much better. (Marx 1960; Meirs 1960)
30	Still confined to bed, resumes work on message to Congress. (Ibid.)

December 1863

1	John Hay writes to president of Union Pacific Railroad: "I have not been permitted until today to present to the President your communication of November 23." (Nicolay & Hay 1905) "Steadily recovering." (Miers 1960)
4	Telegraphs Mrs. Lincoln in New York: "All going well." Still confined to room. (Ibid.)
5	Telegraphs Mrs. Lincoln: "All doing well." (Ibid.)
6	President's face reported "slightly marked." Telegraphs Mrs. Lincoln: "All doing well." (Basler 1971–72; Meirs 1960)
7	Telegraphs Mrs. Lincoln: "All doing well." (Ibid.)

8	Prayers said for president's recovery in House. Receives joint committee from Congress and announces that Annual Message will be sent to Congress next day. Issues Proclamation of Amnesty and Reconstruction. (Sandburg 1939; Meirs 1960)
9	Annual Message read to Congress at 12:30 P.M. (Ibid.)
10	Sees visitors with special business. (Ibid.)
11	Lawyer Browning from Illinois vaccinated while visiting Washington, "smallpox being prevalent." (Sandburg 1939)
12	Sees no visitors because of illness. (Miers 1960)
14	Browning sees president.
15	Cabinet meeting. Welles notes president well, in good spirits. President and family visit Ford's Theater. (Sandburg 1939; Meirs 1960)
17	Justices of Supreme Court pay their annual visit to president. (Miers 1960)
19	Reception at White House by president and Mrs. Lincoln for officers of Russian naval vessels visiting Washington.

January 1864

1	Noah Brooks writes that at White House New Years Day reception president looks better: "his complexion is clearer, his eyes less lack-luster and he has a hue of health to which he has long been a stranger." (Sandburg 1939)
2	United States Senator Lemuel J. Bowden of Virginia dies of smallpox in Washington. (Leech 1941)
8	Chicago Tribune reports "great terror" in Washington because of smallpox. (Basler 1971–72)
12	President says his valet, William H. Johnson, is "at present very bad with the small pox." (Ibid) At evening reception, president appears "in excellent health." (Miers 1960)
19	President sends telegram to son Robert in Boston: "There is a good deal of small-pox here. Your friends must judge for themselves whether they ought to come or not." (Nicolay & Hay 1905)
28	Solomon Johnson appointed in William Johnson's place.

scattered" and no doubt wishing to minimize the gravity of the situation, Lincoln's doctors said he was suffering from "varioloid," a term sometimes used to describe a mild case of smallpox in a previously vaccinated person whose immunity had waned. I have found no reference, however, to Lincoln's having ever been vaccinated.

Mild though his rash apparently was—Lincoln's face was described as only "slightly marked" during his convalescence—the president was ill until mid-December. Meanwhile, the White House was placed under what one person on the staff called "penetrable quarantine." The president worked on his annual message to Congress, and he continued to see selected persons, including members of his Cabinet, when his condition permitted.

Once made, the astonishing correct diagnosis could not be kept secret, though the White House undoubtedly would have preferred for the news not to become public with a war going on. Some of the ever-present crowds of office seekers reportedly fled the White House when they found out what Mr. Lincoln's diagnosis was. Others, apparently mindful that the president "could appoint (them) today and die tomorrow," were more persistent.

How and where Lincoln caught smallpox is uncertain. The most likely possibility is that he was infected by his youngest son, Tad, who lay ill in the White House with an illness and rash that his doctor (presumably Dr. Stone) also called "scarlatina" when the president left Washington for Gettysburg on 17 November. How long ten-year-old Tad had been ill, obviously a critical factor here, I have not been able to determine. Lincoln also might have been infected during an excursion to and from Alexander Gardner's photographic studio on Sunday 8 November, eleven days before his illness began (plate 34). "On Sunday," according to one disgruntled writer in 1861, "the city appears almost entirely to belong to the negroes, for on that day they, and especially their wives, . . . parade in the most elegant costumes, the most glaring colors, the broadest crinolines, rustling in silks and most closely imitating the white ladies and gentlemen" (Bryan, 7). As we have seen, smallpox victims of the black area known as Duff Green's row were not hospitalized, and it is possible that the president may have engaged by chance in a brief casual conversation with an infectious member of an affected community. Lincoln might also have paid a brief visit to one of the numerous military hospitals in the city to see some of "his boys" during his outing to the studio, and there have been inadvertently exposed to an undiagnosed case of smallpox. He often visited hospitals during the war, and there were three temporary hospitals within three or four blocks of Gardner's studio at the corner of Seventh and D Streets.

Wherever he got infected, and whatever the reason for his own relatively mild illness—*V. minor* didn't appear in North America for another thirty years—Lincoln apparently infected William Johnson, his black valet and companion, who accompanied him to Gettysburg and cared for him during the trip back to Washington, and perhaps afterward. According to Lincoln, William Johnson was "very bad with the small pox" on 12 January 1864. That day the president also told a visiting reporter for the *Chicago Tribune* that "He did not catch it from me, however; at least I think not." Johnson died of his infection later that

January and was buried in Arlington National Cemetery at Lincoln's expense.

Although the president survived his infection, such a favorable outcome could not be assumed at all as long as he was still ill, and the scanty news of his dangerous illness caused concern in North America and Europe. China and Japan each lost an emperor to smallpox a few years after the president recovered. As the *New York World* and *Detroit Free Press* editorialized during Lincoln's illness, "His death at this time would tend to prolong the war" (Sandburg 1939, 2: 493). Though the illness almost prevented President Lincoln from delivering his Gettysburg Address, it was not responsible for the classic brevity of that masterpiece. On the way to Gardner's studio on 8 November, Lincoln had told Noah Brooks, a journalist who accompanied him from the White House, that the address he was preparing for the Gettysburg ceremony would be "short, short, short" (ibid., 445). Still, had Lincoln's illness begun only twenty-four hours earlier, one of the world's greatest political orations might never have existed, since Lincoln wrote the last half of his speech in Gettysburg, the night before it was given. All in all, however, apart from the fright it gave the country, President Lincoln's illness apparently had no serious consequences. It did give him a badly needed rest, and an opportunity to display his political instinct and humor. Referring to the still-filled waiting room in the White House at one point during his illness, the president remarked to a visitor, "There is one good thing about this. I now have something I can give everybody" (Sandburg 1954, 448).

Elsewhere, the increased prevalence of smallpox that accompanied the Civil War continued for some time after the war ended. In Mobile, Alabama, an estimated three thousand cases occurred in the winter of 1865–66. Many victims were recently liberated slaves. One physician blamed them for the situation:

> The reason for this extraordinary prevalence of smallpox not only in Mobile, but more or less throughout the whole of our Southern States is very obvious. It is now about 10 months since the close of our civil war, which has thrown our population into great confusion; and the negroes having been suddenly liberated, have from various causes been congregated in the towns, and freed from their accustomed restraint and the fostering care of their former masters. A large proportion of them had never been vaccinated, scarcely any vaccinated, and they therefore afforded an unprecedented amount of material for the disease. Fully nine out of ten of the deaths from small-pox have been among the Freedmen. (Nott 1867, 372).

According to the Stearns (1945), in Tennessee over a hundred Cherokees perished after attending the funeral of an Indian, just returned from service in the United States army, who had died of unrecognized smallpox. Other Indians also still suffered sporadic outbreaks of the disease.

Five years after the end of the Civil War, epidemic smallpox spread from the Missouri to Indians at St. Alberta, Canada, where it killed one hundred and twenty victims in a few weeks. One frantic father caught up in this outbreak threw himself at the feet of the local French bishop, pleading:

> Great Chief of the Prayer, pray for me, for I am indeed wretched. Sickness has taken away six of my children; only this one is left me and even he is in a pitiful state. I havè nobody but him to take care of me and thou seest that he is very sick. I am not angry against the Great Spirit, who has deprived me of my five boys and of my only daughter. In spite of that I thank him; but do pray to Him that he may save me at least this one. (Heagerty 1928, 1: 54)

The boy recovered, but over three thousand Cree and Blackfoot Indians died of the disease that year.

Even as the Union victory in the Civil War ended one source of smallpox by halting the importation of slaves into the United States, increasing immigration of Europeans to North America made up some of the loss. Industrial cities in the North and Midwest were especially affected. Dr. J. L. Smith (1854) reviewed New York City's smallpox epidemics during the first half of the nineteenth century and could already blame a slight increase in prevalence on the influx of unvaccinated Irish immigrants. The disease was introduced into Chicago repeatedly in 1892–93 by a heavy influx of immigrants in connection with preparations for that city's World's Fair. Chicago's health authorities successfully controlled each importation in turn until November 1893, when smallpox re-established itself in the city. By March 1894, Chicago had one-third of all the smallpox reported in the United States (Rauch 1894; Reynolds 1894).

Many immigrants who arrived free of smallpox indignantly refused to be vaccinated, being clearly unwilling, in Waterhouse's phrase, to voluntarily submit "to more restrictions and abridgements of liberty to secure themselves against that terrific scourge than any absolute monarch could have enforced." As one exasperated health officer in Buffalo, New York complained during an epidemic in the 1880s:

> I have experienced a great deal of opposition among the German people to vaccination. This seems strange, for it is very seldom you will ever find a person, born in Germany, who has not been vaccinated, as there it is compulsory. The moment they land on our free soil, they imbibe the spirit of freedom, especially as regards vaccination. (Marcley 1882, 345).

Similar strong sentiments among German and Polish immigrants led to riots in Milwaukee in 1894–95. Here, violent resistance to compulsory isolation of patients was exploited by political opponents of the health commissioner. As a result, the city's health officer was dismissed, a law requiring isolation of patients in hospitals was repealed, and the authority of local health officials to control all infectious diseases, itself a result of earlier nineteenth-century epidemics, was eroded (Leavitt 1976).

Although immigrants from the Orient also brought the virus to the West Coast, immigration from Europe was much heavier, and more important as far as smallpox was concerned, in the later nineteenth century. This was illustrated dramatically in the early 1870s when European immigrants, heavily contaminated by the epidemic fallout of the Franco-Prussian War, triggered epidemics in numerous North American cities.[5] Smallpox killed nearly 2,000 Philadelphians in 1871 and spread from Philadelphia to neighboring New Jersey, where eleven of fifteen counties reported outbreaks the next year. Baltimore reported 1,500 deaths from smallpox in 1872–73, having had no such deaths in the previous five years. In nearby Washington, D.C., over 600 died of smallpox during the same period. Cincinnati reported over 800 deaths in 1869–70, and more than 1,400 others the next year. New York City reported 100 deaths from smallpox in 1870, 533 deaths in 1871, and 444 deaths in the first five months of 1972. More than seventeen hundred persons died of smallpox in New York in 1874–75.

Over one thousand deaths from smallpox occurred in Boston between 1 January 1872 and 1 May 1873. The disease's spread was exacerbated by patients' fearful refusal to take advantage of free care in an isolation hospital on Galloupe's Island, which was associated in the public mind with the neighboring penal institutions. When a new isolation hospital was built in the city, it was burned down the night before it was scheduled to open. From Boston, the disease spread to towns throughout Massachusetts.

Domestic immigrants who came to help rebuild Chicago after the Great Fire in 1871 were blamed for the epidemic of smallpox that began there in October that year and continued until May 1874. In New Orleans, which recorded over 1,400 deaths from smallpox in 1872–75, twenty-three of the first cases in 1872 originated from eight other cities in Europe and North America.

Another, smaller, series of smallpox epidemics occurred across the United States and Canada in 1881–83. Cincinnati, which had not had any cases in 1879 and 1880, recorded 57 deaths from smallpox in the week ending 20 May 1882. That same week, Chicago reported 16 deaths from smallpox and New Orleans reported 23.

One of the patients from this series of outbreaks illustrated again the bizarre ways in which the delirium caused by the virus sometimes contributed to spread of the disease. According to his physician, Dr. Hurd, Patrick Ryan had been isolated at the city hospital in Paterson, New Jersey, on 26 June 1882.

On the 30th of June, Ryan, alias *"The bunch of bad luck,"* during his delirium escaped from the pest-house and wandered over a distance of four miles in his doublings and turnings: I was at once on his track, having been notified from the Almshouse, by telephone, of his escape, but did not succeed in finding him until nearly noon, having had a chase of over four hours. Luckily his wanderings were confined to the open fields and meadows outside of the city limits. I returned him to the pest-house and tied him fast to his bed; but scarcely had reached the city again when word was sent me that he had freed himself from his bonds and was "running amuck" through the most densely populated portion of the city.

I at once notified my senior officer, Dr. Myers, and he, with the police and myself, gave chase and finally captured Ryan in a cellar: he was naked at the time. We clothed him and returned him to the pest-house, and shackled him to the bed. (Hurd 1883, 374)

Hurd attributed twenty-six new infections to this episode.

According to Duffy, one positive result of the epidemic wave of the early 1880s was realized in Massachusetts, where a "statewide outbreak of smallpox . . . shocked local school boards into action" (1978, 345). Massachusetts, it will be recalled, already had a mandatory school vaccination law on the books, but now officials began to enforce it. A similar effect was reported in Atlanta where the secretary of the Board of Health discovered in 1880 that 2,875 of 3,600 children enrolled had never been vaccinated. Regulations requiring all schoolchildren to be vaccinated were enforced a few months before an epidemic broke out in the city in 1882. None of the children in public schools were infected (Slaton 1881–82). Vaccination of Indian children attending schools established for them became compulsory in the United States in 1907.

Railways, an increasingly popular mode of travel, had undoubtedly facilitated the dissemination of infected persons over North America during the epidemics in the early 1870s and before, but their importance in spreading smallpox became more and more apparent as the century progressed. Heagerty (1928) reports that a traveler from Japan became ill on a Canadian railway in May 1900 and planted the seeds of several outbreaks along the line from Winnipeg to Montreal before dying of undiagnosed smallpox. According to Blunt (1900), so great was the risk in Texas, that around 1899, the state health officer sent a circular to all railway managers in the state, warning of smallpox spread by and among railway workers. The circular advised all railway workers who had not been vaccinated in the past three years to be revaccinated. As early as 1837, another medical man reported the chain of infection and death left behind by a woman who carried a young child who had smallpox in her arms while traveling from Quebec to Lowell, Massachusetts, and who then continued by train to Boston and Worcester (Green 1837).

One contemporary described a small epidemic in Baltimore in mid-December 1879 in which "a man was discovered in the line of purchasers of tickets at Camden Station, Baltimore and Ohio Railroad, who seemed to be suffering from some eruptive disease." The man was from Washington, D.C., and left a trail of smallpox among people he'd contacted while seeking shelter and directions en route to the train station that Christmas week. One of the victims who died in this outbreak was a man who was making boxes on a sidewalk near the station when the infected traveler stopped to ask directions. At the time, the man making the boxes remarked to someone else that the fellow "looked like he had the smallpox," but then forgot the whole incident until he himself got sick (Carter 1879). That same month, an immigrant triggered an epidemic in Chicago that lasted until 1882 and was spread to California by a railway passenger in October 1881.

Railway passengers from Chicago were also responsible for Montreal's last great epidemic of smallpox in 1885–86. Many of the Indians in the province of Quebec had been vaccinated by this time, but most of the French-speaking residents were woefully susceptible. Since 1875, French-speaking Quebecois had intensely opposed vaccination after a series of vaccinated persons developed "serious ulcerations, some of them possibly of syphilitic origin" (Heagerty 1928, 1: 90). This opposition to vaccination had caused riots in the decade before 1885.

In February 1885, two men arrived in Montreal by train from Chicago, where smallpox was occurring again. Both were ill on arrival or became ill soon after. One of them stayed home. The other, a Pullman car porter, was admitted to a large general hospital—the Hotel Dieu—with a diagnosis of chickenpox and was discharged three weeks later, still without the correct diagnosis being realized. Two days after the porter was discharged, a servant at the Hotel Dieu developed typical smallpox and was isolated in the same hospital. By mid-April, when there were sixteen cases of smallpox, "the municipal hospital for infectious diseases was made ready for the small-pox patients, and all those not affected, over 100 in number, were sent home in order to thoroughly disinfect and purify the now infected Hotel Dieu" (Brayton 1902, 291). Of course an unknown number of the evicted patients were already incubating the virus, a predictable circumstance which apparently escaped, or was ignored by, hospital authorities. Moreover, two months later, crowds of people participated in a procession of the *Fête Dieu*, and large numbers gathered at the funeral of the Roman Catholic archbishop. Smallpox spread all over the city.

When Montreal authorities began trying to enforce vaccination and compel removal of smallpox victims to the isolation hospital, riots broke out toward the end of September 1885. Two municipal health offices and the office of the *Montreal Herald* were smashed, the chief of police was badly beaten, and troops had to be called out. Eighty thousand residents were vaccinated or revaccinated by December 1885, but by then, the city was almost shut down (Heagerty 1928; Brayton 1902).

A story in the 28 November 1885 issue of the news magazine *Harper's Weekly* illustrates the ordeal of one of the Montreal families that resisted hospitalization of its children:

> The children of Elie Gagnon, living in a rickety tenement-house at No. 19 Rolland Lane, had been taken ill with the small-pox, and a health-officer had been sent to the dwelling. For three days Gagnon, half crazed by the suffering of his poor children, and through his wild fear of the detested health officials, kept the officers of the law at bay, successfully guarding his scourge-ridden residence from all intruders. Finally, however, it was determined that he should be dislodged, and his children removed to the hospital. At one o'clock in the afternoon twenty members of the city police force, under the Assistant Chief of Police, and accompanied by the Mayor of the City in person, approached the tenement in Rolland Lane. Policemen were stationed at each end of the block to keep back the crowd. There was a desperate struggle, followed by an interchange of shots, which, however fortunately failed to take effect. The officers of the law finally succeeded in overpowering Gagnon and his son, and the children were taken away in a van to the hospital.

Accompanying the article was a drawing (plate 35), which the magazine avowed represented "a truthful picture of a scene which seems almost incredible as having occurred on this continent in these enlightened days." The Gagnons' ordeal was repeated many times over before the epidemic ended.

In April 1885, there were 6 deaths from smallpox, followed by 10 in May, 13 in June, 52 in July, 250 in August, 829 in September, and 1243 in October. By the time the epidemic ceased in 1886, more than ten thousand of Montreal's 168,000 inhabitants had been infected, of whom 3,164 died. Eighty-six percent of the dead victims were children less than ten years old. However, the outside world, "and thereafter Montreal itself," it was alleged, began to take notice of the epidemic only after Sir Francis Hicks, a prominent politician, died of smallpox. Provincial health authorities in neighboring Ontario took the unusual step of inspecting railway baggage and passengers in Montreal as well as at their own borders, amid public charges that they were trying to ruin Montreal's trade. The Ontario officials also took advantage of this occasion to establish local health organizations, get health officers appointed, and pass sanitary legislation. Only 15 cases of smallpox occurred in Ontario (Brayton 1902; Bryce 1885).

In the United States all baggage from Canada was fumigated at the bridge crossing into Detroit, an act which caused P. H. Bryce, an Ontario health official, to comment before a meeting of the American Public

Health Association: "but what kind of kinship is it, I ask, which treats Ontario in the manner stated, while New York City, with twice as many cases, is not looked upon with any alarm?"

Despite the epidemic resurgence of the eighteen-sixties, seventies, and eighties, the overall prevalence of smallpox declined greatly in most of the United States toward the end of the nineteenth century For example, according to the 1894 issue of the *Boston Medical Surgical Journal*, in Massachusetts there were an average of 170 deaths from smallpox per million residents annually in 1854–73, but only 8 deaths per million annually from 1874 to 1893. As the overall downward trend continued, importations of smallpox into the United States from Mexico became more important.[6] But the declining trend in the United States was abruptly reversed by a case of smallpox imported into Pensacola, Florida, in 1896. That fateful patient almost certainly did not come from Mexico.

The outbreak of smallpox that began in Pensacola, a small port city on the Gulf of Mexico, in November affected fifty-four people in the city itself by July 1897. Many others were infected in the surrounding county. The feature that distinguished this epidemic from all other preceding outbreaks of smallpox in North America, and that made it a historic watershed, was that none of the patients died. This was the first known appearance of *V. minor* in North America.

It is not known exactly where the new variety of smallpox came from. It may have come from the Caribbean. Refugees were arriving in Florida at that time from Cuba, where the revolt against Spain had recently started. It was rumored to have been brought back by United States soldiers returning from the Spanish-American War, but in fact, the disease had arrived before the soldiers had even left. Dr. Izett Anderson had described a similar epidemic in Jamaica in 1863–64. It might also have come from Africa. Forty vessels from African ports had arrived in Pensacola in 1896, nearly half of them from southern Africa, where a similar or identical infection, called "amaas," had been known for decades (Chapin 1913; Anderson 1886; Chapin 1926).

In 1897, *V. minor* type smallpox spread to six other states in the southeastern United States. By the end of 1898 it had spread as far north as Montana, Michigan, and western Quebec Province. It invaded most of the United States in 1899, reaching Alaska, British Columbia, Nova Scotia, and New Brunswick in 1900 (fig. 14).

The new type of smallpox confused doctors as well as the public. Apart from their low death rate, patients infected with *V. minor* did not appear seriously ill as patients who had *V. major* did, and despite the extensive pustular rash, which was indistinguishable between the two types of smallpox, patients with *V. minor* seemed to have less scarring afterward. Some said the patients with *V. minor* lacked the characteristic "smallpox odor" (Groff 1904). But most of all, it was that the victims

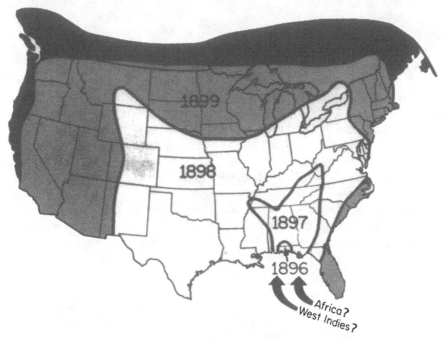

Fig. 14. Spread of *Variola minor* in North America. Adapted from Chapin (1913).

looked like they had smallpox, but didn't die, that bewildered many doctors and laymen as the infection spread beyond Pensacola. This was not the "Destroying Angel" North Americans knew so well.

Some doctors were not perplexed, being convinced that the disease was chickenpox. In Great Falls, Montana, one physician allowed his patient to leave town at the height of the rash and allegedly told the man "to keep out of the way of physicians while on his trip, for the eruption resembled small pox and there was a possibility that he might be removed from the train and placed in a 'pest house' before he should reach his intended destination" (Bracken 1901, 730–31). He was. In St. Augustine, Florida, another physician distinguished patients with the new type of smallpox by noting that in contrast to his previous smallpox patients, these slept well "and never miss a meal, and come out of the hospital looking fat and sleak" (Rainey 1899, 135). In Ohio, one old experienced physician epitomized the dilemma by declaring, "If this disease we are having here is smallpox, then the whole subject of smallpox, as given in our text-books, must be re-written." When he was asked if that wouldn't be equally true if the disease were chickenpox, as it was being called, he said "I guess that's so, too" (Probst 1899, 1589–90).

As the disease spread, many of the names applied to it—"Cuban itch," "Manila Scab," "Spanish Measles," "Filipino itch," "Porto Rico Scratches" —reflected popular beliefs about its source. It was frequently misdiagnosed as chickenpox or impetigo. Other diagnostic terms—"subtropical smallpox," "tropical smallpox," or "pseudo smallpox"—simply reflected the prevailing uncertainty about the disease itself. The diagnostic acrobatics peaked when one patient was said to be suffering from "chicken pox aggravated by secondary syphilis." (Bishop 1898–99).

Since patients with *V. minor* usually did not feel very sick and seldom died, the disease was often not taken very seriously, and that compounded the difficulties of controlling all smallpox, including the more fatal variety. One physician reported that "persons betraying all the external evidences of the disease attended churches, schools and theaters; delivered milk, groceries and other provisions at the houses of their customers; officiated in public stations; and even slept in beds occupied by other non-infected members of the same family" (Hyde 1901, 559).

Typical of the casual disregard of *V. minor*, in 1898 more than two hundred cases of smallpox in six different communities in Ohio derived from a touring production, "Uncle Tom's Cabin Show." Two of the child actors were ill during the tour with what their physician called chickenpox. One of the ill girls was playing the part of Topsy and "[took] her part in the play each night." In one town of nine thousand people, the show caused an outbreak of 203 cases (Probst 1899).

During the same spring the variolous Topsy was spreading smallpox in Ohio, another tour group, the Joshua Simpkins Opera Company, was carrying it through Georgia, West Virginia, Pennsylvania, and New York. Eleven of the twenty-six member group, who lived and traveled together in automobiles, were infected over a two month period. The first patient in the company was thought to have been infected in Richmond, Kentucky. His brother, the company's second case, "continued his duties as actor, musician and ticket collector" throughout his illness. Over one hundred and sixty smallpox cases were attributed to this group in western New York State (Bishop 1898–99).

In some communities, great public pressure built up to force changes in the smallpox laws and regulations fashioned to protect the public against the severe type of smallpox. The danger, of course, was that individuals with *V. major* or *V. minor* were impossible to tell apart reliably, and both diseases were sometimes present in a community at the same time. Moreover, even in communities where the distinct nature of the two strains was recognized, it wasn't known at the time whether one type could revert to the other type. In 1900 or 1901, a joint session of the sections on Practice of Medicine, Hygiene, and Sanitary Science at a meeting of the American Medical Association passed the following resolution with one dissenting vote: "Resolved that the disease now prevailing extensively in the United States, and called in some instances 'pseudo-smallpox' is genuine smallpox, and should be so treated with vaccination and quarantine" (Bracken 1901, 735).

Notwithstanding the AMA resolution and all other efforts, the number of smallpox cases reported annually in the United States rose from an average of about 2,200 cases in 1895–96 to 11,000 cases in 1899; 20,000 in 1900 and 48,000 cases in 1901. The increase occurred despite the fact that cases of *V. minor*, which predominated, were far less likely to be reported than cases of *V. major*.[7] Two hundred and eighty-three thousand cases of smallpox were reported in the decade 1901–10. At the same time, the overall percentage of deaths among the reported smallpox cases dropped from 20 percent in 1895 and 1896, to 6.2 percent in 1897, 4 percent in 1900 and 0.6 percent in 1906. In the southern United States, most of the patients were black. The epidemic of *V. minor* also caused a mild upsurge in smallpox among Indians throughout North America in 1898–1901, but according to the Stearns (1945), smallpox was of little social significance among the Indian population of the United States after 1905.

Twentieth Century

After *V. minor* spread across North America, it remained the predominant type of smallpox until the disease was eliminated from Canada and the United States in the 1940s. Reported cases of *V. minor* outnumbered reported cases of *V. major* twenty to one in the United States during the first three decades of the century, even though persons with *V. minor* were often not reported nor even seen by a physician, because their symptoms were so mild.

V. major continued to occur sporadically, often after importation from Europe or Asia—immigration from Europe was particularly heavy in the early part of the century—or after importation from Mexico into the southwestern United States. Hedrich (1936) reviewed the origins of cases of *V. major* imported into the United States between 1915 and 1929 and found that fourteen of twenty-three outbreaks derived from Mexico. Twice, in 1901–3 and in the early 1920s, smallpox reached epidemic levels reminiscent of the late nineteenth century.

During the first peak, 135,000 cases of mild smallpox were reported in the United States in 1901–02, and 16,000 cases of severe smallpox were reported in 1902–3, when that type was unusually prevalent. Boston, New York City, Philadelphia, New Jersey, and Ohio accounted for two-thirds of the severe smallpox reported in 1902–3. In 1902, when both types of smallpox were widely prevalent, Boston reported 1,024 cases with 190 deaths; New York City 1,516 cases, 310 deaths; Cleveland 1,034 cases, 182 deaths; and Philadelphia 1,342 cases with 231 deaths. Chicago reported 339 cases with only 5 deaths; Cincinnati 162 cases and 1 death; and Ontario 2,797 cases with 12 deaths.

As in Montreal in 1885, hospitals sometimes were the places where patients got, rather than recovered from, smallpox. In the summer of 1901, nearly 50 of 1,450 inmates of an insane asylum in Kalamazoo, Michigan, were infected during an outbreak of *V. minor*. The hospital's medical staff might have been tempted to withhold control measures, since one of them reported later that "some of our insane cases were clearer, mentally, in or following the period of invasion and all, both nurses and patients, seem and profess to be feeling better than before the illness" (MacGugan 1901, 930). No one felt better after an outbreak in New Orleans's Charity Hospital in 1900. Seven hundred and fifty-two patients were infected with smallpox while they were in the hospital, and one-third of them died of it.

The epidemic of 1901–2 was Boston's last great epidemic of smallpox, but it was also notable for two other reasons. Like its many predecessors, this epidemic in Boston was caused by *V. major*, and Councilman and his associates conducted a thorough pathological study of fifty-four of the victims that remains a landmark in the scientific study of the disease. Physicians at Boston's Smallpox Hospital, then located at 112 South-hampton Street, also tested the effectiveness of the red light treatment, or "erythrotherapy," on some of their smallpox patients during this outbreak (plate 36). Elsewhere, the wave of epidemic smallpox provided opportunities for clinical trials of the curious erythrotherapy in Philadelphia, Indianapolis, and Dubuque (see chapter 8).[8]

The next, and last, widespread surge of smallpox in North America came two decades later. Over 200,000 cases of *V. minor* were reported in the United States in 1920–21. This was followed by a smaller wave of *V. major* (about 7,400 cases) in 1924–25, which was still the largest epidemic of *V. major* the United States had experienced since 1904. A third of the *V. major* cases in 1924–25 were reported from only four cities: Cleveland, Pittsburgh, Toledo, and Detroit. In 1925, the United States had "the unenviable distinction of reporting more smallpox cases [43,193] than any other country except India" (Ingalls 1926).

Two outbreaks that struck Detroit in 1923–24 demonstrated how differently medical authorities and the public reacted when faced with *V. minor* as compared to *V. major*. When mild smallpox was present from September 1923 to early March 1924, 710 cases with 4 deaths were reported, and the health department averaged 6,000 vaccinations a month, mostly of children. After severe smallpox became rampant in late March 1924, causing 795 cases and 105 deaths in less than 2 months, "a half million persons were vaccinated in one month, and nearly 800,000 (about 70 percent of the entire population) within 5 months" (Hedrich

1936, 376). The second outbreak spread to Windsor, Ontario, where a third of its victims died. Such differences in control measures were part of the reason *V. minor* predominated.

In Canada, the mild type of smallpox was epidemic in 1924 and in 1927–28, but reported cases declined steadily thereafter. A review of the smallpox situation in 1929–31 published in *Medical Annals of the District of Columbia* (1932) revealed that the total number of cases declined during that three-year period from 43,694 to 26,004 in the United States and in Canada from 1,283 to 865. In eighty-five Canadian cities, there had been "no deaths from smallpox during the past two years, and only one fatal case was reported in 1929." The review concluded:

> There were more smallpox cases (1,112) in the single State of Washington, with a population of but 1,589,000, than occurred among the 48,900,000 inhabitants of the whole Atlantic Coast.... It is hard to realize that in this day, with our knowledge of the ease with which smallpox can be controlled, there are communities like Helena, Arkansas; Fort Scott, Kansas, and Bennington, Vermont, where one out of every hundred of the population has been infected with smallpox during a single year. What this means can best be understood by supposing the same case-rate that was reported for Fort Scott, Kansas, to have prevailed in the City of New York. In that case, there would have occurred in 1931 at least 85,000 cases of smallpox in New York. Actually only one case was reported in the metropolis during that year. (176)

Public resistance to vaccination and to vaccination laws, accentuated by the emergence of mild smallpox in the U.S. at the end of the nineteenth century, continued to build early in the twentieth century. This resistance was partly responsible for wide differences in the incidence of smallpox between different states. The resistance accelerated after a lull during which less than three hundred deaths from smallpox were reported in the entire country between 1906 and 1908. In a flurry of activity reminiscent of late nineteenth century England, antivaccinationists claimed that vaccination was worse than the disease. During an outbreak of mild smallpox in Ohio, one citizen demanded that the state health department place guards on the home of the victims, instead of trying to vaccinate persons who may have been exposed (Schwartz & Kerr 1918) At Niagara Falls, a "well-known anti-vaccinationist center," an observer described "one instance where a case of smallpox was found in a factory [and] the manager offered free vaccination or two weeks lay-off without pay, and only seven out of 97 employees accepted vaccination" (Williams 1915, 426). This was also an outbreak of mild smallpox. Dr. C. V. Chapin, a highly respected epidemiologist in Rhode Island, complained in 1913 that the United States was "the least vaccinated of any civilized country."

California had repealed its law that required compulsory vaccination for schoolchildren, in order to allow freedom of choice for conscientious objectors, two years before Chapin made his remark. As a result, according to an article in the *American Journal of Public Health* in 1921, 37 percent of the smallpox reported in California occurred in children under fifteen years old in 1916, by 1918 the comparable proportion had risen to 57 percent, and in 1919, it was 65 percent. After *V. minor* became rampant again nationwide starting in 1920, the United States Supreme Court ruled in 1922 that school authorities did indeed have the right to require vaccination for admission to school at all times, whether there was an immediate local threat of smallpox or not.

By the 1930s, four states had laws prohibiting compulsory vaccination (North Dakota, Minnesota, Utah, and Arizona). Twenty-nine states had no vaccination laws, six states provided for local option, and ten states (including the District of Columbia) had compulsory vaccination laws. Between 1919 and 1928, the average incidences of smallpox per 100,000 population in these four groups of states, respectively, were: 115.2, 66.7, 51.3, and 6.6. A nationwide survey conducted in 1928–31 revealed that over 40 percent of the population had never been vaccinated. By and large, persons living in Atlantic coast states in the United States accepted vaccination more readily than did residents of central and western United States or Saskatchewan, Canada ("Smallpox in the United States and Canada," 1932).

The human dimensions of multiple tragedies resulting from the controversy over vaccination were illustrated in one of the states that prohibited compulsory vaccination. State law already forbade compulsory vaccination of schoolchildren in 1917, when three Finnish immigrants, exposed to smallpox aboard the ship that took them to New York, started an outbreak in Minnesota. Among those killed in the epidemic were two of four children who had been infected while taking leave of their mother, who lay dying of tuberculosis in a multipurpose isolation hospital. The children carried the smallpox to their new home in the orphanage. Another eighteen-year-old girl, who was admitted to the smallpox isolation ward with what turned out to be chickenpox, contracted smallpox while in the hospital, and infected all eleven members of her family. Her mother, father, and infant sister died. In all, ninety-two persons were infected, of whom seventeen died (Chesley 1919).

Despite the vaccination controversy, in 1927 for the first time no outbreaks of *V. major* were reported in the United States. That milestone may have been partly due to immunity induced by the extensive outbreak of *V. minor* in 1920–21. But smallpox continued to be reported sporadically in the United States during the 1930s and early 1940s. In 1944, Canada became free of smallpox altogether.

In 1945, an American soldier returning from Japan introduced smallpox into Seattle, Washington. An outbreak of sixty-five cases resulted, twenty of them fatal. Much of the early spread occurred while the soldier was hospitalized, even though his illness had been diagnosed before he disembarked. Two years later, a man infected in Mexico died of hemorrhagic smallpox in a Manhattan hospital, but this time the correct diagnosis was not made until typical cases of smallpox began appearing among persons who had been in contact with him in the hospital. Over six million New Yorkers were vaccinated in the panic caused by this outbreak, which ended after twelve persons were infected, two of whom died. Mexico was probably also the source of the last outbreak of smallpox in the United States, in which eight persons were infected (one died) in the lower Rio Grande Valley of Texas in 1949, although the exact source of that outbreak was never established (Palmquist 1947; Weinstein 1947; Irons *et.al.*, 1953).

The last case of smallpox in North America, a fourteen-year-old boy, arrived in Toronto in August 1962, from an endemic area of Brazil, via New York City. He did not infect anyone else. Nine years later, the United States Public Health Service recommended that routine vaccination against smallpox should be discontinued in the United States. An estimated six to eight children were dying each year from rare complications of vaccination, but by then there had been no smallpox in the United States in twenty-two years (McLean et al., 1962; "Eradication of Smallpox in America," 1971).

Eight

Erythrotherapy and Eradication

PEOPLE BELONGING TO DIFFERENT cultures around the world devised innumerable remedies over the years in futile attempts to protect themselves against smallpox, as we have seen. In eighteenth-century Europe, purgatives and bleeding were especially popular therapies employed by physicians to help their patients recover from smallpox. Other treatments included diverse ointments, such as palm oil and other herbal liniments in West Africa, powdered horse excrement in Brazil, and fat from an ass in medieval Arabia. Some Japanese patients who had smallpox were bathed in hot water to which sake, rice water, red beans, and salt were added in hope of a cure. Elsewhere, many victims had special foods prescribed for them to eat, while some other variolous patients were subject to specific taboos or prohibitions. Entire families of some victims in India, for example, were forbidden to fry or season any food during the victim's illness. One fourteenth-century European physician and an eighteenth century Moghul physician in India recommended opening the pustules with a gold or silver needle. Viewed against the background of these and other extraordinary "treatments," one wonders that Jenner's promotion of cowpox to prevent smallpox raised as many European eyebrows as it did.

Of all the various remedies employed through the ages to treat smallpox, however, the most curious and persistent were based on widely held beliefs in the therapeutic efficacy of red objects. The conviction that red substances could help cure smallpox can be traced as far back as tenth-century Japan, when the *I Shinho* first mentioned use of red cloth hangings in the sick room of persons with smallpox. Seven centuries later, a European doctor visiting Japan reported that even then, Japanese physicians believed firmly in the "red treatment": Kaempfer described the red furnishings in the apartments of the emperor's children and noted that even those who came near the smallpox patient had to dress in red.

The treatment was still prevalent in the nineteenth century. In 1818 a Western visitor wrote that Japanese babies suffering from smallpox wore little red caps. When a famous Japanese novelist's grandchildren were ill with smallpox in 1831, they were clothed in red garments, and given red playthings, red confectionaries, and red pictures to ease their convalescence. Red prints of strong Japanese historical figures were especially popular for hanging in rooms of smallpox victims. Among these the most favored were figures of the twelfth-century archer, Chinzei Hachiro Tametomo (plate 17).

Faith in the red treatment was also manifest in ancient China, where physicians swabbed the first smallpox pustules that appeared with cotton soaked in red pigamon; later, fuchsin and scarlet pigments were used. Reverend Justus Doolittle, a veteran of fourteen years missionary work in China who described worship of the Chinese goddess of smallpox in 1865, also observed that infected Chinese children wore a piece of red cloth on their heads when they appeared before a figure of the goddess to appeal for their recovery. According to Dr. Ma Kan Wen of Peking (personal communication, 1981), editor of the *Journal of Traditional Chinese Medicine*, some Chinese used to hang red artifacts such as a red gourd or strip of red paper or cloth in the windows or doorways of smallpox patient's sickrooms to treat the disease and at the same time to warn others of the presence of smallpox. The red treatment was still practiced in Tonkin, Indochina, in the 1890s (Finsen 1901).

In India, where the treatment was reportedly practiced as recently as World War II (McNalty 1971), traditional representation of the Hindu goddess of smallpox in a red sari may have originated in the same colorful conviction. Turkish children who were inoculated in Constantinople late in the eighteenth century had scarlet clothes hung around their beds, because that was believed to be the favorite color of the angel who presided over smallpox. And in Asian Georgia, mothers preferred to use "red rags" to wrap the arm of an inoculated child (Miller 1957).

In Africa, the color red was also specifically associated with Shapona, the Yoruba god of smallpox. After investigating traditional Dahomeyan attitudes toward smallpox, an observer wrote that:

> A smallpox epidemic is "hot earth," and someone who dies is carried away by hot breath. During the dry season Shopona prowls about, wearing red, seeking to vent his anger. For this reason, red is a colour reserved for the god. (Quinn 1968, 157)

Nigerian and Dahomeyan smallpox victims who belonged to this cult and died of the disease were "wrapped in a shroud of red, white, and black dots" (ibid., 160). The same three colors were also associated with worship of the New World version of the same god, Omolu, in northeast Brazil.

In Western countries, the red treatment is first encountered in the twelfth-century writings of Averroes, who also offers the earliest medical explanation of how the treatment was thought to have worked. According to Averroes, the undesirable humors of smallpox needed to be drawn to the surface of the skin so that the body could excrete them. Since white colored objects acted as refrigerants, and red objects had warming properties, red was the treatment of choice for smallpox. Averroes's ideas on this subject may have originated in the writings of Avicenna (980–1037), whose sixth canon was cited by a Portuguese physician, Valescus de Taranta, in 1418 as the source of his own recommendation to "wrap the [smallpox] patient in a woolen cloth of purple or at least of a red color, so that the sight of the red cloth may move the blood to the exterior and may hold it there in a moderate heat" (Handerson 1904, 438). One wonders whether Avicenna's or Averroes's thoughts on hot and cold medicinal properties in relation to color may have derived from contact with China or India. Partly because most European medicine during the Middle Ages was based on the writings of Averroes, Avicenna, and other Moslem physicians, the red treatment for smallpox became popular all over Europe.

In England, Gilbertus Anglicus recommended use of red artifacts for treating victims of smallpox in his *Compendium Medicinae*, published in 1240. He also described how old country women gave smallpox patients burnt purple or red drinks to cure the disease. Three quarters of a century later, John of Gaddesden, Court physician to King Edward II, published an account of how he cured the king's son of smallpox in 1314, using similar methods. Gaddesden's description of the English prince's treatment is reminiscent of Kaempfer's report from Japan:

> Then let a red cloth be taken, and the variolous patient be wrapped in it completely, as I did with the son of the most noble King of England . . . I made everything about his bed red. (Creighton 1894, 1: 447)

Besides being surrounded by red blankets and red curtains, Prince John was made "to suck the juice of a red pomegranate and to gargle his throat with red mulberry wine" (Lebeuf 1900, 493).

Other European royalty were also subjected to the red treatment.[1] King Charles V ("the Wise") of France was dressed in a red shirt, red stockings, and red veils when he was stricken by smallpox. When England's Queen Elizabeth I fell ill with smallpox in 1562, she too was wrapped in a red blanket, as was the Austrian emperor Joseph I in 1711. Empress Maria Theresa of Austria probably also underwent the remedy in 1767, since her personal physician, Van Swieten, is known to have practiced it.

Fourteenth-century French (Bernard de Gordonio of Montpellier) and Italian (Franciscus de Pedemontium) physicians used the red treatment for their smallpox patients, usually by having them wrapped in red blankets. Franciscus de Pedemontium recommended the therapy in order

to excite and assist nature in drawing them to the skin: which is to be done
by warm air and by red bed coverings . . . that the blood should be carried
to the surface of the body, by looking upon red substances. (Moore 1815,
150)

The Italians (Mercurialis and Astiarias) and French (Simon de Vallem-
bert and Ambroise Paré) still employed the red treatment during the
sixteenth century, and smallpox patients in the Swiss canton of Vaud were
so treated during the seventeenth. One writer claimed that certain Italian
doctors who used the treatment "were so successful that they were accused of being in league with the devil, and had to desist" (Emerson 1903,
419). The therapy was used to treat French victims in the eighteenth
century, and it was practiced in Portugal and Rumania in the nineteenth.
Sometime during the eighteenth century it was adopted by Rosen von
Rosenstein of Sweden. There in Northern Europe, the ancient practice
was transformed and given new life at the end of the nineteenth century.

   In 1893, an eminent thirty-two-year-old Danish dermatologist, Professor Niels Finsen (1901), began to claim that treating smallpox victims
with red light reduced scarring among the survivors. Finsen had a well-
established reputation as a result of his pioneering, successful use of
actinic rays of light for treating another skin disease, lupus. However, his
combined series of 150 smallpox patients, whom he said he treated with
red light with only one "failure," was drawn mainly from the populations
of Northern European countries, which were then among the best vaccinated in Europe. Thus, many of Finsen's patients may have had only
milder manifestations of smallpox ("varioloid"), as a result of waning
vaccinal immunity (Schamberg 1903, 1904).

   The fact that Finsen chose red light to treat smallpox apparently was
not fortuitous. He was obviously aware of the long-standing use of red
colored objects to treat smallpox victims when he wrote in 1894 that
"doubtless the red coverlets were arrived at empirically, and, later, it was
sought to explain their utility by saying that the red colour irritated the
blood, and provoked a more intense exanthem, which was regarded,
according to the ideas of the time, as an advantageous result" (1901, 26).
Whether he learned of the historical red treatment before or after under-
taking his own studies is not clear. It seems likely, however, that the idea of
trying red light occurred to him as a result of popular contemporary
beliefs. Finsen's own rationale was that by filtering out the short-wave rays
of natural and artificial light, his red light treatment, or "erythrotherapy,"
reduced formation of pustules, thereby diminishing the secondary fever
and preventing scars.

   Finsen developed several rules for his erythrotherapy. Two of them
required:

1. The exclusion of the chemical rays must be absolute. The thickness of the red material employed to filter the light depends upon its nature. If paper or thin cotton material is used, four to five layers will suffice. It is more convenient to employ red glass, but in that case the glass must be very dark. To put it another way, smallpox patients must be protected from the chemical rays with as much care as the photographer uses for his plates and paper. For artificial light neither electric light nor any too brilliant illuminant must be used. The globes and lamp-glasses should be of a very dark red. A candle is permissible on account of its feeble illuminating power. It may be used to examine the patient and give light while he is having his meals.

2. The treatment should be continued without the least interruption until the vesicles have completely dried up. Even a short exposure to daylight may produce suppuration, with its sequels. It is therefore absolutely necessary to nail up the curtains, to prevent the patients and nurses from allowing the light to penetrate, for it has been found that these people tire of being in the semi-darkness, let in the light, and so reduce to naught the good results hoped for from the treatment. (Hancock 1902, 816–17)

The effects of Finsen's second rule, one suspects, probably were what caused the English physicians Ricketts and Byles (1904) to report that "the tendency to mental symptoms (delirium, headache, restlessness, etc.) seemed more marked" in patients undergoing the red light treatment than in those who didn't.

Over the next decade, clinical trials were set up to evaluate Finsen's method at medical centers in Britain, South Africa, Russia and the United States. The Russian empress ordered erythrotherapy to be thoroughly tested in one of her country's smallpox hospitals. In Indianapolis Dr. Nelson Brayton treated 300 patients with red light therapy and reported negative results early in the twentieth century. Dr. Jay Schamberg gave the therapy up as worthless after treating only two patients in Philadelphia's municipal hospital in 1902. One of Schamberg's patients died, the other was badly pockmarked. What Dr. Schamberg lacked in quantity, however, he made up for in quality:

> Our red room was complete in its appointments. The window panes were of a ruby red color, the gas jet at night was surrounded by a red globe, the walls of the room were painted deep red, and a red curtain covered the inner of two doors so as to completely exclude the light of day. (Schamberg 1903, 1185)

In Dubuque, Dr. J. C. Hancock reported in 1902: "In our smallpox hospital last winter I had the windows and transoms of several rooms covered with five to seven thicknesses of red paper. It was impossible to begin the treatment earlier in the season." Several patients at Boston's

Smallpox Hospital were transferred to that hospital's Red Room, "a room in which the window was covered with red curtain cloth" during an epidemic in 1902 (Bancroft 1902, 548–49). That March, when a young physician who had been caring for others at the hospital contracted smallpox himself, he too was placed in the Red Room, where he recovered (plate 36).

Dr. Finsen died in 1904 at the height of the controversy about erythrotherapy, one year after he was awarded a Nobel prize for his discovery of the efficacy of actinic rays for treating lupus.[2] In an article published in the *British Medical Journal* in 1903 he wrote: "The action of light on the course of smallpox is astonishing, and the effect of the red light treatment is one of the most striking results known in medicine." Commenting on the last article Finsen wrote on behalf of the red light treatment a few weeks before he died, two of his defenders maintained:

> It was in his proposal to treat small-pox patients in rooms from which the chemical rays of daylight are shut out and in the *rationale* of this method that Finsen's genius burst forth beyond all question. . . . The above article, the last from his hand, shows that he to the end maintained an unshakeable confidence in the therapeutic value of this method. (Forchammer & Busck 1902)

Finsen's red light treatment survived him for many years.

According to Renbourn (1972), a Viennese doctor around this time elaborated on Finsen's method by vaccinating his patients in rooms illuminated with red light, then covering the vaccinated area with red bandages. He claimed "excellent results." K. B. Roberts, a Canadian author, said that his father made him "wear a red ribbon band around the upper arm for a few days after [he] was vaccinated or re-vaccinated as a schoolboy in the 1930s!" (1978, 8).

An Austrian soldier reported having seen the red treatment being practiced during World War I, when some Poles in Galicia and Russian Poland "pasted their windows with red tissue-paper. . . . We found this treatment everywhere" (Olbert 1962). In 1925, it was said to still be in vogue in the Caucasus, parts of France, and Rumania. Only four years earlier, Schamberg had felt obliged to end the section on treatment of smallpox in his new textbook, *Disease of the Skin and the Eruptive Fevers*, with the statement, "I concur in the verdict of Ricketts and Bayles, of London, who say: 'We cannot agree that the (red light) treatment has any of the merits which have been claimed for it' " (1921, 510).[3]

ERADICATION

If the red treatment was a therapeutic blind alley, Jennerian vaccination clearly was not. A full account of the global Smallpox Eradication Program (SEP) of 1967–77 is not my intent, but a summary of that successful endeavor is necessary in order to complete our story. Jenner himself foresaw the ultimate result of vaccination. In 1800, only four years after his great discovery, he wrote:

> May I not with perfect confidence congratulate my country and society at large on their beholding . . . an antidote that is capable of extirpating from the earth a disease which is every hour devouring its victims; a disease that has ever been considered as the severest scourge of the human race!

One wonders whether he would have believed in the first decade of the nineteenth century that smallpox would endure for more than one and a half centuries.

Two major impediments to eradicating smallpox globally remained even after Jenner's vaccine had been proven to be effective. In the first place, the vaccine was difficult to preserve and supplies were limited. Second, the very possibility of eradicating smallpox required a faith and foresight that were hard to find so long as the disease seemed to be everywhere, all the time. The former technological problems had to be solved before practical steps toward global eradication could be seriously considered.

Negri of Naples introduced the first improvement in technology when he began producing safe vaccine in large quantities from inoculated cattle in 1842. Half a century later, Britain's Monckton Copeman demonstrated glycerin's beneficial effect as a preservative (MacNalty 1962). Copeman's discovery further improved the quality of vaccine, but excessive bacterial contamination remained a problem until the mid-twentieth century. Persons vaccinated with contaminated vaccines sometimes developed a pustule and a persistent scar caused by the bacteria. The pustules and scars were often confusingly similar to those caused by true vaccina virus, but they conferred no immunity.

Even glycerine-preserved vaccine lost its potency quickly if left at ambient temperatures in tropical climates, where refrigeration was scarce. To obviate that problem, Dutch and French researchers developed a hardier "dried" smallpox vaccine for use in their colonies, beginning in the 1920s. Their dried vaccine, however, was difficult to reconstitute and was of inconsistent quality from batch to batch. Thus, it was only after the costly outbreak of smallpox in New York City in 1947 led to a reconsideration of the method that an improved method of freeze-drying was developed at the Michigan State Laboratories in 1949 and field tested in Peru. It was fully adapted to commercial production in 1954 at the Lister Institute in England. The improved freeze-dried smallpox vaccine maintained its potency in virtually any climate for months without refrigeration, thus eliminating the main technological hindrance to eradication. (Polak 1968; Fasquelle 1971; Soper 1966; Collier 1954, 1978).

As slow as the improvements in, and systematic employment of, Jenner's vaccine may seem to us now, we have seen how knowledge about the disease itself was gained even more slowly, considering how long the disease had been around. Once a safe, effective, practical way to prevent smallpox was in hand, however, detailed knowledge of the responsible microbe wasn't as vital for a successful attack as was knowledge about other characteristics of the disease.

It had long been recognized that persons who once suffered the disease were usually immune to another attack for the rest of their lives. This was the principle underlying inoculation. Nearly all infectious patients had an obvious, easily recognized rash, and by isolating them, one could help keep the disease from spreading to others. In addition, by early in the twentieth century, some would-be eradicators felt fairly confident that there was no reservoir in animals, from which the disease might reinfect people, if it could be eliminated from the human population. However, largely because the surprise discovery in 1932 of a previously unrecognized reservoir of yellow fever in monkeys during a campaign to eradicate the disease in South America had doomed that program to an embarrassing failure, the potential existence of an unrecognized animal reservoir of smallpox virus remained a matter of concern during the early stages of the global Smallpox Eradication Program.

Even as adequate vaccine and sufficient knowledge of the disease's characteristics were becoming available, however, the idea that smallpox might be totally eradicated by concerted international cooperation took hold very slowly. In its own way, the idea was as unnatural to many mid-twentieth century minds as Jenner's revolutionary cowpox vaccine had seemed to many of his contemporaries at the end of the eighteenth century. Malaria, yellow fever, and yaws had each been proposed for eradication campaigns by 1955. Spread of the first two diseases depended on theoretically vulnerable mosquito vectors, which were found in only limited geographic areas, whereas yaws spread relatively slowly by skin-to-skin contact, could be quickly cured by a single injection of penicillin, and usually occurred only in poor, rural tropical areas. Yet none of those diseases had been eradicated by the late 1960s (they still haven't disappeared). Smallpox, on the other hand, occurred everywhere and spread directly and rapidly from person to person. Despite their centuries-long experience with smallpox inoculation, neither the Chinese, Indians, nor Africans had dared to attempt to eliminate the disease altogether. Many knowledgeable public health experts believed it made more sense, and was far less risky, to concentrate on increasing the number of available clinics and other health services, which then could treat many people for many diseases, than to attempt to eradicate one disease, even smallpox, once and for all.

Except for John Haygarth's publication of *A Sketch of a Plan to Exter-*

minate the Casual Small-pox from Great Britain, and to Introduce General Inoculation in London in 1793, virtually all efforts against the disease prior to the twentieth century focused on the personal protection of individuals or groups of individuals, not on eliminating the disease itself. Nevertheless, vigorous control efforts were relatively successful in reducing the threat in the New England colonies of North America in the seventeenth and eighteenth centuries and in Leicester, England, during the late nineteenth century. Several countries that vigorously pursued the personal protection strategy were able to stop smallpox completely. Sweden was the first major country to eliminate indigenous smallpox nationwide, reporting no cases for the first time in 1895 (Zetterberg et al. 1966). A massive vaccination effort eliminated the disease from Puerto Rico in 1899. Endemic smallpox also disappeared from Austria in the 1920s, from England, the Philippines, and the USSR in the 1930s, and from Canada and the United States in the 1940s. But the elimination of smallpox in these and other countries, especially in the earlier part of the twentieth century, was more a by-product of attempts to vaccinate entire populations than the achievement of a national goal in itself. Moreover, except in a few colonial situations, these were not cooperative international efforts.

The first attempts at international cooperation against the disease were cautious and only partly successful. When, for example, in 1926 a Japanese delegate to the Fourteenth International Sanitary Conference of the League of Nations proposed for the first time that smallpox should be made internationally notifiable, as plague, cholera, and yellow fever already were, a Swiss delegate objected that smallpox had "no place in an international convention," since the disease "exists everywhere: there is probably not a single country of which it can be said that there are no cases of smallpox" (Howard-Jones 1975, 4). As a compromise, smallpox was declared an internationally notifiable disease—but only when it was epidemic. Two years before the health functions of the League of Nations were taken over by the World Health Organization (WHO) in 1948, an interim commission stated that it was "impractical as yet" to try to standardize smallpox vaccines (Henderson 1976, 28).

Other abortive efforts to enlist concerted action against smallpox followed the shocking outbreak that panicked New York City in 1947 and an upsurge of the disease in several Asian and African countries ten years later. Smallpox had already disappeared from North and Central America when the Pan American Sanitary Bureau approved a regional smallpox eradication campaign in the Americas using the new freeze-dried vaccine, in 1949–50. At the time, some ninety-one countries around the globe were still reporting smallpox, which was constantly present in about two-thirds of them. The World Health Organization was aware of the limited success of eradication campaigns in Latin America and a few other tropical countries, as well as of the upsurge in smallpox in several other countries in 1957, when in 1958 it adopted a resolution sponsored by the Soviet Union that called for a global push to eradicate the disease, starting the next year. In 1959, an additional stimulus was provided when an artist carried the virus into Moscow from India, causing the first outbreak in the Soviet capital in many years (Baroyan & Serenko 1961). However, this first, half-hearted attempt at a global campaign had little discernable impact on the worldwide problem.·

The final call to arms came in 1966 when the Nineteenth World Health Assembly, meeting in Geneva, adopted a resolution cosponsored by several countries, including the United States and the USSR, that called for intensified efforts to eradicate smallpox, starting the following January. This resolution differed from previous ones, however, in that it set a specific deadline—ten years—for achieving global eradication. At that time, forty-four countries were still reporting smallpox, and the disease was endemic in thirty-three of them (fig. 15).

Despite the earlier efforts, the disease was still greatly underreported when the global campaign began. According to Dr. Donald A. Henderson (1978), whereas some 131,000 cases of smallpox were officially reported in 1967, the first year of the global Smallpox Eradication Program, an estimated 10 to 15 million cases actually occurred that year. Thus, on the average, for every reported case, there were about 99 unreported cases. Under the adroit leadership of Henderson, a medical epidemiologist lent to the WHO by the United States Public Health Service, the new WHO program moved quickly to improve international reporting of smallpox. By designating International Reference Laboratories in Canada and the Netherlands to monitor the quality of vaccine used in the worldwide campaign, the program resolved what had been another serious problem. During the early stages of the campaign, the USSR donated over 140 million doses of vaccine a year as the new global program gathered momentum.

One of the most important challenges to the Smallpox Eradication Program was the need to prove, as quickly as possible, that the disease could be eradicated from poorer countries in spite of their inadequate health services. Many thoughtful public health specialists doubted that could be done to the end of the campaign, but such doubts were especially prevalent during the SEP's early stages. This crucial psychological victory was first achieved in West and Central Africa, where twenty contiguous countries, with advisors, equipment, and vaccine provided by the United States, eradicated smallpox in their region in less than three and a half years (Foege et al. 1975). Although a few of the twenty countries were already free of the virus when the regional program began, six of them had been among the twelve most highly endemic countries in the world.

In addition to proving that smallpox could be eradicated under the most difficult conditions expected, the regional effort in Africa was important to the SEP for another reason. It provided the basis for a significant change in the global campaign's strategy. The SEP's initial strategy emphasized surveillance and mass vaccination, relying upon newly developed jet injectors, each capable of vaccinating up to a thousand persons per hour. The program had not been underway a year when a delay in arrival of vaccine for the mass vaccination program in eastern Nigeria forced the local advisor, Dr. William Foege (1975), to set priorities for what little vaccine he did have. This led to a major discovery: the disease could be eliminated without vaccinating the entire population, if case-finding and containment efforts were concentrated instead on the much smaller number of households and villages that actually had smallpox. Where mass vaccination had required as its target 80 to 100 percent of a country's population, the new "surveillance-containment" strategy focused attention on the much smaller fraction of the population that had or had recently been exposed to smallpox at any one time. The efficacy of this new strategy was quickly confirmed in other West African countries, Brazil, and Indonesia. In retrospect, earlier evidence that such a strategy could work was available in Leicester's experience late in the nineteenth century. C. W. Dixon had suggested such a strategy in his textbook on smallpox published in 1962: "If more study were given to the foci of smallpox, it might be possible to eradicate the disease from an area by vaccinating a far smaller proportion of the total population" (359).

A few months later, WHO-inspired research at Wyeth Laboratories complemented the efficient new surveillance-containment strategy by introducing the bifurcated needle (Henderson 1976). Simple, cheap, and highly appropriate for the new strategy, when dipped in vaccine the bifurcated needles automatically collected the correct amount of liquid needed for a vaccination between the twin points at one end. Moreover, the needles could be easily sterilized for reuse by boiling, and unlike the jet injectors they required no upkeep or spare parts. In two or three minutes, anyone could be taught how to give perfect vaccinations. Few doubted now that smallpox would be eradicated within a few years.

Only eleven months after the disease was eliminated from West and Central Africa in May 1970, Brazil, the last endemic country in the Americas, became smallpox-free. Indonesia recorded its last case in January 1972, nine months after Brazil. By the end of 1972, the disease was confined to only six countries: four in Asia (India, Pakistan, Bangladesh, and Nepal) and two in East Africa (Ethiopia and Sudan) (see fig. 15).

There were also unexpected setbacks. Civil wars in Nigeria, Sudan, and Bangladesh, and fighting between Ethiopia and Somalia delayed operations or caused the reintroduction of disease into areas previously freed of smallpox. The disease staged deadly, surprise appearances "behind the lines" at Meschede, West Germany, in 1970, in Yugoslavia in

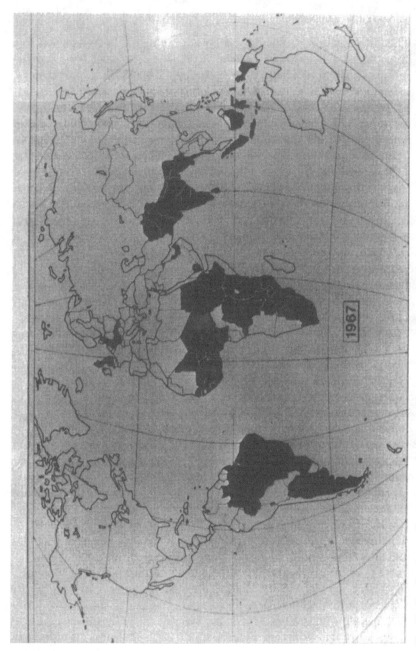

Fig. 15. Decline in smallpox-endemic countries. Courtesy World Health Organization. The global Smallpox Eradication Program began in 1967.

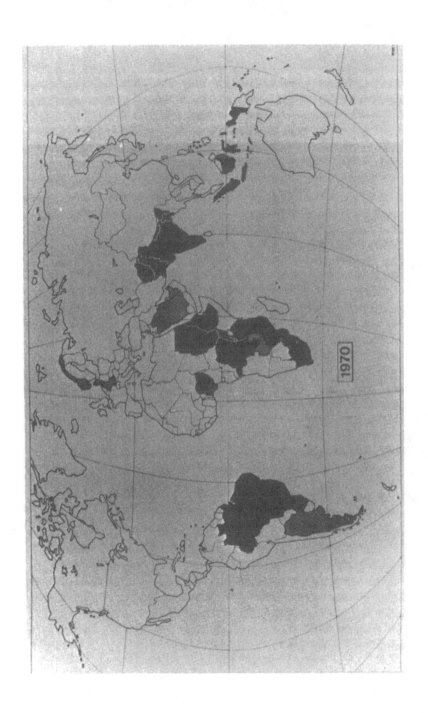

1970

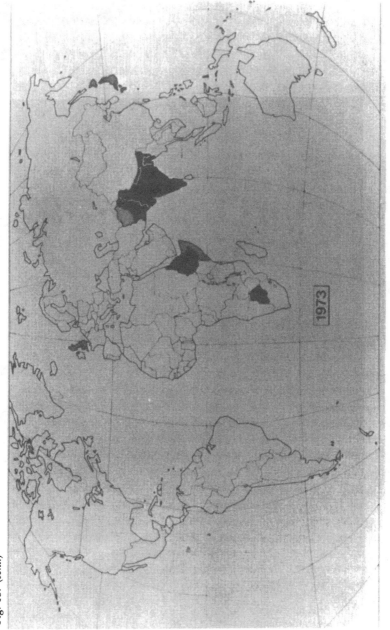

Fig. 15. (*cont.*)

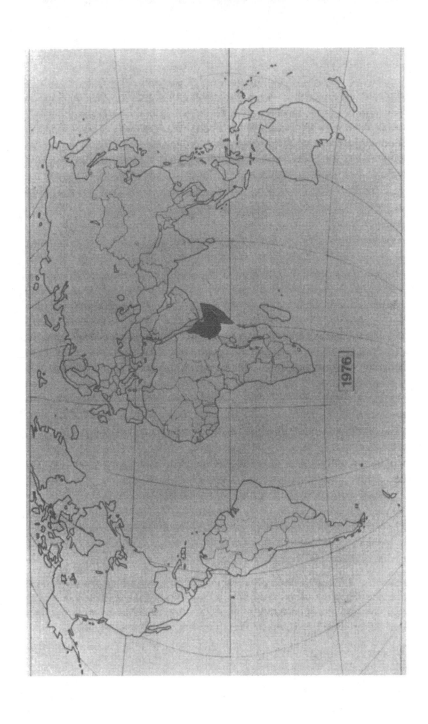

1972, and in London in 1973. In the spring of 1974, an awesome epidemic in Northeast India killed over twenty-five thousand persons.

Asia finally became smallpox free after 16 October 1975, when the rash appeared on a young girl in Bangladesh who was the last known case of endemic *V. major* in the world (plate 25). Less than a year later, just as *V. minor* was eliminated in August 1976 from Ethiopia, the elusive virus turned up in neighboring Somalia. After a protracted thirteen month struggle in Somalia, smallpox was eliminated from that final stronghold in October 1977 (plate 28). But "Variola Rex" still had one more surprise in store for mankind.

Ten months after the last case of smallpox recovered in Somalia, the world prepared to celebrate completion of its first year without the disease. Then, almost as if in defiance, the virus escaped from a research laboratory in Birmingham, England, and infected a photographer's assistant, who subsequently infected her mother. They were the world's last cases of smallpox. In this ultimate salute, the virus also drove one of the world's foremost authorities on smallpox, Professor Henry Bedson, to suicide. Bedson, who had led the team that differentiated *V. intermedius* fifteen years earlier, had been in charge of the laboratory from which the virus escaped.

As the struggle against smallpox drew to a close, the WHO organized a blue-ribbon International Commission to document and certify eradication. Formerly endemic nations were searched intensively for evidence of recent smallpox in order to assure the world that it was really gone. During the certification process, two consultants to the World Health Organization visited Rhodesia (now Zimbabwe) eight years after that country had reported its last case of smallpox to the WHO. In the same country where Chief Lobengula and much of his army had perished from smallpox while resisting British colonizers in 1894, and where 194 cases of smallpox had been reported as recently as 1964, Drs. Grasset and Meikle-john observed in 1978 that

> there was a remarkable lack of knowledge about smallpox among people less than 25 years of age. Almost without exception they failed to recognize the smallpox pictures on the recognition cards and stated that they had never seen or known of the presence of the disease. (13)

Thus, Thomas Jefferson's prophecy was fulfilled. In 1806 the man who drafted the United States of America's Declaration of Independence declared in a letter to Jenner:

> You have erased from the calendar of human afflictions one of its greatest. Yours is the comfortable reflection that mankind can never forget that you have lived. Future nations will know by history only that the loathsome smallpox has existed. (Baron 1838, 2: 95)

May it always be so.

Chronology

c.1500 B.C.– 1 B.C.	Description of smallpox and of worship of smallpox goddess in India.
c.1350 B.C.	Fatal contagious epidemic spreads from Egyptians to Hittites in Syria.
1157 B.C.	Egyptian pharaoh Ramses V dies with smallpoxlike rash.
430–29 B.C.	Plague of Athens spreads to Greece from Egypt, Libya, and Ethiopia; then from Greece to Persia.
395 B.C.	Epidemic spreads to Syracuse from Libya.
c.250–243 B.C.	"Hunpox" introduced into China. Epidemic throughout the empire.
48–49 A.D.	General Ma-yuan's army introduces "captive's pox" into China's Hunan Province. Ma-yuan and half his army die.
165–80	Plague of Antonius spreads to Rome from Mesopotamia; kills Roman emperor Marcus Aurelius at Vienna.
c.185	Cult of goddess of smallpox introduced into Ceylon from India.
302	Bishop Eusebius describes smallpoxlike illness in Syria.
c.340	Ko Hung describes smallpox in China.
450	Bishop Nicaise of Rheims, France, recovers from smallpox; becomes patron saint of the disease.
447, 452	Epidemics and famine cause Huns to retreat from France and Italy.
541	Plague of Justinian (bubonic plague and perhaps smallpox) at Byzantium. Pustular disease in France.
570	Elephant War epidemic defeats Ethiopian soldiers at Mecca; spreads back (?) to Ethiopia, (?) to Italy.
580–81	Bishop Gregory of Tours describes smallpox epidemic in France and Italy.
583	Smallpox introduced into Korea from China.
585–87	Smallpoxlike pestilence introduced into Japan from Korea; kills two Japanese emperors.
622	Aaron describes smallpox at Alexandria.
675–778	*Galrabreac* described in Ireland.
710	Arabs carry smallpox to Spain and Mauritania.
735–37	Smallpox introduced into Japan from Korea; kills four Fujiwara brothers; emperor orders construction of *Nara Daibutsu*.
754	Caliph Abul-al-Abbas, "the blood shedder," dies of smallpox at Damascus.

c.925	Rhazes publishes *A Treatise on the Smallpox and Measles*, at Baghdad.
907	Alfreda, daughter of Alfred the Great, has "smallpox" in England.
977	Smallpox blinds four-year-old Syrian boy, Abul-Ala al-Ma'arri, he becomes reknowned poet.
982	*I Shinho* published in Japan; mentions special isolation hospitals for smallpox victims and red treatment for first time.
c.1240	Gilbertus Anglicus publishes *Compendium Medicinae*, describing varieties of smallpox in England; recommends red treatment.
1241	Smallpox spreads to Iceland for first time.
1257	First reported outbreak of smallpox in Denmark.
1368	King Thadominbya of Burma dies of smallpox.
c.1430	Smallpox spreads to Greenland from Iceland, exterminates the colony.
c.1438	Epidemic in Paris kills fifty thousand.
c.1450	Spread to Sweden.
1507	First outbreak in New World on island of Hispanola.
1518	Epidemic on Hispanola, apparently brought by slaves from West Africa, spreads to Cuba.
1520	Smallpox invades Mexico, kills Aztec emperor Cuitláhuac and hundreds of thousands of Indians.
c.1524–27	Smallpox invades Peru, kills Inca Hyana Capac and an estimated two hundred thousand of his subjects.
1534	King Boramaraja IV of Siam dies of smallpox.
1545	Epidemic in Goa kills eight thousand Indian children and two princes from Ceylon.
1546	Italy's Girolamo Fracastoro publishes book stating doctrine of specific contagion for smallpox and measles.
1554	Smallpox introduced into Chili.
1555	Epidemic in Brazil.
1562	Queen Elizabeth I of England recovers from smallpox. Epidemic kills over thirty thousand Indians in Brazil.
1576	Two million Aztecs die of smallpox.
1577	General Chilarai of Koch Bihar, India, dies of smallpox.
1580	Authorities in Geneva begin to keep records of deaths from smallpox.
1582	King and queen of Kandy (Ceylon) and all their sons die of smallpox.
1583	Maharajah Vijoy Manikya of Tripura dies of smallpox.
1588	Pandemic across South America.
1589	Epidemic along East African coast.
1591	Severe epidemic in Manila, Philippines.
1612	Duke of Mantua and infant son die of smallpox. Question of Mantuan Succession.
1613	Epidemic kills over two thousand six hundred in Nagasaki, Japan.
1614	Widespread epidemic in Europe, Egypt, Turkey, Persia.

c.1617–19	Epidemic kills nine-tenths of Indian population along Massachusetts coast.
1619	Fifty thousand die of smallpox in Chili.
1623	Russian word for smallpox seen for first time, in physician's letter from Moscow.
1630	Large epidemics reported in Siberia.
1634	Large epidemic in Connecticut River valley almost destroys Huron Indians.
1639	Hospital Hotel-Dieu founded at Quebec.
1646	Spanish Habsburg heir, Prince Balthazar Carlos dies of smallpox.
1647	Boston authorities begin quarantining ships with smallpox in harbor.
1650	Smallpox spreads to Faroe Islands from Denmark; Prince William II of Orange dies of smallpox.
1654	Habsburg emperor-elect Ferdinand (IV) and Emperor Gokomyo of Japan die of smallpox.
1660	Duke of Gloucester and his sister, Princess Mary of Orange, die of smallpox. Forty-four thousand Brazilian Indians die.
1661	First Manchu ruler of China, Emperor Fu-lin, dies of smallpox; his third son (K'ang Hsi) elected to succeed him because he is immune.
1665–66	Epidemic along entire coast of Brazil.
1666–67	Maharaja of Tripura, Chattra Manikya, dies of smallpox.
1667	Virginia legislates mandatory isolation of victims at home.
1670	Epidemic around Luanda, Angola.
1677–78	Epidemic in Boston leads to first medical pamphlet in North America.
1680	Epidemic in Ecuador kills more than sixty thousand.
1683	Epidemic at Sennar, Sudan.
1685	Epidemic devastates Elmina, on West Africa's Gold Coast.
1687	Shippers at Bahia, Brazil, threaten to suspend slave traffic because of smallpox in Angola.
1689	Rajah Virappa of Madura dies of smallpox. Death of English physician Thomas Sydenham. Russians send mission to China to study inoculation.
1690	Smallpox thwarts British-Iroquois attack on Quebec.
1694	Queen Mary II of England dies of smallpox.
1699	Governor of Gerri in Sudan regularly examines caravans from Egypt to prevent importation of smallpox.
1700	Duke of Gloucester dies of smallpox, ending Stuart line. King Nagassi of Shoa, Ethiopia, dies of smallpox.
1702–3	Epidemic kills almost one-fourth of population of Quebec City.
1706	West African slave, Onesimus, tells Cotton Mather in Boston, Massachusetts, of inoculation.
1707	Epidemic kills eighteen thousand of fifty thousand Icelanders.
1709	Japanese shogun Tsunayoshi and former emperor Higashiyama die of smallpox.

1711	Habsburg emperor Joseph I and heir to French throne die of smallpox.
1713	Smallpox imported into South Africa for first time at Capetown; decimates Hottentots.
1718	Epidemic kills Ethiopian nobles.
1719	Epidemic kills fourteen thousand Parisians. Epidemic in Sennar kills local notables and former king Ounsa III.
1721	Smallpox inoculation introduced into Europe and North America.
1724	King Luis I of Spain dies of smallpox. Chinese emperor sends inoculation team to assist in controlling epidemic in "Tartary" (Siberia).
1728	Roman Catholic missionaries introduce inoculation into Brazil.
1730	Tsar Peter II of Russia dies of smallpox.
1741	Swedish Queen Ulrica Eleonora dies of smallpox.
1744	Inoculation introduced into Japan.
1746	London Smallpox Hospital founded.
1749	Epidemic in Sumatra.
1750	Epidemic around Belém, Brazil, kills forty thousand.
1755	Smallpox imported into Capetown completes devastation of Hottentots. "Year of the Great Smallpox Epidemic" in Canada.
1762	Development of "Suttonian method" of inoculation. French parliament bans inoculation in towns. Mexico City epidemic kills ten thousand.
1761–63, 1767	Epidemics at court of Empress Maria Theresa of Austria.
1764–65	Pandemic in South America.
1768	Herberden distinguishes smallpox and chickenpox. Dimsdale inoculates Catherine the Great.
1769	Epidemic kills sixty-three thousand in Murshidabad, including nawab of Bengal, Syefuddowla; three million die in India. Epidemic attacks Ethiopian royal family.
1774	King Louis XV of France dies of smallpox.
1775–76	Siege of Boston prolonged because of smallpox.
1776	Smallpox disrupts colonial army at Quebec, preventing United States' capture of Canada. General Thomas dies.
1777	Washington orders Continental army inoculated.
1779	Smallpox cripples powerful Spanish-French armada before it can attack England. Epidemic in Mexico City kills eighteen thousand; inoculation introduced into Mexico.
1780	Tibetan Panchen Lama dies of smallpox at Yellow Temple in Peking.
1785	Inoculation introduced into Burma.
1789	Smallpox introduced into Australia. King of Dahomey, Adahoonzou II (Kpengla) dies of smallpox.
1796	Edward Jenner discovers vaccination.
1797	King Agonglo of Dahomey is poisoned while suffering from smallpox. Epidemic in Mexico kills over fourteen thousand.

1800	Vaccination introduced into North America, India, France, Greece, Turkey. King of Nepal's mistress commits suicide because of scarring from smallpox.
1801	President Jefferson initiates vaccination of American Indians.
1801–2	Pandemic among North American Indians; kills two-thirds of Omaha tribe and their chief, Blackbird.
1803	Spanish king issues order for Balmis Salvany Expedition to take vaccine to all his dominions around the world.
1805	Vaccination introduced into China. King of Kandy recovers from smallpox, is moved to seek peace.
1807	Vaccination made legally compulsory in Bavaria.
1808	National Vaccine Establishment founded in England.
1811	Maharajah of Assam, Kamaleswar Singha, dies of smallpox.
1813	United States Congress passes Act to Encourage Vaccination.
1816	King Girvana Shah of Nepal dies of smallpox.
1824	Crown Prince Oomed Singh of Gujarat, India, dies of smallpox.
1824–29	European pandemic.
1829	Revaccination introduced at Wurtemberg, Germany.
1836–40	Pandemic among North American Indians; destroys the Mandan tribe and their chief, Ma-to-toh-pa.
1837–40	European pandemic.
1840	Vaccination introduced into Siam from Boston Massachusetts.
1840s	Caravans spread smallpox in East Africa.
c.1845	Negri of Naples begins propagating cowpox from cow to cow to use as vaccine.
1849	Vaccination introduced into Japan.
1849–50	Over six thousand die of smallpox in Calcutta.
1858	King Guezo of Dahomey dies of smallpox.
1863	President Lincoln has smallpox.
1863–64	*V. minor* described in Jamaica.
1864–65	Angola suffers its worst smallpox epidemic of nineteenth century.
1865	Governor-General Musa Pasha Hamdi of Sudan dies of smallpox.
1865	Seven thousand die of smallpox in Lahore, India.
1866–67	Epidemic in Indochina.
1867	Emperor Komei of Japan dies of smallpox.
1868–69	Epidemic throughout India kills eight out of every ten children in Hardoi District.
1869	Severe epidemic in coastal China and Japan.
1870–75	European pandemic triggered by Franco-Prussian War; estimated five hundred thousand die of smallpox.
1871	Nearly two thousand die of smallpox in Philadelphia.
1872–74	Pandemic in India.
1875	T'ung Chih, emperor of China, dies of smallpox. Emperor and empress of Japan are vaccinated.
1877–79	Pandemic in India.

1878	Nearly eleven thousand deaths reported from smallpox in India's Allahabad District. Epidemic at Fortaleza, Brazil, kills over fifty-six thousand.
1883	Kimberly Mines Scandal in South Africa.
1884–85	Pandemic in India and Indochina.
1884	Asantehene Kwaku Dua II dies of smallpox.
1885–86	Epidemic in Montreal kills 3,164 persons.
1891	Monckton Copeman demonstrates germicidal effect of adding glycerine to smallpox vaccine.
1893	Finsen introduces red light treatment in Denmark.
1894	Vaccination introduced into Kashmir, India. Chief Lobengula of Matabele dies of smallpox while fleeing British South Africa Company.
1895	Sweden reports no smallpox for first time. *V. minor* described in South Africa.
1896	*V. minor* introduced into North America at Pensacola, Florida.
1898	Emperor Menelik II of Ethiopia issues decree making vaccination compulsory in Addis Ababa.
1899	Epidemic forces Kikuyu to abandon their land, facilitating British settlement of Kenyan highlands. Smallpox eradicated in Puerto Rico.
1901–3	Epidemic in United States. Red treatment tested in Boston, Philadelphia, Indianapolis, and Dubuque.
1904	Epidemic in Rio de Janeiro kills three thousand six hundred.
1905	Epidemic kills three thousand eight hundred in Recife, Brazil. Five thousand six hundred die in Valparaiso, Chili.
1907–8	Epidemic in Kobe, Japan, kills nearly five thousand persons.
1908	Epidemic kills six thousand five hundred in Rio de Janeiro.
1909	Experimental dried smallpox vaccine tested in Guinea, West Africa.
1910	*V. minor* reported for first time in Brazil.
1918–19	Epidemic kills sixty-four thousand Filipinos.
c.1920	Otten develops room-dried stable vaccine for use in Netherlands East Indies.
1924	*V. minor* reported in Europe for first time. Over eleven thousand die in Bombay epidemic.
1930	Epidemics in all of India's major ports cause restrictions on Indian shipping worldwide.
1934	Last case of smallpox in Madagascar.
1939	Great Britain free of smallpox for first time.
c.1943	Vaccination introduced into Tibet.
1944	Canada reports no smallpox for first time.
1947	Twelve persons infected in New York City outbreak; over six million New Yorkers vaccinated.
1949	Freeze-dried smallpox vaccine introduced. Pan American Sanitary Bureau calls for eradication of smallpox in the Americas. Last cases of smallpox in United States (imported).
1957	Pandemic of smallpox in Asia, Africa.

1960   Last cases of smallpox in China.

1962   India begins National Smallpox Eradication Program.

1966   World Health Assembly votes global Smallpox Eradication Program.

1967   Global Smallpox Eradication Program begins; India reports two-third's of world's smallpox.

1968   Bifurcated needle introduced. Surveillance-containment strategy introduced.

1970   Last case of smallpox in West Africa.

1971   Last case of smallpox in South America.

1972   Smallpox imported into Yugoslavia for first time since 1930. Smallpox reintroduced into Bangladash.

1973   Smallpox escapes from laboratory in London, kills two persons.

1974   Massive epidemic in Northeast India kills over ten thousand persons in Bihar State in one month.

1975   Last case of smallpox in India. World's last case of endemic *V. major* in Bangladesh.

1977   World's last case of endemic smallpox, *V. minor*, in Somalia.

1978   Smallpox escapes from laboratory in Birmingham, England, kills two persons—one by suicide.

1979   Global Commission certifies the eradication of smallpox.

1980   Thirty-third World Health Assembly accepts the Final Report of the Global Commission for the Certification of Smallpox Eradication.

Notes

Chapter 1

1. King Suppiluliumas declared war on Egypt when one of his sons was assassinated soon after he arrived in Egypt. The prince had been sent to Egypt in response to an unprecedented appeal from the young widow of Tutankhamun for a Hittite prince to become her consort and succeed to the Egyptian throne.

Chapter 2

1. William II lay in state at the Binnenhof in the Hague for four months. In March his body was moved to Delft, where he was buried in the House of Orange's royal crypt at New Church (Van der Zee & Van der Zee 1973).

2. The queen's state bed chamber in which Mary II died, and the ornate writing cabinet that contained her papers may still be seen at Kensington Palace. The letter she wrote to her husband the night of 20 December, to be opened after her death, informed him of the pain he had caused her by his supposedly secret affair with one of the ladies at court. Another note instructed that her body should not be opened, and forbade an elaborate funeral, but it was discovered too late to be observed. The queen's body lay in state at Whitehall "in a bed of Purple all open" before her burial in Westminster Abbey. The lord-mayor and aldermen of London, both Houses of Parliament, judges, sergeants at law, "and all her majesty's household" joined the funeral procession in March 1695 (Noorthouck 1773, 282). Henry Purcell composed a special funeral anthem, and Sir Christopher Wren constructed a passageway covered with black cloth between Whitehall and Westminster Abbey for the occasion.

3. Most accounts say that the duc de Borgogne, his wife, and son died of measles, which it probably was, rather than smallpox. But according to Lavisse (1911), the diagnosis of their atypical rashes was disputed at the time of their deaths early in 1712. The grand dauphin's death from smallpox is not disputed.

4. Circassian women were avidly sought for the Turkish sultan's harem at Constantinople because of their legendary beauty. Indeed, Barber believed that the demand for Circassian girls in Constantinople may itself have "encouraged [Circassian] parents to preserve their girl children from the disfigurement of the widespread smallpox by inoculation" (1973, 69).

5. A volume of her letters published in London in 1767 included a drawing of "Lady M-y W-r-t-l-y M-nt-g-e The Female Traveller, in the Turkish Dress," facing the title page, with the following words of advice below:

Let Men who glory in their better sense,
Read, hear, and learn Humility from hence,
No more let them Superior Wisdom boast,
They cannot but equal M-nt-g-e at most.
(Montague 1767, frontispiece)

6. Statistics are drawn from Creighton 1894; Cardenas 1976; Kübler 1901; Lersch 1896; Miller 1957; Edwardes 1902b; and Minor 1882.

7. The room where Luis lay in state still exists at Madrid's Museum of the Army, near the Prado.

8. Ulrica Eleonora, Federick I, and her brother Charles XII share the Carolinian burial chapel in Stockholm's Riddarholmen Church. The timing of her early symptoms suggests that the physician who bled her, or a member of his entourage, might have carried the infection to the palace.

9. This was a widespread phenomenon in Europe. In France, Sainte-Beuve noted, "Several of the young ladies who became the outstanding nuns of Port-Royale had had smallpox, which at an early age had disfigured their faces.... I do not wish to say that we give to God only that which no longer has value in the world" (Durant 1963, 50–51).

10. This method of facilitating acceptance of a new practice was echoed during the Smallpox Eradication Program two centuries later, as any number of Third World mayors, prime ministers, and chiefs were vaccinated first as an encouraging example to their constituents.

11. The state bed and bedroom in which he died are on view at Versailles.

12. British statistics are taken from Creighton 1894; Edwardes 1902b; Razzell 1977a; Moore 1815. Continental statistics are also drawn from Edwardes, as well as from Rosenthal 1959; Baron 1827; Haygarth 1793; Lersch 1896; Hirsch 1883; Sandwith 1910; Tyson 1901; and Seely 1871.

13. Statistics for the Franco-Prussian War pandemic are taken from the following sources: Prinzing 1916; Rolleston 1933; Low 1918; Kübler 1901; Newsholme 1902; Burke 1872; Howard 1962; and Kraechenko 1970.

14. Smallpox declined sharply in Paris soon after the siege ended. The Paris correspondent of the London paper *Medical Times and Gazette* wrote in its issue of 2 June 1872, "It is very perverse of unvaccinated Paris to be free from smallpox, while the disease rages in vaccinated London ... " Three weeks later, a London physician wrote wondering "whether the combination of thousands of tons of gunpowder purified the atmosphere of Paris," and went on to suggest that "an experiment on a small scale, if it could be performed with safety, might be worth a trial."

15. Interested readers are referred to Macleod's comprehensive article "Law, Medicine, and Public Opinion: The resistance to compulsory Health Legislation, 1870–1907," on the background and consequences of this crisis.

16. Statistics for the late nineteenth and the twentieth centuries are from the following sources: Minor 1882; "Smallpox at Milan," 1888; Kraechenko 1970; Rahts 1887; Zetterberg et al. 1966; Low 1918; Jones 1914; McVail 1902; Moller-Christensen & Simonsen 1962; Hedrich 1936; Frey 1924–25; Do Amaral 1960; Gantt 1924; Dixon 1962; Cardenas 1976; and Mack 1972.

Chapter 3

1. Several religious statues, "said to have been presented in the 6th century by the King of Korea to the Emperor of Japan," are preserved in the Zenkoji temple at Nangano on the island of Honshu (Harrison 1978, 638).

2. Right nostril for boys, left for girls. In 1869, a traveler reported that in the Indian Himalayas, inoculation for smallpox was performed at the base of the thumb on the right wrist for males and on the left wrist for females (Pringle 1869, 44–45).

3. Yoshimitsu, the shogun who ended the schism of the northern and southern emperors was attacked by a fatal disease in the summer of 1408, within weeks of his adolescent son's sudden death following an illness of "a few days" on 1 June (Sansom 1974, 2: 157, 173). Whether these deaths were related and due to poison or contagion I do not know.

4. In June 1981, this run-down but still striking temple was being restored and was temporarily closed to visitors.

5. One of the Kalmuck leaders, Amursana, helped the Chinese to capture the region of Sungaria in Chinese Turkestan. He later rebelled, and escaped being captured by the Chinese three times before fleeing to Siberia, where his surrender became the cause of a dispute between China and Russia in 1756. When Amursana finally died of smallpox in Siberia the following autumn, the Chinese refused to believe he was dead until the Russians agreed to exhibit his corpse (Hummel 1943; Parker 1907).

6. Statistics for the twentieth century are drawn from the following sources: Dold 1915; Low 1918; MacDonald 1944; Korns 1921; Garrison 1914; Irwin 1910; Amako 1909; Bowers 1981; Dixon 1962; McVail 1924; Heiser 1936; Tregonning 1958; Tarling 1971; Polak 1968; Cumpston 1914; WHO 1980; WHO 1979a, 1979c; WHO 1974a.

7. In 1916, a United States Foreign Service officer, Charles P. McKiernan, died of smallpox in Chung Kiang, China—one of five such deaths in the twentieth century of United States Foreign Service officers while on active duty. According to a memorial plaque at the Department of State (C Street entrance) the others died in Mexico (in 1910, 1914, and 1921) and in Bolivia (in 1918).

8. It was graciously brought to my attention by Dr. Olaf K. Skinsnes of the University of Hawaii.

Chapter 4

1. On his deathbed, this young king commanded an officer to return to the palace and kill the queen, so that she would not pass to another man. When the officer arrived at the palace and announced his mission to the queen, she married him on the spot (Harvey 1925, 80–81).

2. Ceylonese statistics drawn from Selkirk (1844) and De Silva (1953).

3. Indian statistics are compiled from Hirsch 1883; Aiya 1906; Vaughn 1907; Das 1895; Hunter 1881; Pringle 1869; Nevill 1904; Moore 1869.

4. During the comparatively mild period of food shortages just before the harvest in West Bengal in 1973, I encountered a hungry middle-aged man in a

village where several people had already died of smallpox and the epidemic was still in progress who angrily refused to be vaccinated, saying he would rather die quickly from smallpox than starve to death.

5. Statistics for the twentieth century are compiled from Low 1918; Dixon 1962; Govt. of India 1925, 1931a; Bhore 1946, Hedrich 1936; Govt. of Thailand 1978; Gelfand 1966; Basu et al. 1979; Davis 1951; WHO 1979b, 1970; Koko 1970; WHO 1974b, 1975; WHO & Min. Hlth. 1977; WHO 1976.

6. In Ceylon, a carved pillar "unsurpassed in delicacy and beauty," which is dedicated to the goddess of smallpox and chastity, was described much more recently at Medagoda, near Ruanwelli (Williams 1950, 444).

7. Bang said Shitala is described as a "beautiful maiden in a yellow sari" (1973, 82–83). According to Nicholas, the goddess is "invariably dressed as a married woman in red cloth or a red-bordered sari." In all of the anthropomorphic figures I saw in West Bengal (about a dozen), the goddess wore red.

Chapter 5

1. The year of the Elephant War is variously given as A. D. 568–72. Arab tradition ascribes the birth of the Prophet to the "Year of the Elephant" (Willis 1971, 139).

2. Such was the reputed splendor of the old capital, Damascus, that tradition says the young Mohammed "hesitated to enter [it] because he wished to enter paradise only once" (Hitti 1964, 215).

3. Adahoonzu II and Agonglo are buried in the royal compound at Abomey, Republic of Benin (Burton 1966, 308).

4. Statistics are from the following sources: Hirsch 1883; Theal 1903; Burrows 1958; Peterson 1969; Gardner 1852.

5. Pankhurst's 1965 article is most useful for Ethiopia's smallpox history, and I rely largely on his research in this discussion.

6. I have relied on the following sources for twentieth-century statistics: Roberts 1967; Junod 1962; Low 1918; Sery 1973; Imperato 1968; Glokpor 1970; Kuczynski 1939; Scott 1965; Hopkins 1971a; Price et al. 1960; Hedrich 1936; Hartwig 1981; Weidner 1962; Külz 1907; Rudin 1938; Seymour-Price et al. 1960; Henderson 1933; Islam 1978; Cockburn 1966; Fasquelle 1971; Foege et al. 1975; Tekeste 1979; Weithaler & De Quadros 1973; Deria et al. 1980.

7. In some societies it was taboo even to speak the word for smallpox. Among the Afar of Djibouti, its name was also used as a curse word (WHO 1979d, 2).

Chapter 6

1. My statistics are drawn from the following sources: Moll 1944; Magner 1942; D'Ardois 1961; Cameron 1968; Rippy 1938; Spence 1878; Hemming 1978; Dixon 1962; Clissold 1972; Bowser 1974; McNeill 1976.

2. If the Chilean Indians became a little paranoid about Spaniards and smallpox, it is not surprising. In his *Memoirs of the War of Chili*, Jeronimo Quiroga reported an incident in which the mere suspicion that Spaniards were deliberately introducing smallpox among the Indians was enough to start a war:

"Sometime since, the viceroy of Peru sent as a present to the governor, Juan Xaraquemada, from Lima to Chili, several jars of powder, honey, wine, olives, and different kinds of seed; one of these being accidentally broken in unloading, the Indians who were in the service of the Spaniards having noticed it, imagined that it was the purulent matter of the small-pox, which the governor had imported in order to disseminate among their provinces, and exterminate them by this means. They immediately gave notice to their countrymen, who stopped all communication and took up arms, killing forty Spaniards who were among them in full security of peace. The governor, to revenge this outrage, entered the Araucanian territory, and thus, owing to the suspicion of these barbarians, was a war excited, which was continued until Don Alonzo de Rivera returned a second time to assume the government of the kingdom." (Molina 1809, 2: 159–60).

3. Eighteenth-century statistics for all of South America are compiled from Moll 1944; Cooper 1965; Lastres 1954; Elliot 1911; Moses 1919; Hirsch 1883; Starkey 1939; Pittman 1917; Phelan 1967; Crow 1946; Scott 1939; Clavigero 1937; Cook 1939a; D'Ardois 1961.

4. In 1729, smallpox broke out among 300 Indian boatmen traveling with a Jesuit from Buenos Aires up the Rio de la Plata to Misiones, six hundred miles away. The epidemic began when they were midway between their origin and destination, without any available assistance. When the outbreak ended, 179 of the boatmen were dead, and only 40 escaped infection (Moses 1914, 1: 393–95).

5. Nineteenth-century statistics are drawn from Moll 1944, Hirsch 1883, Low 1918; Penna 1885; Nicholson 1869; Miller 1867; Parsons 1930.

6. Twentieth-century statistics compiled from Moll 1944; Low 1918; Chapin 1913; De Carvalho Filho et al. 1970; Carini 1911; Jones 1922; Dixon 1962; Hedrich 1936; Fredericksen 1962.

Chapter 7

1. Early in the eighteenth century, the virus also had a small role in the founding of the state of Georgia. When a friend died of smallpox in a London debtors prison, James E. Oglethorpe, then a member of Parliament, launched a highly publicized inquiry into the British penal system that resulted in many prisoners being freed. To provide employment for the released prisoners, Oglethorpe "conceived the idea of sending a hundred or more of these people . . . to America" (Amsaschbach 1936, 110). Parliament agreed, and King George II signed a charter on 9 June 1732. So far as is known, none of these colonists brought smallpox to Savannah in February 1733, although one of the Indians who escorted Oglethorpe back to England died of the disease there the next year (Harris 1841, 96).

2. Increase, Cotton, and Samuel Mather are buried in the same tomb in the Cobb Hill Cemetery near Old North Church.

3. Statistics from Blake 1959; Razzell 1977a; Wolman 1978; Duffy 1953.

4. The autographed copy now rests in the Francis A. Countway Library of Medicine in Boston, along with an inscribed silver case Jenner sent to Benjamin Waterhouse in 1801.

5. Statistics from Wells 1872; Vasselli 1951; Greenwood 1935; Smart 1879; Minor 1881–82; MacDonald 1872; Webb 1873; Rauch 1894; White 1881–82; Bryce 1885.

6. One of the most unusual importations from Mexico occurred after black laborers recruited from Alabama and Georgia to grow cotton began to develop what their employers called "cottonpox" months after their arrival in Mexico. Hundreds of the laborers deserted because of the outbreak, and returned to the Texas border, where they were realized to have smallpox. They were isolated at "Camp Jenner" near Eagle Pass, Texas. Fifty-one died (Rosenau 1896, 234–35).

7. Statistics for the late nineteenth and early twentieth centuries are from Chapin 1913; Chapin & Smith 1932; Henderson 1906; Ball 1903; Low 1918; Heagerty 1928; Kohnke 1900; Hedrich 1936; Pierce 1925; Woodward & Feemster 1933; Dixon 1962.

8. A resident of Prineville, Oregon, Mrs. Lorene Lakin (1972) recalled a different type of "red light treatment" when smallpox broke out in that community in 1903: "Prineville's leading House of Ill-repute was just around the corner from the Poindexter Hotel. If desired, a person could step out the back door of one building into the back door of the other. The red light district was across the creek but this downtown establishment was for the high class clientele. The word SMALLPOX swept the town like a tidal wave. The Madam went into action while others froze with fear. She made her beds available for hospital use—she and her girls standing-by to help nurse. This was Dr. Hutchinson's suitable house. All of the community was grateful but never publicly acknowledged its debt."

Chapter 8

1. References for use of the red treatment in Europe before 1893 are from Cumston 1925; Sitwell 1962; Coxe 1820; Morris 1937; Archer 1893; Moore 1815; Laignel-Lavastine & Molinery 1934; Oliver 1939; Emerson 1903; Finsen 1901; Bleichsteiner 1954.

2. A research institute (Finseninstituttet) named after him and devoted to research on radiobiology and effects of ultraviolet light stands at Strandboulevard 49 in Copenhagen.

3. As late as 1962, three European physicians—Moller-Christensen, Simonsen, and Jopling—still refused to dismiss the red-light treatment. They complained that Finsen's method had never been properly tested and described how a properly controlled trial should be arranged.

Bibliographical Note

BECAUSE OF THE WIDE TEMPORAL, geographical, and thematic scope of this book, it necessarily depends heavily, although not entirely, upon secondary scources. Chief among the pitfalls inherent in engaging such a wide-ranging topic are errors that almost inevitably creep into secondary sources and works based on them. I have tried to avoid such errors, by cross-checking data and depending on what is in my judgment the more reliable source whenever possible. Specific sources of various data or material are provided in the references, as a starting point for verification of facts and further investigation of subjects mentioned here. The purpose of this note is to indicate for interested readers the main types of sources used in this study.

Medical aspects of the disease are thoroughly described in C. W. Dixon's *Smallpox* (London, 1962). A good supplementary source of photographs of patients and discussion of the disease's symptoms and pathology exists in the two volume *Diagnosis of Smallpox* by Thomas F. Ricketts and John B. Byles (reprinted in 1966 by the United States Department of Health, Education, and Welfare from the 1908 London edition). Dixon's book also includes an appendix in which he gives the numbers of officially reported cases of smallpox and deaths by country from 1920 to 1957. More reliable data on numbers of cases of smallpox reported from each country between 1920 and 1979 are given in a table in the World Health Organization's final report of the Global Commission for the Certification of Smallpox Eradication, *The Global Eradication of Smallpox* (Geneva, 1980).

The best general history to date is James Moore's *History of the Smallpox* (London, 1815), which concentrates mainly on Britain and Europe, with some information on Asia and North Africa, and little on the Americas. Other histories by J. J. Paulet, *Histoire de la Petite Vérole* (Paris, 1768); P. Kübler, *Geschichte der Pocken* (Berlin, 1901); and Edward J. Edwardes, *A Concise History of Small-Pox and Vaccination in Europe* (London, 1902) are similarly eurocentric in approach. Charles Creighton's two volume *History of Epidemics in Great Britain* (Cambridge, 1891, 1894), provides much useful information about the history of smallpox in Britain, and his translation of A. Hirsch's *Handbook of Geographical and Historical Pathology*, vol. 1 (London, 1883) provides English-speaking readers with a chapter on smallpox's history that encompasses all the major geographic regions of the world. It should be noted that the eurocentric bias of most studies to date can be attributed to the simple fact that so much data pertaining to the history of smallpox in Britain and Europe are available compared to the rest of the world.

Other outstanding sources that provide good, reliable overviews of the disease's impact in specific periods or places include the chapter on smallpox in John

Duffy's *Epidemics in Colonial America* (Baton Rouge, 1953), several sections in John B. Blake's *Public Health in the Town of Boston* (Cambridge, 1959), and E. Wagner Stearn and Allen E. Stearn's *The Effect of Smallpox on the Destiny of the Amerindian* (Boston, 1945). For South America, the closest but less satisfactory equivalent is the appropriate sections of A. A. Moll's *Aesculapius in Latin America* (Philadelphia, 1944).

In Asia, there is a Japanese equivalent of Creighton in Yu Fujikawa's *Nihon Shippeshi* (History of Diseases in Japan), published in 1911, but to my knowledge it unfortunately has not been translated into English or any other Western language. Indeed, the history of smallpox in Japan, China, and India almost certainly rivals the more accessible story of smallpox's impact in Europe. Because of the language barrier, however, I have had to depend heavily on articles or books published in Western languages by missionaries, physicians, historians, and others, which provide a less complete view of our subject in those countries. In that part of the world, only in Australia is a reasonable overview of smallpox's history available, in J. H. L. Cumpston's *The History of Smallpox in Australia, 1788–1908* (Melbourne, 1914).

In Africa as in Asia, there are no good overviews of what smallpox did and meant on that continent. Here, sources of information about the history of smallpox range from various paleopathologic studies of Egyptian mummies—of which those by Marc Ruffer, G. Elliot Smith, and the recent studies edited by James E. Harris and E. F. Wente (*Atlas of the Royal Mummies* [Chicago, 1980]) are most reliable—to descriptive works such as those by Richard Pankhurst, "The History and Traditional Treatment of Smallpox in Ethiopia" (1965), which trace facets of the disease's history in a single country. There are also analytical studies such as Gerald Hartwig's "Demographic Considerations in East Africa during the Nineteenth Century" (1979), which include information about smallpox as part of a broader historical analysis, and eye-witness accounts by missionaries or travelers, such as James Bruce's *Travels to Discover the Source of the Nile* (London, 1805), from which one can obtain incidental glimpses of the disease's impact in Africa. As a representative of the latter group, Bruce had the advantage for our purposes of being a physician.

Of several excellent studies that focus on specific episodes in the history of smallpox and analyze them thoroughly, Genevieve Miller's meticulous, now classic study, *The Adoption of Inoculation for Smallpox in England and France* (Philadelphia, 1957) remains the standard. Of comparably focused works by medical authors, Dr. Derrick Baxby's recent *Jenner's Smallpox Vaccine* (London, 1981) provides a similarly thorough, detailed explanation of the controversy over the origins of vaccines introduced by Jenner and his successors. Other excellent works of this type include Michael M. Smith's "The 'Real Expedición Marítima de la Vacuna' in New Spain and Guatemala" (1974), which describes the mission sponsored by the king of Spain to send Jennerian vaccine to his colonies around the world; two articles by John B. Blake, "The Inoculation Controversy in Boston, 1721–1722" (1952), and "Smallpox Inoculation in Colonial Boston" (1958); and "The Judgement of the Smallpox" in Perry Miller's *The New England Mind from Colony to Province* (Cambridge, 1953). The last three articles all describe the introduction of inoculation into Boston.

A fuller perspective of the history of ideas regarding contagion may be found in George Rosen's *A History of Public Health* (New York, 1958), chapter 9 of Miller's *The Adoption of Inoculation for Smallpox in England and France*, and in Lise Wilkinson's "The Development of the Virus Concept as Reflected in Corpora of Studies on Individual Pathogens: 5. Smallpox and the Evolution of Ideas on Acute (Viral) Infections" (1979).

The main sources of information on the progress of the global Smallpox Eradication Program itself, pending the appearance of the definitive account of that campaign, are the Global Commission's final report published by the World Health Organization, *The Global Eradication of Smallpox* (Geneva, 1980); the series of articles, "Smallpox Surveillance," published periodically in WHO's *Weekly Epidemiological Record* throughout the global campaign; and other summary articles in WHO's *Bulletin of the World Health Organization*, such as Foege, Millar, and Henderson's "Smallpox Eradication in West and Central Africa" (1975). Numerous articles, among them my own (with Lane, Cummings, and Millar) "Smallpox in Sierra Leone" (1971), have been published in various medical journals over the past decade or so, describing recent aspects of the disease and its eradication in different countries. In two key instances, the WHO has published extensive basic information on the conduct of eradication programs: *The Eradication of Smallpox from India* by R. N. Basu, Z. Jezek, and N. A. Ward (New Delhi, 1979) and *The Eradication of Smallpox from Bangladesh* by A. K. Joarder, D. Tarantola, and J. Tulloch (New Delhi 1980).

The most reliable sources of data in preparing this book are the primary sources cited, for example, the periodical reports published by the World Health Organization, chronicles like the *Wiener Diarium*, which provides a record of some of Joseph I's activities during the fortnight preceding his fatal illness, and first hand accounts from newspaper articles or published letters concerning smallpox in different parts of the world. Critical studies of specific episodes such as Genevieve Miller's, or of the disease in certain geographic areas such as in Blake's Boston study are almost as reliable as many primary sources, and much more helpful for obtaining an overview and perspective of the events in question. General histories of medicine or medical histories of regions or countries are generally not as dependable as primary sources or authoritative microanalyses. Articles by medically trained persons are usually not the most reliable source of historical facts, although some are. On the other hand, professional historians aren't always as careful about recording accurate diagnoses or complete medical descriptions as one would like.

Unlike most others once smallpox was recognized as a separate disease, it was usually distinctive and visible enough that eye witnesses' diagnoses were probably correct, especially where several patients were seen. But numbers of cases and deaths during epidemics were subject to exaggeration from time immemorial, as well as to underreporting in official statistics gathered in more recent centuries. In general, however, the more recent the event, the more complete is the information available to us about it.

References

Ackerknecht, E. H. 1965. *History and Geography of the Most Important Diseases*. New York: Hafner Publishing Co.

Adamson, P. B. 1970. "The 'Bubu Tu' Lesion in Antiquity." *Med. Hist.* 14: 313–18.

Aiya, V. N. 1906. *The Travancore State Manual*. Trivandrum: Travancore Government Press.

Akinjogbin, I. A. 1965. "Dahomey and Yoruba in the Nineteenth Century." In *A Thousand Years of West African History*, edited by J. F. A. Ajayi and I. Epsie. Ibadan: Ibadan University Press.

Alivizatos, G. P. 1950. *The Early Smallpox Epidemics in Europe and the Athens Plague after Thucidides*. Athens.

Amako, T. 1909. "Studien über die Variolaepidemie in Kobe." *Archiv. f. Schiff. u. Tropen Hygiene* 13: 109–21.

Amsaschbach, E. 1936. *Edward Oglethorpe: Imperial Idealist*. Oxford: Clarendon Press.

Anderson, I. 1866. "On Epidemic Varioloid Varicella in Jamaica." *Trans. Epidemiol. Soc. Lond.* 2: 414–18.

Archer, S. 1893. "Smallpox: An Historical Sketch." *Liverpool Medico-Chirurgical J.* 13: 120–34.

Arita, I., and Henderson, D. A. 1976. "Monkeypox and Whitepox Viruses in West and Central Africa." *Bull. Wld. Hlth. Org.* 53: 347–53.

Arnold, J. 1931. *The Legacy of Islam*. Oxford: Clarendon Press.

Arseniev, K. 1839. *The Reign of Tsar Peter II*. Translated by P. Gerstein. St. Petersburg: Imperial Russian Academy.

Asiegbu, J. U. J. 1969. *Slavery and the Politics of Liberation, 1787–1861*. London: Longmans, Green and Co.

Aston, W. G., trans. 1896. *Nihongi: Chronicles of Japan from the Earliest Times to A.D. 697*. London: Kegan Paul, Trench, Trübner and Co.

"The Bacteriology of Vaccinia and Variola Virus in Its Theoretical and Practical Aspects." 1902. *Brit. Med. J.* 2: 52–67.

Balfour, A., and Scott, H. H. 1924. "Health Problems of the Empire." In *The British Empire*, vol. 4, edited by H. Gunn. New York: Henry Holt and Co.

Ball, J. D. 1904. *Things Chinese*. 4th ed. London: John Murray.

Ball, M. V. 1903. "Death Rate from Smallpox in Various Cities and States." *Amer. Med.* 5: 450.

Bamzai, P. N. K. 1962. *A History of Kashmir*. Delhi: Metropolitan Book Co.

Bancroft, H. H. 1883. *History of Mexico*, Vol. 1. In *The Works of Hubert Howe Bancroft*. San Francisco: A. L. Bancroft and Co.

Bancroft, I. 1902. *Clinical Records of the Smallpox Hospital at 112 Southhampton Street.* 23 January 1902 to April 1902. Boston: Francis A. Countway Library of Medicine.

Bang, B. G. 1973. "Current Concepts of the Smallpox Goddess Sitala in Parts of West Bengal." *Man in India* 53: 79–104.

Bantug, J. P. 1953. *A Short History of Medicine in the Philippines during the Spanish Regime, 1565–1898.* Manila: Colegio Medico-Pharmaceutico de Filipinas.

Barber, N. 1973. *The Sultans.* New York: Simon and Schuster.

Bardell, D. 1976. "Smallpox during the American War of Independence." *ASM News* 42: 526–30.

Barnes, J. 1848. "Case of Variola Nigra, or Black Smallpox." *St. Louis Med. Surg. J.* 5: 533–46.

Baron, John. (1827, 1838) *The Life of Edward Jenner.* 2 vols. London: Henry Colburn.

Baroyan, O. V., and Serenko, A. F. 1961. "The Smallpox Outbreak in Moscow in 1959–1960." *Zh. Mikrob. Epid. Immun.* 32: 672–80.

Barrett, J. J. 1942. "The Inoculation Controversy in Puritan New England." *Bull. Hist. Med.* 12: 169–90.

Bartlett, M. S. 1957. "Measles Periodicity and Community Size." *J. Roy. Stat. Soc.*, ser. A, 120: 48–59.

———. 1960. "The Critical Community Size for Measles in the United States." *J. Roy. Stat. Soc.*, ser. A, 123: 37–44.

Basler, R. P. 1971–72. "Did President Lincoln Give the Smallpox to William H. Johnson?" *Huntington Library Quarterly* 35: 279–84.

Bastin, J. 1957. *The Native Policies of Sir Stamford Raffles in Java and Sumatra.* Oxford: Clarendon Press.

Basu, R. N.; Jezek, Z.; and Ward, N. A. 1979. *The Eradication of Smallpox from India.* New Delhi: World Health Organization.

Baxby, D. 1977. "The Origins of Vaccinia Virus." *J. Inf. Dis.* 136: 453–55.

———. 1981. *Jenner's Smallpox Vaccine.* London: Heinemann Educational Books.

Bayoumi, A. 1976. "The History and Traditional Treatment of Smallpox in the Sudan." *J. East Afr. Rsch. Devel.* 6: 1–10.

Beall, O. T., Jr., and Shryock, R. H. 1954. *Cotton Mather: First Significant Figure in American Medicine.* Baltimore: Johns Hopkins Press.

Bedson, H. S.; Dumbell, K. R.; and Thomas, W. R. G. 1965. "Variola in Tanganyika." *Lancet* 2: 1085–88.

Bell, C. 1928. *The People of Tibet.* Oxford: Clarendon Press.

Bell, R. 1836. *History of Russia.* Vol. 2. London: Longman, Rees, Orme, Brown, Green and Longman.

"Benjamin Waterhouse and Gilbert Stuart." 1962. *New Engl. J. Med.* 267: 624–25, 675–77.

"Benjamin Waterhouse (1754–1846)—The American Jenner." 1964. *J. Amer. Med. Ass.* 188: 929–31.

Bergamini, J. 1969. *The Tragic Dynasty: A History of the Romanovs.* New York: G. P. Putnam's Sons.

———. 1974. *The Spanish Bourbons.* New York: G. P. Putnam's Sons.

"Bericht über die Pockenepidemie des Jahres 1858 in Berlin." 1859. *Archiv der Deutschen Medicinal Gesetzgebung u. Öffentl. Gesundsheitspflege*, pp. 124–27.

Bernstein, S. S. 1951. "Smallpox and Variolation: Their Historical Significance in the American Colonies." *J. Mt. Sinai Hosp.* 18: 228–44.

Bhore, Sir Joseph, Chairman. 1946. *Report of the Health Survey and Development Committee*. Delhi: Manager of Publications.

Bhuyan, S. K. 1933. *Tungkhungia Buranji; or, A History of Assam, 1681–1826*. London: Oxford University Press.

Biscoe, C. E. T. 1922. *Kashmir*. Philadelphia: J. B. Lippincott Co.

Bishop, E. R. 1898–99. "The Epidemic of Smallpox in Western New York." *Buffalo Med. J.* 38: 420–23.

Bishop, W. J. 1932. "Thomas Dimsdale and the Inoculation of Catherine the Great of Russia." *Ann. Med. Hist.*, n.s., 4: 321–38.

Black, F. L. 1966. "Measles Endemicity in Insular Populations: Critical Community Size and Its Evolutionary Implication." *J. Theoret. Biol.* 11: 207–11.

Blake, J. B. 1952. "The Inoculation Controversy in Boston, 1721–1722." *New Engl. Quart.* 25: 489–506.

———. 1953. "Smallpox Inoculation in Colonial Boston." *J. Hist. Med. Allied Sci.* 8: 284–300.

———. 1957. *Benjamin Waterhouse and the Introduction of Vaccination*. Philadelphia: University of Pennsylvania Press.

———. 1958. "Benjamin Waterhouse: Harvard's First Professor of Physic." *J. Med. Educ.* 33: 771–82.

———. 1959. *Public Health in the Town of Boston, 1630–1822*. Cambridge: Harvard University Press.

Bland, J.O. P., and Blackhouse, E. [1910] 1921. *China under the Empress Dowager*. Reprint. London: William Heinemann.

Blanton, W. B. 1931. *Medicine in Virginia in the Eighteenth Century*. Richmond: Garrett and Massie.

Bleichsteiner, R. 1954. "Die Blatternogottheiten und die Hl. Barbara in Volksglauben der Georgier." In *Beiträge zur Volkskunde aus Österreich Bayern und der Schweiz: Festschrift für Gustav Gugitz*, pp. 63–83. Vienna: Öst. Ms. f. Volkskunde.

Bloch, H. 1973. "Rev. Thomas Thacher 1620 to 1678." *N.Y. State J. Med.* 73: 700–702.

———. 1974. "Benjamin Waterhouse (1754–1846)." *Amer. J. Dis. Child.* 127: 226–9.

Bloomfield, A. L. 1958. *A Bibliography of Internal Medicine: Communicable Diseases*. Chicago: University of Chicago Press.

Blunt, W. F. 1900. "Circular to All the Railroad Managers of the State." *Texas Med. J.* 15: 479.

Bonner, A., ed. 1964. *The Complete Works of François Villon*. New York: Bantam Books.

Boorstin, D. J. 1958. *The Americans: The Colonial Experience*. New York: Vintage Books.

Bose, K. C. 1890. "The Prevalence of Smallpox in Calcutta and How to Arrest Its Spread." *Ind. Med. Gaz.* 25: 77–85.

Bosman, W. 1958. "The Coast, 1700." In *Pageant of Ghana*, edited by E. Wolfson. London: Oxford University Press.

Boutry, M. 1903. "La variole à la cour de Marie Thérèse d'Autriche." (Translated by E. Hopkins.) *Chron. Med.* (Paris) 10: 305–18.

Bovill, E. W. 1968. *The Golden Trade of the Moors.* 2d ed. London: Oxford University Press.

Bowers, J. Z. 1981. "The Odyssey of Smallpox Vaccination." *Bull. Hist. Med.* 55: 17–33.

Bowser, F. P. 1974. *The African Slave in Colonial Peru, 1524–1650.* Stanford: Stanford University Press.

Boxer, C. R. 1962. *The Golden Age of Brazil, 1695–1750.* Berkeley: University of California Press.

Boyd, A. 1864. *Washington and Georgetown Directory.* Washington: Hudson Taylor.

Bracken, H. M. 1901. "The Present Epidemic of Smallpox in America." *St. Paul Med. J.* 3: 723–37.

Bradby, G. F. 1906. *The Great Days of Versailles.* New York: Charles Scribner's Sons.

Brandon, W. 1974 *The Last Americans.* New York: McGraw-Hill Book Co.

Brau, S. 1969. *La Colonización de Puerto Rico.* San Juan: Instituto de Cultura Puertor-riquena.

Brayton, A. W. 1902. "Smallpox: A Consideration of the Present Mild Type in the Mississippi Valley." *St. Louis Med. Rev.* 45: 289–97.

Breasted, J. H. 1964. *A History of Egypt.* New York: Bantam Books.

Brede, H. D. 1979. "Die Ausrottung der Pocken." *Forum Mikrobiol.* 4: 172–76.

Bredon, J., and Mitrophanow. I. 1927. *The Moon Year: A Record of Chinese Customs and Festivals.* Shanghai: Kelly and Walsh.

Breman, J. G. et. al. "Human Monkeypox, 1970–79." *Bull. Wld. Hlth. Org.* 58: 165–82.

Breman, J. G., and Arita, I. 1980 "The Confirmation and Maintenance of Smallpox Eradication." *New Engl. J. Med.* 303: 1263–73.

Brinkley, F., and Kikuchi, B. 1915. *A History of the Japanese People.* New York: Encyclopaedia Britannica Co.

Brinton, S. 1927. *The Gonzanga: Lords of Mantua.* London: Methuen and Co.

Broadbeut, J. F. H. 1934. "Acute Infectious Diseases." In *A Short History of Some Common Diseases,* edited by W. R. Bett. London: Humphrey Milford.

Brown, J. R., and McLean, D. M. 1962. "Smallpox—A Retrospect." *Canad. Med. Ass. J.* 87: 765–67.

Bruce, J. 1805. *Travels to Discover the Source of the Nile.* London: Longman, Hurst, Rees and Orme.

———. 1812. *Travels between the Years 1765 and 1773.* London: James Robins and Co., Allison Press.

Bryan, W. B. n.d. "Washington on the Eve of the Civil War." In *Washington during War Time,* edited by M. Benjamin. Washington: National Tribune Co.

Bryce, P. H. 1885. "Smallpox in Canada and the Methods of Dealing with It in the Different Provinces." *Pub. Hlth. Papers & Rep.* 11: 166–81.

Buckley, C. B. 1965. *An Anecdotal History of Old Times in Singapore.* Kuala Lumpur: University of Malaya Press.

Budgeii, E. A. W. 1907. *The Egyptian Sudan.* London: Keagan Paul, Trench, Trübner and Co.

Bulkey, J. W. n.d. "The War Hospitals." In *Washington during War Time,* edited by M. Benjamin. Washington: National Tribune Co.

Burke. 1872. "On the Present Epidemic of Smallpox." *Dublin J. Med. Soc.* 53: 146–59, 219–34.

Burrows, E. H. 1958. *A History of Medicine in South Africa.* Capetown: A. A. Balkema.

Burton, R. [1860] 1961. *The Lake Regions of Central Africa.* Reprint. New York: Horizon Press.

———. 1966. *A Mission to Gelele King of Dahome.* London: Routledge and Kegan Paul.

Cabanes, 1897 *The Secret Cabinet of History.* Paris: Charles Carrington.

Cameron, R. 1968. *Vice Royalties of the West.* London: Weidenfeld and Nicolson.

Cardenas, E. A. 1976. "Datos para la Historia de la Viruela en España." *Rev. San. Hig. Pub.* 50: 485–98.

Carini, A. 1911. "A-propos d'une épidémie très bénigne de variole." *Bull. Soc. Path. Exot.* 4: 35–39.

Carp, L. 1970. "Mozart: His Tragic Life and Controversial Death." *Bull. N.Y. Acad. Med.* 46: 271–80.

Carr, C. E. 1909. *Lincoln at Gettysburg.* Chicago: A. C. McClurg and Co.

Carter, A. R. 1879. "Report on Smallpox in Baltimore." *Nat. Bd. of Hlth. Bull.* Washington 1: 243.

Cartwright, F. F. 1972. *Disease and History.* London: Rupert Hart-Davis.

Cash, P. 1973. *Medical Men at the Siege of Boston.* Philadelphia: American Philosophical Society.

Castiglioni, A. 1941. *A History of Medicine.* New York: Alfred A. Knopf.

Catlin, G. 1841. *North American Indians.* London: Chatto and Windus.

Cerny, J. 1975. "Egypt: From the Death of Ramses II to the End of the Twenty-first Dynasty." In *The Cambridge Ancient History,* Vol. 2., edited by I. E. S. Edwards et.al., pp. 606–57. Cambridge: At the University Press.

Cha, J. H. 1976. "Epidemics in China." In *Plagues and Peoples,* edited by W. H. McNeill, pp. 293–302. Garden City, N. Y.: Anchor Press, Doubleday.

Challenor, B. D. 1971. "Cultural Resistance to Smallpox Vaccination in West Africa." *J. Trop. Med. Hyg.* 74: 57–59.

Chapin, C. V. 1913. "Variation in Type of Infectious Disease as Shown by the History of Smallpox in the United States, 1895–1912." *J. Infect. Dis.* 13: 171–96.

———. 1926. "Changes in Type of Contagious Disease." *J. Prev. Med.* 1: 1–29.

Chapin, C. V., and Smith, J. 1932. "Permanency of the Mild Type of Smallpox." *J. Prev. Med.* 6: 273–320.

Charnock, J. 1795. *Biographia Navalis.* London: R. Faulder.

Chen, C. Y. 1969. "Names of Diseases Engraved on Carapaces and Bones More than Three Thousand Years Ago." *Hist. Chinese Med. Science,* pp. 24–25.

Chesley, A. J. 1919. "Smallpox, Benign and Virulent, in Minnesota." *Minn. Med.* 2: 92–95.

Chizynski, Z., and Rozewska-Chizynska, M. 1972. "The History of Smallpox Immunizations in Poland." (Translated by E. Belansky.) *Bull. Military Acad. Med.* 15, no. 1: 173–78.

Clarac. 1904a. "Causes du developpement et de la propagation de la variole a Madagascar avant l'occupation française." (Translated by E. Hopkins.) *Ann. Hyg. Med. Colon.* (Paris) 7: 286–94.

———. 1904b. "Epidémies de variole a Madagascar." (Translated by E. Hopkins.) *Ann. Hyg. Med. Colon.* (Paris) 7: 434–45.

———. 1904c. "Prophylaxie de la variole sous les rois malagaches jusqu'a l'occupation française." (Translated by E. Hopkins.) *Ann. Hyg. Med. Colon.* (Paris) 7: 20–28.

Claridge, W. W. 1964. *A History of the Gold Coast and Ashanti.* London: Frank Cass and Co.

Clark, C. U. 1955. "The Treatment of Smallpox in Peru in 1589." *J. Hist. Med.* 10: 327–31.

Clavigero, F. J. 1937. *The History of California.* Stanford: Stanford University Press.

Clement, E. W. 1915. *A Short History of Japan.* Chicago: University of Chicago Press.

Clendenning, P. H. 1973. "Dr. Thomas Dimsdale and Smallpox Inoculation in Russia." *J. Hist. Med.* 28: 109–25.

Clissold, S. 1972. *Latin America.* London: Pall Mall Press.

Cockburn, A. 1963. *The Evolution and Eradication of Infectious Diseases.* Baltimore: Johns Hopkins Press.

Cockburn, W. C. 1966. "Progress in International Smallpox Eradication." *Amer. J. Pub. Hlth.* 56: 1628–33.

Codellas, P. S. 1946. "The Case of Smallpox of Theodorus Prodromus." *Bull. Hist. Med.* 20: 207–15.

Cohen, I. B. 1949. "Edward Jenner and Harvard University," *Harvard Libr. Bull.* 3: 347–58.

Collier, L. H. 1954. "The Preservation of Vaccinia Virus." *Bact. Rev.* 18: 78–79.

———. 1978. "The Preservation of Smallpox Vaccine." *Trends in Biological Science* 3: 27–29.

Colville, H. 1895. *The Land of the Nile Springs.* London: Edward Arnold and Co.

Colvin, I. 1922. *The Life of Jameson.* London: Edward Arnold and Co.

Cone, T. E., Jr. 1974. "Cotton Mather Anguishes over the Consequences of His Son's Inoculation against Smallpox." *Pediatrics* 53: 756.

———. 1976. "Highlights of Two Centuries of American Pediatrics, 1776–1976." *Amer. J. Dis. Child.* 130: 762–65.

———. 1978. "The Reverend Francis Higginson Describes His Young Daughter's death from Smallpox on Board a Ship Bound for Massachusetts in 1629." *Pediatrics* 61: 192.

Congo Free State Government, 1906. *Report of the Commission of Inquiry Appointed by the Congo Free State Government: The Congo.* New York: Knickerbocker Press.

Connecticut Courant. 2 August 1774.

Cook, A. R. 1945. *Uganda Memoirs.* Kampala: Uganda Society.

Cook, S. F. 1939a. "The Smallpox Epidemic of 1797 in Mexico." *Bull, Hist, Med.* 7: 937–69.

———. 1939b "Smallpox in Spanish and Mexican California, 1770–1845." *Bull. Hist. Med.* 7: 153–91.

Cooper, D. B. 1965. *Epidemic Disease in Mexico City, 1761–1813.* Austin: University of Texas Press.

Cooray, M. P. M. 1965. "Epidemics in the Course of History." *Ceylon Med. J.* 10: 88–91.

Cordiner, J. 1807. *A Description of Ceylon.* London: Longman, Hurst, Rees and Orme.

Corlett, W. T. 1935. *The Medicine Man of the American Indian.* Springfield: Charles C. Thomas.

Corlieu, A. 1892. *La Mort des rois de France*. Paris: Honore Champion.

Cornevin, R. 1962. *Histoire du Dahomey*. (Translated by D. Morens.) Paris: Editions Berger-Levrault.

Cory, G. E. 1910. *The Rise of South Africa*. London: Longmans, Green and Co.

Coughlan, R. 1974. *Elizabeth and Catherine: Empresses of All the Russias*. New York: G. P. Putnam's Sons.

Coulanges, P. 1976. "Variole et vaccine a Madagascar et aux Comores." (Translated by E. Hopkins.) *Arch. Inst. Pasteur Madagascar* 45: 127–71.

Coulter, L., and Coulter, J. L. S., eds. 1961. *Medicine and the Navy, 1200–1900*. Edinburgh and London: E. and S. Livingstone.

Cowles, V. 1971. *The Romanovs*. London: William Collins Sons and Co.

Cox, G. W. 1888. *The Life of John William Colenso*. London: W. Ridgway.

Coxe, W. 1815. *Memoirs of the Kings of Spain - 1700–1788*. Longman, Hurst, Rees, Orme, and Brown, Paternaster Row.

———. 1820. *History of the House of Austria*. 2d ed. London: Longman, Hurst, Rees, Orme, and Brown.

Crankshaw, E. 1969. *Maria Theresa*. London: Longman Group.

———. 1971. *The Habsburgs*. New York: Viking Press, 1971.

Cranmer-Byng, J., ed. 1963. *An Embassy to China*. Hamden: Aschon Books.

Crantz, D. 1820. *The History of Greenland*. London: Longman, Hurst, Rees, Orme and Brown.

Crawford, J. 1820. *History of the Indian Archipelago*. Edinburgh: Archibald Constable and Co.

Crawford, O. G. S. 1951. *The Fung Kingdom of Sennar*. Gloucester: John Bellows.

Creighton, Charles. 1887. *The Natural History of Cowpox and Vaccinal Syphilis*. London: Cassell and Co.

Creighton, C. [1891, 1894] 1963. *A History of Epidemics in Britain*. 2 vols. Reprinted. London: Frank Cass and Co.

———. 1892. *Jenner and Vaccination*. Providence: Snow & Farnham.

Cronin, V. 1965. *Louis XIV*. Boston: Houghton Mifflin Co.

———. 1974. *Louis and Antoinette*. New York: William Morrow and Co.

Crooke, W. 1906. *Things Indian*. New York: Charles Scribner's Sons.

———. 1921. *Islam in India*. London: Oxford University Press.

———. 1925. *Religion and Folklore of Northern India*. New Delhi: S. Chand and Co.

Crosby, A. W. 1967. "Conquistador y Pestilencia: The First New World Pandemic and the Fall of the Great Indian Empires." *Hisp. Amer. Hist. Rev.* 47: 321–37.

Crow, J. A. 1946. *The Epic of Latin America*. New York: Doubleday and Co.

Crowder, M. 1977. *West Africa: An Introduction to its History*. London: Longman Group.

Cumston, C. G. 1925. "Under the Red Light." *Med. J. and Rec.* 121: 112–13.

Cumpston, J. H. L. 1914. *The History of Smallpox in Australia, 1788–1908*. Melbourne: Albert J. Mullett, Government Printer.

Curtin, P.; Feierman, S.; Thompson, L.; and Vansina, J. 1978. *African History*. Boston: Little, Brown and Co.

Dalzel, A. [1793] 1967. *The History of Dahomey*. Reprint. London: Frank Cass and Co.

D'Angerville, M. 1924. *The Private Life of Louis XV*. New York: Boni and Liverright.

Dann, J. C., ed. 1980. *The Revolution Remembered*. Chicago: University of Chicago Press.

Danvilla, A. 1902. *Luisa Isabel de Orleans y Luis I*. Madrid: Libreria de Fernando Fe.

D'Ardois, G. S. 1961. "La Viruela en la Nueva España." *Gac. Med. Mex.* 91: 1015–24.

Das, A. K., and Raha, M. K. 1963. *The Orarons of Sunderban*. Calcutta: Government of West Bengal.

Das, S. C. 1902. *Journey to Lhasa and Central Tibet*. London: John Murray.

Das, S. M. 1895. "Smallpox in Calcutta." *Med. Reporter* (Calcutta) 6: 114–15.

Davidson, B. 1961. *Black Mother*. London: Victor Gollancz.

Davies, J. W. 1970. "A Historical Note on the Reverend John Clinch, First Canadian Vaccinator." *Canad. Med. Ass. J.* 102: 957–61.

Davis, F. H. 1916. *Japan*. London: T. C. and E. C. Jack.

Davis, K. 1951. *The Population of India and Pakistan*. Princeton: Princeton University Press.

"Death of Benjamin Waterhouse, M.D." 1846. *Bost. Med. Surg. J.* 35: 206.

De Carvalho Filho, E. S., et al. 1970. "Smallpox Eradication in Brazil, 1967–69." *Bull. Wld. Hlth. Org.* 43: 797–808.

De Gamboa, P. S. 1907. *History of the Incas*. Translated by C. Markham. Cambridge: Hakluyt Society.

De Haro y Peralta, A. N. 1797. Circular letter, 31 October. Resumen General de las Sociedades de Caridad, 1797. Library of the Wellcome Institute for the History of Medicine, London.

De la Vega, G. 1971. *The Incas: The Royal Commentary of the Inca*, edited by Alain Gheerbrant. Translated by Maria Jolas. New York: Avon Books, Orion Press.

Del Castillo, B. D. 1956. *The Discovery and Conquest of Mexico*. New York: Farrar, Straus and Giroux.

Del Perugia, P. 1939. *La tentative d'invasion de L'Angleterre de 1779*. Paris: Alcan Presses Universitaires de France.

Denis, P. 1911. *Brazil*. London: T. Fisher Unwin.

Dent, H. C. 1886. *Year in Brazil*. London: Kegan Paul, Trench and Co.

Deria, A.; Jezek, Z.; Markvart, K.; Carrasco, P.; and Weisfeld, J. 1980. "The World's Last Endemic Case of Smallpox: Surveillance and Containment Measures." *Bull. W. H. O.* 58: 279–83.

De Sahagun, B. 1905. *Codex Florentino: Historia General de las Cosas de Nueva España*, edited by Francisco de Paso y Troncoso. Vol. 5, box 12, Pl. 153, no. 114. Madrid: Fototipia de Hauser.

De Silva, C. R. 1953. *Ceylon under the British Occupation, 1795–1833*. Colombo: Colombo Apothecaries Co.

———. 1972. *The Portuguese in Ceylon, 1617–1638*. Colombo: H. W. Cave and Co.

Destenay, A. 1980. *Nagel's Encyclopedia Guide: China*. Geneva: Nagel Publishers.

DeVillalba, J. 1802. *Epidemiologica Española*. Madrid: La Imprenta de Don Mateo Repullés.

DeVoto, B. 1947. *Across the Wide Missouri*. Boston: Houghton Mifflin Co.

Diffie, B. W. 1945. *Latin American Civilization: Colonial Period*. Harrisburg: Stackpole Sons.

"The Diffusion of Vaccination: History of its Introduction into Various Countries." 1896. *Brit. Med. J.* 1: 1267–69.

Dixon, C. W. 1962. *Smallpox*. London: J. and A. Churchill.

Do Amaral, Carlos. 1960. "Historia da Variola." *A. Medicina Contemporanea* 78: 537–71.

Dobyns, H. F. 1963. "An Outline of Andean Epidemic History to 1720." *Bull. Hist. Med.* 37: 493–515.

Dodwell, H. 1920. *Calendar of the Madras Dispatches, 1744–1755*. Madras: Madras Government Press.

Dold, H. 1915. "Periodisches Auftreten der Pocken in Schanghai." *Ztschr. f. Hyg. u. Infektionskrankh.* 80: 467–80.

Doolittle, J. 1865. *Social Life of the Chinese*. New York: Harper and Brothers.

Downie, A. W. 1951. "Jenner's Cowpox Inoculation." *Brit. Med. J.* 2: 251.

———. 1965. "Poxvirus Group." In *Viral and Rickettsial Infections of Man*, 4th ed., edited by F. L. Horsfall, Jr., and I. Tamm, Philadelphia: J. B. Lippincott Co.

Drake, S. A. 1971. *Old Landmarks and Historic Personages of Boston*. Rev. ed. Rutland, Vt.: Charles E. Tuttle Co.

Drake-Brockman, D. L., ed. 1911. *District Gazetteers of the United Provinces* 27 (Mirzapur): 38–9; 28 (Jaunpur); 33 (Azamgarh): 25–6. Allahabad: Government Press. 27

du Chaillu, P. B. 1871. *A Journey to Ashango-Land*. New York: Harper and Brothers.

Dudgeon, J. 1871. "Report on the Health of Peking for the Half Year Ended 31st March 1871." *Customs Gazette Med. Rep.* (Shanghai) 1: 114–23.

Dudgeon, J. A. 1963. "Development of Smallpox Vaccine in England in the Eighteenth and Nineteenth Centuries." *Brit. Med. J.*, pp. 1367–72.

Duffy, J. 1951. "Smallpox and the Indians in the American Colonies." *Bull. Hist. Med.* 25: 324–41.

———. 1953. *Epidemics in Colonial America*. Baton Rouge: Louisiana State University Press.

———. 1968. *A History of Public Health in New York City, 1625–1866*. New York: Russell Sage Foundation.

———. 1978. "School Vaccination: The Precursor to School Medical Inspection." *J. Hist. Med.* 33: 344–55.

Duncan, J. 1968. *Travels in Western Africa in 1845 and 1846*. London: Frank Cass and Co.

Durant, W. 1950. *The Age of Faith*, New York: Simon and Schuster.

Durant, W., and Durant, A. 1963. *The Age of Louis XIV*. New York: Simon and Schuster.

———. 1967. *Rousseau and Revolution*. New York: Simon and Schuster.

Eccles, W. J. 1973. *France in America*. New York: Harper and Row.

Edwardes, E. J. 1885. "Smallpox in Germany." *J. Stat. Soc. London* 48: 670–74.

———. 1902a. "A Century of Vaccination: Small-Pox Epidemics and Small-Pox Mortality before and since Vaccination Came into Use." *Brit. Med. J.* 2: 27–30.

———. 1902b. *A Concise History of Small-Pox and Vaccination in Europe*. London: H. K. Lewis.

Edwardes, M. 1969. *Everyday Life in Early India*. London: B. T. Batsford.

Elliot, G. F. S. 1911. *Chile*. London: T. Fisher Unwin.

Ellis, W. 1869. *History of Madagascar*. London: Fisher, Son and Co.

Elwin, V. 1955. *The Religion of an Indian Tribe*. London: Oxford University Press.

Emerson, J. B. 1903. "The Red Light Treatment of Smallpox." *Med. Times and Hosp. Gaz.* 31: 419.

"The Epidemic of Smallpox in Trinidad." 1871–72. *Med. Times and Gaz.* (London) 1: 633, 444, 263–64, 171; 2: 721.

"Une épídemie de variole en Cournonterrel, Obs. de syphilis vaccinal." 1871. *Montpel. Med.* 26: 257; 28: 303, 414.

"Epidemiological Study of Smallpox in California." 1921. *Amer. J. Publ. Hlth.* 11: 119–25.

"Eradication of Smallpox in the Americas." 1972. *Boletin de la OSP*, English ed. 6: 91–94.

Evans, I. H. N. 1953. *The Religion of the Tempasuk Dusuns of North Borneo.* Cambridge: At the University Press.

Fadeyi, S. O. 1967. "Yoruba Beliefs Regarding Smallpox Prevention and Folklore." In *Handbook for Smallpox Eradication Programmes in Endemic Areas*, SE/67.5 Rev. 1, Annex 2, V–20. Geneva: World Health Organization.

Farr, W. 1840–41. "Note on the Present Epidemic of Smallpox, and on the Necessity of Arresting its Ravages." *Lancet* 1: 351–54.

Fasquelle, R., and Fasquelle, A. 1971. "A-propos de l'histoire de la lutte contre la variole dans les pays d'afrique francophone." (Translated by E. Hopkins.) *Bull. Soc. Path. Exot.* 64: 734–54.

Fawcett, C. 1936. *The English Factories in India.* Oxford: Clarendon Press.

Fenner, F. 1948. "The Pathogenesis of the Acute Exanthems." *Lancet* 2: 915–20.

Ferrars, M., and Ferrars, B. 1900. *Burma.* London: Sampson Low, Marston and Co.

Fiedler, A. 1872. "Statistische Mittheilungen u. Ephoristische Bemerkungen über die Pockenepidemie zu Dresden in den Jahren 1870 u. 1871." *Jahresbericht d. Gellesch. f. Nat. u. Heilk. in Dresd*, pp. 44–71.

Finney, J. M. T. 1940. *A Surgeon's Life.* New York: G. P. Putnam's Sons.

Finsen, N. R. 1901. *Phototherapy.* Translated by James H. Sequeira. London: Edward Arnold and Co.

———. 1903. "Remarks on the Red-Light Treatment of Smallpox." *Brit. Med. J.* 1: 1297–98.

Fisher, H. J. 1975. "The Central Sahara and Sudan." In *The Cambridge History of Africa*, edited by R. Gray. Cambridge: At the University Press.

Fitz, R. 1942. "Something Curious in the Medical Line." *Bull. Hist. Med.* 11: 239–64.

Fitz, R. H. 1911. "Zabdiel Boylston, Inoculator, and the Epidemic of Smallpox in Boston in 1721." *Bull. Johns Hopkins Hosp.* 22: 315–27.

Fluker, J. L. 1972. "Mozart, His Health and Death." *Practitioner.* 209: 841–45.

Foege, W. H.; Millar, J. D.; and Henderson, D. A. 1975. "Smallpox Eradication in West and Central Africa." *Bull. World Hlth. Org.* 52: 209–22.

Forbes, A. K. 1973. *Ras Mala: Hindu Annals of Western India.* New Delhi: Heritage Publishers.

Forbes, J. 1832. "Report of a Recent Irruption of Smallpox in Ceylon." *Lond. Med. Gaz.* 10: 17–19.

———. 1841. *Eleven Years in Ceylon.* London: Richard Bentley.

Forchammer, H., and Busck, G. 1902. Postscript. *Lancet* 2: 1272.

Forrer, E. O. 1937. "The Hittites in Palestine II." *Pal. Expl. Quart.* 69: 100–15.
Foster, E. A. 1950. *Motolinia's History of the Indians of New Spain.* Berkeley: Cortes Society, 1950.
Foster, S. O., et. al. 1972. "Human Monkeypox." *Bull. Wld. Hlth. Org.* 46; 569–76.
Fox, R. H. 1919. *Dr. John Fothergill and his Friends.* London: Macmillan and Co.
Fracastoro, H. 1930. *De Contagione et Contagiosis Morbis.* Translated by W. C. Wright. New York: G. P. Putnam's Sons.
Fraser, A. 1979. *Royal Charles.* New York: Alfred A. Knopf.
Fraser, S. M. F. 1980. "Leicester and Smallpox: The Leicester Method." *Med. Hist.* 24: 315–32.
Frey. 1924–25. "Die Pockenepidemie in der Schweiz in den Jahren 1921 bis 1924." *Deutsche Ztshr. f. offentl, Gesundsheitspflege* 1: 169–77.
Frederiksen, H. 1962. "Strategy and Tactics for Smallpox Eradication." *Publ. Hlth. Repts.* 77: 617–22.
Freeman-Grenville, G. S. P. 1965. *The French at Kilwa Island,* Oxford: Clarendon Press.
Freyre, G. 1970. *Order and Progress,* New York: Alfred A. Knopf.
Frobenius, L. 1926. *Die Atlantische Götterlehre.* Jena: Eugen Diederichs.
Fryatt, N. R. 1972. *Boston and the Tea Riots.* Princeton: Auerbach Publishers.
Fryer, J. 1909. *A New Account of East India and Persia.* Edited by W. Crooke. London: Hakluyt Society.
Fujikawa, Y. 1911. *Nihon Shippeishi* (History of diseases in Japan). Translated by T. Kitamura.
———. 1934. *Japanese Medicine.* Clio Medica, vol. 12, edited by E. B. Krumbhaar. New York: Paul B. Hoeber.
Furman, B. *A Profile of the United States Public Health Service, 1798–1948.* Washington D.C.: U.S. Government Printing Office.
Furukawa, A. 1971. "History of Variolation in Europe, Especially the Introduction of the Turkish Method in the West." *Nihon Ishigaku Zasshi.* 17: 272.
Gait, E. 1926. *A History of Assam.* Calcutta: Thacker, Spink and Co.
Gantt, W. H. 1924. "A Review of Medical Education in Soviet Russia." *Brit. Med. J.* 1: 1055–58.
———. 1937. *Russian Medicine.* Clio Medica, vol. 20, edited by E. B. Krumbhaar. New York: Paul B. Hoeber.
Gardner, W. H. 1852. "History of an Epidemic of Smallpox in the Mauritius." *London J. Med.* 4: 38–44.
Garrison, F. H. 1914. *An Introduction to the History of Medicine.* Philadelphia: W. B. Saunders Co.
Geil, W. E. 1926. *The Sacred Five of China.* London: John Murray.
Gelfand, H. M. 1966. "A Critical Examination of the Indian Smallpox Eradication Program." *Amer. J. Publ. Hlth.* 56: 1634–51.
Gelfand, H., and Posch, J. 1971. "The Recent Outbreak of Smallpox in Meschede, West Germany." *Amer. J. Epid.* 93: 234–37.
Gibb, G. D. 1855. "Epidemic of Smallpox in Quebec." *J. Publ. Hlth.* (London) 1: 113–17.
Gibson, J. E. 1937. *Dr. Bodo Otto and the Medical Background of the American Revolution.* Springfield: Charles C. Thomas.

Gie, S. F. N. 1963. "The Cape Colony under Company Rule, 1708–1795." In *The Cambridge History of the British Empire*, vol. 8, edited by E. A. Walker. Cambridge: At the University Press.

Glokpor, G. F. 1970. "Notes on Variolation." In *The SEP Report: Seminar on Smallpox Eradication and Measles Control in Western and Central Africa* 4, no. 1 (Jan. 7): 59–61.

Gomes, E. H. 1911. *Seventeen Years among the Sea Dyaks of Borneo*. London: Seeley and Co.

Gottfried, R. S. 1978. *Epidemic Disease in Fifteenth-Century England*. New Brunswick: Rutgers University Press.

Government of Gujarat. 1965. *Gujarat State Gazetteers: Rajkot District*. Ahmedabad.

Government of India. 1885. *Gazetteer of the Bombay Presidency*. Poona: Government Central Press.

———. 1901. *Gazetteer of the Bombay Presidency*. Bombay: Government Central Press.

———. 1925. *Bombay, 1923–24*. Bombay: Government Central Press.

———. 1931a. *Annual Report of the Public Health Commissioner with the Government of India for 1928*. Calcutta.

———. *India in 1930–31*. Calcutta.

———. 1931b. *India in 1929–30*. Calcutta.

Government of India. Imp. Rec. Dept. 1919. *Calendar of Persian Correspondence*. Calcutta: Government Printing.

Government of Sweden. 1741. *Story of the Cause of Death of Her Queenly Majesty, Ulrica Eleonora*. (Translated from Swedish by M. Barron.) Stockholm: Royal Press.

Government of Thailand, Ministry of Public Health, and World Health Organization. 1978. "Smallpox Eradication in Thailand." WHO/SE/78.113.

Grasset, N., and Meiklejohn, G. 1978. "Report on a Visit to Southern Rhodesia, 10–30 January 1978." WHO/SE/78.108.

Gray, R., ed. 1975. *The Cambridge History of Africa*. Cambridge: Cambridge University Press.

Gregory of Tours. 1977. *The History of the Franks*. Translated by L. Thorpe. Hardmondsworth: Penguin Books.

Green, C. M. 1962. *Washington: Village and Capitol, 1800–1878*. Princeton: Princeton University Press.

Green, J. O. 1837. "Smallpox in Lowell, Mass." *Boston Med. Surg. J.* 17: 321–29.

Greenfield, M. 1962. *A History of Public Health in New Mexico*. Albuquerque: University of New Mexico Press.

Greenwood, M. 1935. *Epidemics and Crowd Diseases*. London: Williams and Norgate.

Groff, G. G. 1904. "Observations on Smallpox Prevailing in Pennsylvania Since 1898." *Am. Med.* 8: 106–9.

Gupta, A. C. D. 1959. "Report on Vaccination in Bengal." In *The Days of John Company: Selections from Calcutta Gazette, 1824–1832*. Calcutta: West Bengal Government.

Gurdon, P. R. T. 1914. *The Khasis*. 2d ed. London: MacMillan and Co.

Guy, W. A. 1882. "Two Hundred and Fifty Years of Small Pox in London." *J. Roy. Stat. Soc.* 45: 399–437.

Halbrohr, J. G. 1973. "Smallpox Surveillance in Venezuela." Unpublished.

Hale-White, W. 1935. *Great Doctors of the Nineteenth Century*. London: Edward Arnold and Co.

Halliday, F. E. 1955. "Queen Elizabeth I and Dr. Burcot." *History Today* 5: 542–44.

Halsband, R. 1953. "New Light on Lady Mary Wortley Montagu's Contribution to Inoculation." *J. Hist. Med.* 8: 390–405.

———. 1956. *The Life of Lady Mary Wortley Montagu*. Oxford: Clarendon Press.

Hancock, J. C. 1902. "Some Aspects of the Present Smallpox Epidemic." *Medicine* (Detroit) 8: 807–18.

Handerson, H. E. 1904. "John of Gaddesden, Variola and the Finsen Light-Cure." *Cleveland Med. J.* 3: 433–41.

Hardwick, A. A. 1903. *An Ivory Trader in North Kenya*. London: Longmans, Green and Co.

Hare, R. 1954. *Pomp and Pestilence*. London: Victor Gollancz.

———. 1967. "The Antiquity of Diseases Caused by Bacteria and Viruses." In *Diseases in Antiquity*, edited by D. Brothwell and A. T. Sandison. Springfield: Charles C. Thomas.

Hargreaves-Mawdsley, W. N., ed. 1973. *Spain under the Bourbons, 1700–1833*. London: Macmillan and Co.

Harke, T. H. 1891. *My Personal Experiences in Equatorial Africa*. 3d ed. London: Sampson Row, Marston and Co.

Harper, G. J. 1961. "Airborne Micro-Organisms: Survival Tests with Four Viruses." *J. Hyg.* (Cambridge) 59: 479–86.

Harris, J. E., and Weeks, K. R. 1973. *X-raying the Pharoahs*. New York: Charles Scribner's Sons.

Harris, T. M. 1841. *Biographical Memorial of James Oglethorpe*. Boston: Freeman and Bolles.

Harrison, H. S. B. 1978. *Nagel's Encyclopedia Guide: Japan*. Geneva: Nagel Publishers.

Hartwig, G. W. 1979. "Demographic Considerations in East Africa during the Nineteenth Century." *Int. J. Afr. Hist. Stud.* 12: 653–72.

———. 1981. "Smallpox in the Sudan." *Int. J. Afr. Hist. Stud.* 14: 5–33.

Harvey, G. E. 1925. *History of Burma*. London: Longmans, Green and Co.

Haslip, J. 1977. *Catherine the Great*. New York: G. P. Putnam's Sons.

Hauptman, L. M. 1979. "Smallpox and American Indian." *N.Y. State J. Med.* 79: 1945–49.

Hawes, L. E. 1974. *Benjamin Waterhouse, M.D.* Boston: Francis A. Countway Library of Medicine.

Haygarth, John. 1793. *Sketch of a Plan to Exterminate the Casual Small-Pox from Great Britain*. London: J. Johnson.

Heagerty, J. J. 1928. *Four Centuries of Medical History in Canada*. Bristol: John Wright and Sons.

Heaton, C. E. 1945. "Medicine in New York during the English Colonial Period." *Bull. Hist. Med.* 17: 9–37.

Hedrich, A. W. 1936. "Changes in the Incidence and Fatality of Smallpox in Recent Decades." *Publ. Hlth. Repts.* 51: 363–92.

Heiser, V. 1936. *An American Doctor's Odyssey*. New York: W. W. Norton and Co.

Helleiner, K. F. 1967. Chapter 1. In *The Cambridge Economic History of Europe*, vol. 4. edited by E. E. Rich and C. H. Wilson. Cambridge: At the University Press.

Helps, A. 1904. *The Spanish Conquest of America*. London: John Lane.

Hemingway, F. R. 1907. *Madras District Gazetteers: Trichinopoly.* Madras: Government Press.

Hemming, J. 1978. *Red Gold.* Cambridge: Harvard University Press.

Henderson, D. A. 1976. "The Eradication of Smallpox." *Sci. Amer.* 235 (October): 25–33.

———. 1978. "Smallpox—Epitaph for a Killer?" *Nat. Geogr.* 154: 796–805.

———. 1980. "Smallpox Eradication." *Publ. Hlth. Repts.* 95: 422–26.

Henderson, K. D. D. 1933. *The Making of Sudan.* London: Faber and Faber.

Henderson, P. 1965. "Smallpox and Patriotism: The Norfolk Riots, 1768–69." *Virginia Magazine of Historical Biography* 73: 413–24.

Henderson, S. C. 1906. "Smallpox, as Observed in Alabama in Recent Years." *Mobile Med. and Sur. J.* 9: 19–23.

Henschen, F. 1966. *The History and Geography of Diseases.* New York: Delacorte Press.

Herbert, Eugenia W. 1975. "Smallpox Inoculation in Africa." *Journal of African History* 16: 539–59.

Herrick, S. S. 1888. "Review of Smallpox in San Francisco." *Pacific Med. Surg. J.* 31: 207–10.

Herskovits, M. J. 1938. *Dahomey: An Ancient West African Kingdom.* New York: J. J. Augustin.

Hervieux, M. 1899. "La Variole en Indo-Chine." (Translated by E. Hopkins.) *Bull. Acad. de Med.* (Paris), 3d 542: 61–67.

Hes, H. S., and Rutkovska, C. 1973. "Smallpox Prevention during the Ming Dynasty." *Koroth* 6: xxxiii.

Hill, R. 1970. *On the Frontiers of Islam.* Oxford: Clarendon Press.

Hinde, S. L. [1897] 1969. *The Fall of the Congo Arabs.* Reprint. New York: Negro Universities Press.

Hirsch, A. 1883. *Handbook of Geographical and Historical Pathology.* Vol. 1. London: New Sydenham Society.

The History of Inoculation and Vaccination. 1913. London: Burroughs Wellcome and Co.

"The History of Smallpox." 1871. *Clinic Cincin.* 1: 229–32.

Hitti, P. K. 1964. *History of the Arabs.* 8th ed. London: Macmillan and Co.

"H. M. Alexander, M.D." 1894. *Portrait and Biographical Record of Lancaster County, Pennsylvania.* Chicago: Chapman Publishing Co.

Hobson, W. 1963. *World Health and History.* Bristol: John Wright and Sons.

Hodge, G. P. 1977. "A Medical History of the Spanish Habsburgs." *J. Amer. Med. Ass.* 238: 1169–74.

Hookham, H. 1969. *A Short History of China.* New York: New American Library.

Hopkins, E. W. 1901. *India Old and New.* New York: Charles Scribner's Sons.

Hopkins, D. R. 1977. "Benjamin Waterhouse (1754–1846): The 'Jenner of America.' " *Am. J. Trop. Med. Hyg.* 26: 1060–64.

Hopkins, D. R.; Lane, J. M.; Cummings, E. C.; and Millar, J. D. 1971a "Smallpox in Sierra Leone. I. Epidemiology." *Amer. J. Trop. Med. Hyg.* 20: 689–96.

———. 1971b. "Two Funeral-Associated Smallpox Outbreaks in Sierra Leone." *Amer. J. Epidemiol.* 94: 341–347.

Hose, C. 1926. *Natural Man: A Record From Borneo.* London: MacMillan and Co.

Howard, M. 1962. *The Franco-Prussian War.* London: Rupert Hart-Davis.

Howard-Jones, N. 1975. "Thousand Year Scourge." *World Health* (Feb.-Mar.): 4–11.

Howell, W. B. 1933. *Medicine in Canada.* Clio Medica, vol. 9, edited by E. B. Krumbhaar. New York: P. B. Hoeber.

Huard, P., and Wong, M. 1968. *Chinese Medicine.* New York: McGraw-Hill Book Co.

Huc, M., and Gabet, M. 1928. *Travels in Tartary, Thibet and China, 1844–46.* London: George Routledge and Sons.

Hucker, C. O. 1975. *China's Imperial Past.* Stanford: Stanford University Press.

Hudson, E. H. 1964. "Treponematosis and African Slavery." *Brit, J. Vener. Dis.* 40: 43–52.

Hummell, A. W., ed. 1943,1944. *Eminent Chinese of the Ch'ing Period.* 2 vols. Washington, D.C.: U.S. Government Printing Office.

Hunter, R. W. 1876. *A Statistical Account of Bengal.* London: Trübner and Co.

Hunter, W. W. [1881] 1887. *The Imperial Gazetteer of India.* 2d ed. London: Trübner and Co.

Hurd, W. L. 1883. "Report of an Epidemic of Smallpox at Paterson." *Trans. Med. Soc. N.J.* 9: 373–80.

Hutchinson, J. C. 1854. "On Vaccination and the Causes of the Prevalence of Small-Pox in New York in 1853–4." *N.Y. J. Med.,* n.s. 12: 349–68.

Hyde, J. N. 1901. "The Late Epidemic of Smallpox in the U. S." *Pop. Sci. Mon.* 59: 557–67.

Immerman, H.; Jurgensen, T.; Liebermeister, C.; Lenhartz, H.; and Sticker, G. 1902. *Variola, Vaccination, Varicella, Cholera, Erysipelas, Whooping Cough, Hay Fever.* Philadelphia: W. B. Saunders and Co.

Imperato, P. J. 1968. "The Practice of Variolation among the Songhai of Mali." *Trans. Roy. Soc. Trop. Med. Hyg.* 62: 868–73.

Imperato, P. J.; Sow, O.; and Fofana, B. 1973. "The Persistence of Smallpox in Remote Unvaccinated Villages during Eradication Program Activities." *Acta. Trop.* (Basel) 30: 261–68.

Imperato, P. J., and Traore, D. 1968. "Traditional Beliefs about Smallpox and Its Treatment in the Republic of Mali." *J. Trop. Med. Hyg.* 71: 224–28.

Ingalls, A. G. 1926. "Smallpox." *Sci. Amer.* 135: 55.

"L'inoculation (Variolisation) et Louis XV." 1971. *Arch. Int. Claude Bernard* 1: 3–4.

Ions, V. 1967. *Indian Mythology.* London: Paul Hamlyn.

Irons, J. V., et. al. 1953. "Outbreak of Smallpox in the Lower Rio Grande Valley of Texas in 1949." *Amer. J. Publ. Hlth.* 43: 25–29.

Irwin, F. 1910. "Smallpox in Japan." *Pub. Hlth. Rep.* 25: 1205–8.

Ishwaran, K. 1968. *Shivapur: A South Indian Village.* London: Routledge and Kegan Paul.

Isichei, E. 1976. *A History of the Igbo People.* London: MacMillan and Co.

Islam, Z. 1978. "Report on Smallpox Situation in Madagascar." WHO/SE/78.124.

Ives, E. 1773. *A Voyage From England to India.* London: Edward and Charles Dilly.

Jaggi, O. P. 1977. *Medicine in Medieval India.* History of Science and Technology in India, vol. 8. Delhi: Atma Ram and Sons.

James, M. 1933. *Andrew Jackson: The Border Captain.* Indianapolis: Bobbs-Merrill Co.

James, S. P. 1909. *Smallpox and Vaccination in British India*. Calcutta: Thacker, Spink and Co.

Janssens, U. 1981. "Matthieu Maty and the Adoption of Inoculation for Smallpox in Holland." *Bull. Hist. Med.* 55: 246–56.

Japan Biographical Research Dept (JBRD). 1918. *Japan Biographical Encyclopedia and WHO'S WHO* 3d. ed. Tokyo: Rengo Press.

Jenkins, E. H. 1973. *A History of the French Navy*. London: MacDonald and Jane's.

Jenkins, E. 1958. *Elizabeth the Great*. New York: Coward-McCann.

Jenner, E. 1800. *A Continuation of Facts and Observations Relative to the Variolae Vaccine, or Cow Pox*. London: Sampson Low, Marston and Co.

Jezek, Z., and Hardjotanojo, W.1978. "Residual Skin Changes in Patients Who Have Recovered from *Variola minor*." WHO/SE/78.131.

Jochman, G. 1914. *Lehrbuch der Infektionskrankheiten*. Berlin: Springer Verlag.

Johnson, S. 1973. *The History of the Yorubas*. London: Routledge and Kegan Paul.

Johnston, H. 1902. *The Uganda Protectorate*. New York: Dodd Mead and Co.

———. 1906. *Liberia*. London: Hutchinson and Co.

———. 1908. *George Grenfell and the Congo*. London: Hutchinson and Co.

Joly, A., and Maroteaux, P. 1961. "A-propos de la mort de Louis XV." *Presse Med.* (Paris) 69: 2235–37.

Jones, E. R. 1914. "Smallpox in Germany." *Pub. Hlth. Rep.* 29: 164–68.

Jones, S. B. 1922. "Outbreak of Smallpox in Anguilla, B. W. I." *J. Trop. Med. Hyg.* 25: 321–26.

Jopling, W. H. 1962. Letter to the Editor. *Lancet* 1: 746.

Junod, H. A. 1962. *The Life of a South African Tribe*. New Hyde Park, N.Y.: University Books.

Kaempfer, E. 1906. *The History of Japan*. Glasgow: James MacLehose and Sons.

Kahn, C.1963. "History of Smallpox and Its Prevention." *Amer. J. Dis. Child.* 106: 597–609.

Kalidos, R. n.d. *History and Culture of the Tamils*. Dindigul: Vijay Publications.

Kati, M. 1913. *Tarik el-Fettah*. Paris: Ernest Leroux.

Kieman, M. C. 1973. *The Indian Policy of Portugal in the Amazon Region, 1614–1693*. New York: Octagon Books.

Kingsley, M. H. 1897. *Travels in West Africa*. London: Macmillan and Co.

Kirkpatrick, F. A. 1934. *The Spanish Conquistadores*. London: A. and C. Black.

Kitching, A. L. 1912. *On the Backwaters of the Nile*. London: T. Fisher Unwin.

Kjekshus, H. 1977. *Ecology Control and Economic Development in East African History*. London: Heinemann.

Klebs, A. C. 1913. "The Historic Evolution of Variolation." *Bull. Johns Hopkins Hosp.* 24: 69–83.

———. 1914. *Die Variolation in Achtzehnten Jahrhundert*. Giessen: Verlag von Alfred Töpelmann.

Klein, J. 1974. "Zur Geschichte der Pocken—Inokulation in Russland." Diss. Freien Universität, Berlin.

Klengel, E., and Klengel, H. 1970. *Die Hethiter*. Vienna: Verlag Anton Schroll and Co.

Kobischchanov, Y. M. 1979. *Axum*. University Park: Pennsylvania State University Press.

Kohnke, Q. 1900. "Some Recent History of Smallpox in New Orleans." *New Orleans Med. Surg. J.*, n.s. 27: 699–706.

Koko, U. 1970. "Strategy in National Smallpox Eradication Programme of Burma." *Trans. Roy. Soc. Trop. Med. Hyg.* 64: 444–53.

Korns, J. M. 1921. "Incidence of Vaccination and Smallpox in North China." *China Med. J.* (Shanghai) 35: 561–63.

Kraechenko, A. T. "History of Smallpox Eradication in the USSR." (Translated by G. Kipya.) *Zh. Mikrobiol. Epidemiol. Immunobiol.* 49: 3–8.

Krogman, W. M., and Baer, M. J. 1980. "Age at Death of Pharaohs of the New Kingdom, Determined from X-ray Films." In *Atlas of the Royal Mummies*, edited by J. E. Harris and E. F. Wente, pp. 188–212. Chicago: University of Chicago Press.

Kübler, P. 1901. *Geschichte der Pocken und der Impfung.* Berlin: Verlag von August Hirschwald.

Kuczynski, R. R. 1939. *The Cameroons and Togoland.* London: Oxford University Press.

Külz. 1905. "Pockenbekämpfung in Togo." *Archiv. für Schiffs u. Trop. Hyg.* 9: 241–53.

———. 1907. "Über Pocken und Pockenbekämpfung in Kamerun." *Archiv. für Schiffs u. Trop. Hyg.* 11: 447–48.

Labaree, L. W., ed. 1961. *The Papers of Benjamin Franklin.* New Haven: Yale University Press.

Laidler, P. W., and Gelfand, M. 1971. *South Africa: Its Medical History, 1652–1898.* Capetown: C. Struik.

Laignel-Lavastine, M., and Molinery, M. R. 1934. *French Medicine.* Clio Medica, vol. 15, edited by E. B. Krumbhaar. New York: Paul B. Hoeber.

Lakin, L. 1972. "My Recollection of the 1903 Epidemic," as told to Mrs. Ruth French. Edited by S. A. Washburn. *Oregon Hlth. Bull.* 50, no. 10, (Oct.): 2.

Landau, M. 1889. *Geschichte Kaiser Karls VI. als König von Spanien.* Stuttgart: Verlag der T. G. Cotta schen Buchhandlung. 1889.

Langer, W. L. 1976. "Immunization against Smallpox before Jenner." *Sci. Amer.* 234: 112–17.

Lastres, J. B. 1954. *Historia de la Viruela en el Peru.* Lima: Ministerio de Salud Publica.

Latourette, K. S. 1934. *The Chinese: Their History and Culture.* New York: Macmillan Co.

Laval, E. 1967–68. "La Viruela en Chile." *An. Chil. Hist. Med.* 9–10: 203–76.

Lavisse, E. 1911. *Histoire de France.* Vol. 8, part 1. Paris: Librairie Hachette.

Law, E. *The History of Hampton Court Palace.* Vol. 1. London: George Bell and Sons.

Law, J. 1976. *Fleur de Lys.* London: Hamish Hamilton.

Lawrence, A. W. 1963. *Trade Castles and Forts of West Africa.* London: Jonathan Cape.

Leavitt, J. W. 1976. "Politics and Public Health: Smallpox in Milwaukee, 1894–1895." *Bull. Hist. Med.* 50: 553–68.

Lebeuf, L. G. 1900. "History of Smallpox." *Indian Lancet* (Calcutta) 15: 492–94.

Lee, S. 1829. *The Travels of Ibn Batua.* London: John Murray.

Lee, Y. K. 1973. "Smallpox and Vaccination in Early Singapore: Part I." *Singapore Med. J.* 14: 525–31.

Leech, M. 1941. *Reveille in Washington, 1860–1865.* New York: Harper and Brothers.

LeFanu, W. R. 1951. *A Bio-Bibliography of Edward Jenner.* London: Harvey and Blythe.

Leikind, M. C. 1940. "Colonial Epidemic Diseases." *Ciba Symposia* 1: 372–78.

Leikind, M. C. 1942. "Variolation in Europe and America." *Ciba Symposia,* ser. 1, 3: 1090–1102.

Lersch, B. M. 1896. *Geschichte der Volksseuchen.* Berlin: S. Karger Verlag.

Levine, D. N. 1965. *Wax and Gold.* Chicago: University of Chicago Press.

Lievin, A. 1873. "Die Pockenepidemie der Jahre 1871 u. 1872 in Danzig." *Deutsche Vrtljschr. f. öff. Gsndhtspflg.* 5: 365–74.

Little, H. W. 1884. *Madagascar: Its History and People.* Westport: Negro Universities Press.

Littman, R. J., and Littman, M. L. 1969. "The Athenian Plague: Smallpox." *Proc. Amer. Philol. Assoc.* 100: 261–75.

———. 1973. "Galen and the Antonine Plague." *Amer. J. Philol.* 94: 243–55.

Livingstone, D. 1860. *Missionary Travels and Researches in South Africa.* New York: Harper and Brothers.

Long, D. 1955. "Smallpox in North Carolina." *North Carolina Med. J.* 16: 496–99.

Long, E. B., ed. 1962. *Personal Memoirs of U.S. Grant.* New York: Universal Library.

Long, J. 1978. *Rajamala; or, An Analysis of the Chronicles of the Kings of Tripura.* Rev. ed. Calcutta: Firma KLM.

Lord, J. 1971. *The Maharajas.* New York: Random House.

Low, R. B. 1918. "The Incidence of Small-Pox throughout the World in Recent Years." *Reports to the Local Government Board on Public Health and Medical Subjects,* n.s. no. 117. London: His Majesty's Stationery Office.

Lucas, J. O. 1948. *The Religion of the Yorubas.* Lagos: C. M. S. Bookshop.

Ludowyk, E. F. C., ed. 1948. *Robert Knox in the Kandyan Kingdom.* London: Oxford University Press.

———. 1966. *The Modern History of Ceylon.* London: Weidenfeld and Nicolson.

Ludwig, E. 1904. *Visit of the Teshoo Lama to Peking-Ch'ien Lung's Inscription.* Peking: Tsientsin Press.

Macaulay, Lord Thomas B. 1914. *The History of England.* Edited by C. H. Firth. London: Macmillan and Co.

MacDonald. A. E. 1872. "Smallpox Statistics, 1871." *Med. Rec. New York* 7: 142–43.

MacDonald, D. 1944. *The Land of the Lama.* Philadelphia: J. B. Lippincottt Co.

MacGowan, D. J. 1884. "Introduction of Smallpox and Inoculation into China." *Imp. Customs Med. Rep.* (Shanghai) 27: 16–18.

MacGowan, J. [1897] 1973. *The Imperial History of China.* 2d ed. Reprint. London: Curzon Press.

MacGugan, A. 1901. "An Epidemic of Smallpox at the Michigan Asylum for the Insane." *Kalamazoo Med. News* 79: 927–30.

Mack, T. M. 1972. "Smallpox in Europe, 1950–1971." *J. Inf. Dis.* 125: 161–69.

MacKinney, L. C. 1937. *Early Medieval Medicine.* Baltimore: Johns Hopkins Press.

Maclean, C. M. 1965. "Traditional Medicine and Its Practitioners in Ibadan, Nigeria." *J. Trop. Med. Hyg.* 68: 237–44.

MacLeod, R. M. 1967. "Law, Medicine and Public Opinion: The Resistance to Compulsory Health Legislation, 1870–1907." In *Public Law*, edited by J. A. G. Griffith. London: Stevens and Sons.

MacMunn, G. 1933. *The Underworld of India*. London: Jarrolds.

MacNalty, A. S. 1968. "The Prevention of Smallpox: From Edward Jenner to Monckton Copeman." *Med. Hist.* 12: 1–18.

———. 1971. "The Medical History of Queen Elizabeth I of England." *Hist. of Med.* 3: 9–12.

Maekawa, K. 1976a. "Changes of Sasayu Ceremony with the Lapse of Time in the Edo Era." *Nihon Ishigaku Zasshi* 22: 48.

———. 1976b. "Prevailing Custom of Smallpox Treatment from the Diary of Bakin Takizawa." *Nihon Ishigaku Zasshi* 22: 391.

Maenchen-Helfen, J. O. 1973. *The World of the Huns*. Berkeley: University of California Press.

Magner, J. A. 1942. *Men of Mexico*. Milwaukee: Bruce Publishing Co.

Mahoney, I. 1975. *Madame Catherine*. New York: Coward, McCann and Geoghegan.

Major, R. H. 1936. *Disease and Destiny*. New York: D. Appleton Century Company.

———. 1954. *A History of Medicine*. Oxford: Blackwell Scientific Publications.

Majumdar, M. R. 1965. *Cultural History of Gujarat*. Bombay: Popular Prakashan.

Majumdar, P. C. 1905. *The Musnud of Murshidabad, 1704–1904*. Calcutta: Kuntaline Press.

Majumdar, R. C., ed. 1974. *The Mughul Empire*. Vol. 7 of *The History and Culture of the Indian People*. Bombay: Bharatiya Vidya Bhavan.

Makpeace, W.; Brooke, G. E.; and Braddell, R. St. J. 1921. *One Hundred Years of Singapore*. London: John Murray.

Marbaniang, I. 1970. *Assam in a Nutshell*. Shillong: Chapala Bookstall.

Marcley, J. I. 1882. "Variola in Buffalo." *Med. and Surg. J.* 21: 337–46.

Marcus, H. G. 1975. *The Life and Times of Menelik II*. Oxford: Clarendon Press.

Markens, E. W. 1922. "Lincoln and His Relation to Doctors." *J. Med. Soc. New Jersey* 19: 44–47.

Marks, G., and Beatty, W. K. 1976. *Epidemics*. New York: Charles Scribner's Sons.

Marsden, W. 1966. *The History of Sumatra* 3d ed. Kuala Lumpur: Oxford University Press.

Martin, H. A. 1881. "Jefferson as a Vaccinator." *North Carolina Med. J.* 7: 1–34.

Marx, R. 1960. *The Health of the Presidents*. New York: G. P. Putnam's Sons.

Mason, H. 1975. *Voltaire*. New York: St. Martins Press.

Massie, R. K. 1980. *Peter the Great*. New York: Alfred A. Knopf.

Mather, R. J., and John, T. J. 1973. "Popular Beliefs about Smallpox and Other Common Infectious Diseases in South India." *Trop. Geogr. Med.* 25: 190–96.

Mathews, J. W. 1887. *In Wadi Yami; or, 20 Years Experience in South Africa*. London: Sampson, Low, Marston, Searle and Rivington.

Matsuki, A. 1970. "A Brief History of Jennerian Vaccination in Japan." *Med. Hist.* 14: 199–201.

———. 1971. "The History of Epidemics and Scurvy in Hokkaido before the Meiji Era." *Nihon Ishigaku Zasshi* 17: 162.

Mayer, A. C. 1960. *Caste and Kinship in Central India*. London: Routledge and Kegan Paul.

McCarry, C., and Mobley, G. F. 1976. "Kyoto and Nara: Keepers of Japan's Past." *Nat. Geogr.* 149: 836–59.

McDonald, N. A. 1871. *Siam: Its Government, Manners, Customs, etc.* Philadelphia: Alfred Martien.

McFarland, G. B., ed. 1928. *Historical Sketch of Protestant Missions in Siam, 1828–1928.* Bangkok: Bangkok Times Press.

McGilvary, D. 1912. *A Half Century among the Siamese and the Lao.* New York: Fleming H. Revell Co.

McGinty, L. 1979. "Smallpox Laboratories, What Are the Risks?" *New Scientist* 81: 8–14.

McGuigan, D. G. 1976. *The Habsburgs.* Garden City: Doubleday and Co.

McLean, D. M., et. al. 1962. "Smallpox in Toronto, 1962." *Canad. Med. Assoc. J.* 87: 772–3.

McNeill, W. H. 1965. *The Rise of the West.* New York: New American Library.

———. 1976. *Plagues and Peoples.* Garden City, N.Y.: Anchor Press, Doubleday.

McVail, J. C. 1902. "Smallpox in Glasgow, 1900–1902." *Brit. Med. J.* 2: 40–43.

———. 1923–24. "Small-Pox and Vaccination in the Philippines." *Brit. Med. J.* 1: 158–62; 2: 281–82.

"M D Remembers: An Anniversary of Variolation." 1971. *MD* 15, no. 6: 97.

"Medicine, Past and Present, in Russia." 1897. *Lancet* 2: 348.

Med. Times and Gaz. 1872. 1: 661.

Meek, C. K. 1931. *A Sudanese Kingdom.* London: Kegan Paul, Trench, Trübner and Co.

Meigs, P. 1935. *The Dominican Mission Frontier of Lower California.* Berkeley: University of California Press.

Mellanby, E. 1949. "Jenner and His Impact on Medical Science." *Brit. Med. J.* 1: 921–26.

Merriman, R. B. 1962. *The Rise of the Spanish Empire.* New York: Cooper Square Publishers.

Meyer, H. 1891. *Across East African Glaciers.* London: George Philip and Son.

Miers, Earl S. 1960. *Lincoln Day by Day.* Washington: Lincoln Sesquicentennial Commission.

Military Journal of the American Revolution. [1862] 1969. Reprint. New York: New York Times and Arno Press.

Millard, C. K. 1916–17. "The Passing of Smallpox in Britain: To What Is It Due." *Publ. Hlth.* 30: 112–20, 128–34.

Miller, D. 1867. "Small-Pox and its Prevention in Jamaica." *Med. Times & Gaz.* (London) 1: 441–42.

Miller, G. 1957. *The Adoption of Inoculation for Smallpox in England and France.* Philadelphia: University of Pennsylvania Press.

———. 1981. "Putting Lady Mary in Her Place: A Discussion of Historical Causation." *Bull. Hist. Med.* 55: 2–16.

Miller, P. *The New England Mind from Colony to Province.* Cambridge: Harvard University Press, 1953.

Minor, T. C. 1881–82. "Small-pox at Cincinnati." *Nat. Bd. of Hlth. Bull.* 3: 207–29.

———. 1882. "Smallpox. Historical Notes on the Epidemics of 1879, 1880 and 1881." *Cinn. Lancet and Clin.* 8: 99–112.

Mitford, N. 1966. *The Sun King: Louis XIV at Versailles*. New York: Harper and Row.

Miyajima, M. 1922–23. "The History of Vaccination in Japan." *Proc. Roy. Soc. Med.* (London) 16: 23–26.

Moffat, M. M. 1911. *Maria Theresa*. London: Methuen and Co.

Molina, J. I. 1809. *History of Chile*. London: Longman, Hurst, Rees, and Ormes, Paternaster Row.

Moll, A. A. 1944. *Aesculapius in Latin America*. Philadelphia: W. B. Saunders Co.

Moller-Christensen, V., and Simonsen, M. 1962. "Red-Light Treatment of Smallpox." *Lancet* 1: 584–85.

Molloy, F. 1906. *The Russian Court in the Eighteenth Century*. 3d ed. London: Hutchinson and Co.

Montafakis, G. J. 1966. "Colonial Heritage of East Africa." In *The Transformation of East Africa*, edited by S. Diamond and F. G. Burke. New York: Basic Books.

Montague, Lady Mary Wortley. 1767. *Letters of the Right Honourable Lady M----y W----y M----e*. London: S. Payne, A. Cook and H. Hill.

Moor, J. H. 1837. *Notices of the Indian Archipelago and Adjacent Countries*. Singapore.

Moore, F. D. 1971. "Muddy River and Boylston's 250th." *New Engl. J. Med.* 284: 1438–39.

Moore, James. 1815. *The History of the Smallpox*. London: Longman, Hurst, Rees, Orme, and Brown, Paternaster Row.

Moore, W. J. 1869. "Smallpox in India and as it Might be in England." *Med. Times and Gaz.* (London) 2: 634–35.

Moorehead, A. 1966. *The Fatal Impact*. London: Hamish Hamilton.

Morgan, E. L. 1898. "Ancient Customs and Treatment of Variola in the Orient." *N. Amer. Med. Rev.* 6: 146–54.

Morgan, K. W. 1953. *The Religion of the Hindus*. New York: Ronald Press Co.

Morley, S. G. 1946. *The Ancient Maya*. Stanford: Stanford University Press.

Morris, C. L. 1937. *Maria Theresa: The Last Conservative*. New York: Alfred A. Knopf.

Morse, E. S. 1917. *Japan Day by Day*. Boston: Houghton Mifflin Co.

Moses, B. 1914. *The Spanish Dependencies in South America*. New York: Harper and Brothers.

———. 1919. *Spain's Declining Power in South America, 1730–1806*. Berkeley: University of California Press.

Mundy, R. 1848. *Narrative of Events in Borneo and Celebes*. London: John Murray.

Mungeam, G. H. 1966. *British Rule in Kenya, 1895–1912*. Oxford: Clarendon Press.

Musgrove, G. C. 1896. *To Kumasi with Scott*. London: Wrightman and Co.

Murdoch, J. 1910. *A History of Japan*. London: Kegan Paul, Trübner and Co.

Nagler, F. P. O., and Rake, G. 1948. "The Use of the Electron Microscope in Diagnosis of Variola, Vaccinia, and Varicella." *J. Bact.* 55: 45–51.

Neale, J. E. 1934. *Queen Elizabeth*. New York: Harcourt, Brace and Co.

Needham, J. 1954. *Science and Civilization in China*. Cambridge: At the University Press.

Needham, J., and Gwei-Djen, L. 1962. "Hygiene and Preventive Medicine in Ancient China." *J. Hist. Med.* 17: 464–66.

Nelson, J. H. 1968. *The Madura Country*. Madras: Government Printing.

Nepali, G. S. 1965. *The Newars*. Bombay: United Asia Publications.

Nevill, H. R., ed. 1904. *District Gazetteers of the United Provinces*. Naini Tal: Government Press.

————. 1903–11. *District Gazetteers of the United Provinces*. 2 (Saharanpur): 38–39; 3 (Muzaffarnagar): 22–23; 4 (Meerut): 33; 5 (Bulandshahr): 30; 6 (Aligarh): 30; 15 (Budaun): 28–29; 17 (Shahjahanpur): 26–27; 19 (Cawnpore): 27–28; 20 (Fatehpur): 30; 23 (Allahbad): 27–28; 31 (Gorakhpur): 36–37; 32 (Basti): 32; 40 (Sitapur): 21; 41 (Hardoi): 23–24; 44 (Gonda): 29. Allahabad: Government Press.

Nevin, A. and Commager, H. S. 1964. *A Pocket History of the United States*, New ed. New York: Washington Square Press.

Newsholme, A. 1902. "The Epidemiology of Small-Pox in the Nineteenth Century." *Brit. Med. J.* 2: 17–26.

Nicholas, R. W. 1970. "Sitala and the Art of Printing: The Transmission and Propagation of the Myth of the Goddess of Smallpox in Rural West Bengal." Draft manuscript for presentation at Duke University Symposium on Language, Arts and Man Cultures in India, 13–15 March.

Nicholas, R. 1981. "The Goddess Sitala and Epidemic Smallpox in Bengal." *Journal Asian Studies* 31: 21–44.

Nicolay, J. G., and Hay, J., eds. 1905. *Complete Works of Abraham Lincoln*. New York: Tandy–Thomas Co.

Nicholson, T. 1869. "On Small-Pox and Vaccination in the Island of Antigua." *Trans. Epidemiol. Soc. Lond.* 3: 48–52.

Noorthouck, J. 1773. *A New History of London*. London: R. Baldwin.

North, A. W. 1908. *The Mother of California*. San Francisco: Paul Elder and Co.

Nott, J. C. 1867. "Small-Pox Epidemic in Mobile during the Winter of 1865–6." *Nashville J. Med. Surg.*, n.s. 2: 372–80.

Olbert, T. 1962. Letter to the Editor. *Lancet* 1: 746.

Oliver, E. 1939. *Medecine et sante dans le pays de vaud au XVIII⁰ siecle*. Lausanne: Editions la Concorde.

Ozaki, Y. T. 1909. *Warriors of Old Japan*. Boston: Houghton Mifflin Co.

Packard, F. R. 1926. *Life and Times of Ambroise Paré*. 2d ed. New York: Paul B. Hoeber.

Palmquist, E. M. 1947. "The 1946 Smallpox Epidemic in Seattle." *Canad. J. Publ. Hlth.* 38: 213–18.

Pankhurst, R. 1961. *Introduction to the Economic History of Ethiopia from Early Times to 1800*. Addis Ababa: Lailibela House.

————. 1965. "The History and Traditional Treatment of Smallpox in Ethiopia." *Med. Hist.* 9: 343–55.

Parker, E. H. 1907. "Smallpox and Inoculation in China." *Brit. Med. J.* 1: 88–90.

Parry, J. H. 1971. *Trade and Dominion*. New York: Praeger Publishers.

Parsons, R. P. 1930. *History of Haitian Medicine*. New York: Paul B. Hoeber.

Paschen, E. 1924. "Die Pocken." In *Jochmann's Lehrbuch der Infektionskrankheiten*. 2d ed. Berlin: Springer Verlag.

Patterson, A. T. 1960. *The Other Armada*. Manchester: Manchester University Press.

Paulet, J. J. 1768. *Histoire de la petit vérole*. Paris: Chez Ganeau.

Pelzer, K. J., 1963. "Physical and Human Resource Patterns," In *Indonesia,* edited by R. T. McVey, pp. 1–23. New Haven: Hraf Press.

Pendle, G. 1969. *A History of Latin America.* Baltimore: Penguin Books.

Penna, J. 1885. *Epidemiologia: La Viruela en la America del Sud y Principalmente en la Republica Argentina.* Buenos Aires: Librairie Generale.

Perrenoud, A. 1980. "Contribution a l'histoire cyclique des maladies: Deux cents ans de variole à Genève (1580–1810)." In *Mensch und Gesundheit in der Geschichte,* edited by A. E. Imhof. Husum: Matthiesen Verlag.

"The Pestilence in Montreal." 1885. *Harper's Weekly* 29: 779, 781.

Peterson, J. 1969. *Province of Freedom: A History of Sierra Leone.* Evanston: Northwestern University Press, 1969.

Phadke, A. M.; Samant, N. R.; and Dewal, S. D. 1973. "Smallpox as an Etiologic Factor in Male Sterility." *Fert. and Steril.* 24: 802–4.

Phelan, J. L. 1967a. *The Hispanization of the Philippines.* Madison: University of Wisconsin Press.

———. 1967b. *The Kingdom of Quito in the Seventeenth Century.* Madison: University of Wisconsin Press.

Pierce, C. C. 1925. "Prevalence of Smallpox." *Am. J. Publ. Hlth.* 15: 855–59.

Pieris, P. E. 1913. *Ceylon: The Portuguese Era.* Colombo: Colombo Apothecaries.

———. 1918. *Ceylon and the Hollanders.* Tellipalai: American Ceylon Mission Press.

———. n.d. *Tri Sinhala: The Last Phase, 1796–1815.* Cambridge: W. Heffer and Sons.

Pierson, D. 1967. *Negroes in Brazil.* Carbondale: University of Southern Illinois Press.

Pittman, F. W. 1917. *Development of the British West Indies, 1700–1763.* New Haven: Yale University Press.

"Plagues and the Fortunes of Men." 1949. *Lancet* 1: 68–69.

Polak, M. F. 1968. "Smallpox Control in Indonesia during the Second Quarter of the Century and Re-establishment of Endemic Smallpox." *Trop. Geogr. Med.* 20: 243–50.

Poma de Ayala, F. G. 1956. *La Nueva Cronica y Buen Gobierno.* Lima: Talleres del Servicio de Prensa, Propaganda y Publicaciones Militares.

Ponsonby-Fane, R. A. B. 1959. *The Imperial House of Japan.* Kyoto: Ponsonby Memorial Society.

Prescott, W. H. 1843. *History of the Conquest of Mexico.* New York: Modern Library.

———. 1847. *History of the Conquest of Peru.* New York: Modern Library.

Price, R. 1982. "State Church Charity and Smallpox: An Epidemic Crisis in the City of Mexico, 1797–98." *J. Roy. Soc. Med.* 75: 356–67.

Pringle, R. 1869. "On Small-pox and Vaccination in India." *Lancet* 1: 44–45.

———. 1970. *Rajahs and Rebels.* London: Macmillan and Co.

Prinzing, F. 1916. *Epidemics Resulting from Wars.* Oxford: Clarendon Press.

Probst, C. O. 1899. "Smallpox in Ohio." *J. Amer. Med. Assoc.* 33: 1589–90.

Quinn, F. 1968. "How Traditional Dahomian Society Interpreted Smallpox." *Abbia* 20: 151–66.

Raghavan, M. D. 1969. *India in Ceylonese History, Society and Culture.* 2d ed. Bombay: Asia Publishing House.

Rahts. 1887. "Ergebnisse einer Statistik der Pockentodesfälle im Deutschen

Reiche für das Jahr 1886." *Arb. aus dem Kaiserlichen Gesundheitsamte* (Berlin) 2: 223–31.

Rainey, J. K. 1899. "An Epidemic at St. Augustine." *Trans. Fla. Med. Assoc.* 131–5.

Randall, R. P. 1955. *Lincoln's Sons.* Boston: Little, Brown and Co.

Rappaport, A. S. 1907. *The Curse of the Romanovs.* London: Chatto and Windus.

Raska, K. 1976. "Measures for Smallpox Eradication in the Czech Countries at the Beginning of the Nineteenth Century." *Int. J. Epid.* 5: 227–29.

Rasmussen, I. Fleming. 1963. "Die Medizinische Fakultät der Universität Kopenhagen." *Grünthal Waage* 3: 124.

Rauch, J. H. 1894. "The Smallpox Situation in the U.S." *J. Amer. Med. Ass.* 22: 471–74.

Razzell, P. 1965. "Population Change in Eighteenth-Century England." *Economic Hist. Review* 18: 317.

———. 1977a. *The Conquest of Smallpox.* Firle: Caliban Books.

———. 1977b. *Edward Jenner's Cowpox Vaccine: The History of a Medical Myth.* Firle: Caliban Books.

Regöly-Merei, G. 1966. "Paläopathologische und Epigraphische Angaben zur Frage der Pocken in Altägypten." *Sudhoff. Arch.* 50: 213–14.

Reich, J. P. 1948. "Smallpox in Medals." *Ciba Symposium* 9: 818–22.

Reira, J. 1977. "Noticia de una Epidemia Segoviana de Viruela (1740–1741)." *Asclepio* 29: 309–17.

Reischauer, R. K. 1937. *Early Japanese History: circa 40 B.C.-A.D. 1167.* Princeton: Princeton University Press.

Renbourn, E. T. 1972. *Materials and Clothing in Health and Disease.* London: H. K. Lewis and Co.

Reusch, R. 1954. *History of East Africa.* Stuttgart: Evangel. Missionsverlag.

Reynolds, A. R. 1894. "Remarks on the Epidemic of Smallpox in Chicago." *Ann. Hyg.* 9: 507–13.

Rhazes. 1848. *A Treatise on the Small-pox and Measles.* Translated by W. A. Greenhill. London: Sydenham Society.

Richardson, H. E. 1962. *Tibet and Its History.* London: Oxford University Press.

Richter, p. 1912. "Beiträge zur Geschichte des Pocken bei den Arabern." *Sudhoffs Arch. Gesch. Med.* 5: 311–31.

Ricketts, T. H., and Byles, J. B. 1904. "The Red Light Treatment of Smallpox." *Lancet* 2: 287–90.

Rippy, J. F., ed. 1938. *History of Colombia.* Chapel Hill: University of North Carolina Press.

Roberts, C. J. 1967. "The Origins of Smallpox in Central Africa." *Centr. Afr. J. Med.* 13: 31–3.

Roberts, K. B. 1978. "Smallpox, an Historic Disease." *Occasional Papers in Medical History,* no. 1. St. John's: Memorial University of Newfoundland.

Rodrigues, R. A. 1975. "Smallpox Eradication in the Americas." *Pan Amer. Hlth. Org. Bull.* 9: 53–68.

Rogers, F. B. 1962. *A Syllabus of Medical History.* Boston: Little, Brown and Co.

———. 1968. " 'Pox Acres' on Old Cape Cod." *New Engl. J. Med.* 278: 21–23.

———. 1972. "Dr. Samuel Gelston, Variolator and His Son, Dr. Robert Gelston, Vaccinator, from Nantucket." *J. Hist. Med.* 27: 81–85.

Rolleston, J. D. 1933. *The Smallpox Pandemic of 1870–1874*. London: John Bale Sons and Danielsson. Reprinted from *Proc. Roy. Soc. Med.* 27: 15–30.

———. 1937. *The History of the Acute Exanthemata*. London: William Heineman Medical Books.

Ronen, D. 1975. *Dahomey: Between Tradition and Modernity*. Ithaca: Cornell University Press.

Roscoe, J. 1924. *The Bagosu*. Cambridge: At the University Press.

Rosen, G. 1958. *A History of Public Health*. New York: M. D. Publications.

Rosenau, M. J. 1896. "Smallpox—Some Peculiarities of the Camp Jenner Epidemic." *Ann. Rep. Superv. Surg.: Gen. Mar. Hosp.* 234–44.

Rosenthal, R. 1959. "The History and Nature of Smallpox." *Journal-Lancet* (Minneapolis) 79: 498–505.

Roth, H. L. 1968. *Natives of Sarawak and British North Borneo*. Kuala Lumpur: University of Malaya Press.

Rubin, S. 1974. *Medieval English Medicine*. London: David and Charles Newton.

Rudin, H. R. 1938. *Germans in the Cameroons (1884–1914)*. London: Jonathan Cape.

Rudolph, R., and Musher, D. M. 1965. "Inoculation in the Boston Smallpox Epidemic of 1721." *Arch. Int. Med.* 115: 692–96.

Ruffer, M. A. 1921. "Pathological Note on the Royal Mummies of the Cairo Museum." In *Studies in the Palaeopathology of Egypt*, edited by R. L. Moodie, pp. 175–76. Chicago: University of Chicago Press.

Ruffer, Marc A., and Ferguson, A. R. 1910. "Note on an Eruption Resembling That of Variola in the Skin of a Mummy of the Twentieth Dynasty (1200–1100 B. C.)" *J. Path. and Bact.* 15: 1–4.

Rupp, J.-P. 1974. "Die Hundertjährige Geschichte des Deutschen Impfgesetzes." *Die Gelben Hefte* 14: 23–30.

Russell-Wood, A. J. R. 1968. *Fidalgos and Philanthropists*. Berkeley: University of California Press.

Rutter, O. 1929. *The Pagans of North Borneo*. London: Hutchinson and Co.

Ryder, A. F. C. 1969. *Benin and the Europeans, 1485–1897*. London: Longmans, Green and Co.

Saigal, O. 1978. *Tripura: Its History and Culture*. Delhi: Concept Publishing Co.

Sakhokia, M. 1903. "Le culte de la petite vérole en Georgie." (Translated by E. Hopkins.) *Bull. et. Mem. Soc. d'Anthr. de Paris.* 5th series, 4: 262–75.

Sandburg, C. 1939. *Abraham Lincoln: The War Years*. New York: Harcourt Brace and Co.

———. 1954. *Abraham Lincoln*. New York: Harcourt Brace and Co.

Sandwith, F. M. 1910. "Smallpox and Its Early History." *Clin. J.* 36: 294–302.

Sansom, G. 1974. *A History of Japan*. Tokyo: Charles E. Tuttle Co.

Sarafian, W. L. 1977. "Smallpox Strikes the Aleuts." *The Alaska History and Arts of the North* 7 (Winter): 46–49.

Sarton, G. 1927. *Introduction to the History of Science*. Baltimore: Williams and Wilkins Co.

Saunders, P. 1982. *Edward Jenner: The Cheltenham Years*. Hanover: University Press of New England.

Schamberg, J. F. 1903. "An Examination into the Claims of the Red-Light Treatment of Smallpox." *J. Amer. Med. Assoc.* 40: 1183–86.

————. 1904. "The Passing of the Red Light Treatment of Smallpox." *J. Amer. Med. Assoc.* 43: 1641–42.

————. 1921. *Diseases of the Skin and the Eruptive Fevers.* Philadelphia: W. B. Saunders Co.

Schmid, H. E. 1896. "Notes from Japan." *Med. Rec.* (N. Y.) 5: 314.

Schram, R. 1971. *A History of the Nigerian Health Services.* Ibadan: Ibadan University Press.

Schultz, M. G. 1968. "A History of Bartonellosis (Carrion's Disease)." *Amer. J. Trop. Med. Hyg.* 17: 503–15.

Schwartz, E. J., and Kerr, S. 1918. "Ohio's Investment in Smallpox." *Ohio Publ. Hlth. J.* 9: 247–53.

Scott, D. 1965. *Epidemic Disease in Ghana, 1901–1960.* London: Oxford University Press.

Scott, F. D. 1972. *Sweden: The Nation's History.* Minneapolis: University of Minnesota Press.

Scott, H. H. 1939. *A History of Tropical Medicine.* London: Edward Arnold and Co.

Seely, W. W. 1871. "Eye Complications of Smallpox." *The Clinic (Cincinnati)* 1: 234–35.

Sekelj, T. 1959. *Window on Nepal.* London: Robert Hale.

Selkirk, J. 1844. *Recollections of Ceylon.* London: J. Hatchard and Son.

Sengupta, J. C. 1969. *West Bengal District Gazetteers: Malda.* Calcutta: Government of West Bengal.

Serruys, H. 1980. "Smallpox in Mongolia during the Ming and Ch'ing Dynasties." *Zentralasiatische Stud.* 14: 41–63.

Sery, V. 1973. "Smallpox and Traditional Medicine in the Developing Countries of Africa and Asia." *Z. Tropenmed. Parasit.* 24: 105–18.

Seward, D. 1973. *Prince of the Renaissance.* New York: Macmillan Co.

————. 1976. *The Bourbon Kings of France.* London: Constable and Co.

Seymour-Price, M.; Cadria, C.; and Fendall, N. R. E. 1960. "Smallpox in Kenya." *E. Afr. Med. J.* 37: 670–75.

Shakabpa, T. W. D. 1967. *Tibet: A Political History.* New Haven: Yale University Press.

Shapiro, S. L. 1968. "Medical History of W. A. Mozart." *Eye Ear Nose Throat Monthly* 37: 17–20.

Sherring, M. A. 1868. *The Sacred City of the Hindus: An Account of Benares.* London: Trübner and Co.

Shorter, A. 1972. *Chiefship in Western Tanzania.* Oxford: Clarendon Press.

Shrestha, P. N. 1972. "History of Smallpox." *J. Nep. Med. Ass.* 10: 107–11.

Shrewsbury, J. F. D. 1949. "The Yellow Plague of A. D. 664." *J. Hist. Med.* 4: 5–47.

————. 1956. "The Saints and Epidemic Disease." *Bgham. Med. Rev.*, n.s., 19: 209–24.

Shutes, M. H. 1933. *Lincoln and the Doctors.* New York: Pioneer Press.

Skeat, W. W., and Blogden, C. O. 1906. *Pagan Races of the Malay Peninsula.* London: MacMillan and Co.

Silverstein, A. M., and Bialasiewicz, A. A. 1980. "A History of Theories of Acquired Immunity." *Cell. Immunol.* 51: 151–67.

Simpson, H. N. 1954. "The Impact of Disease on American History." *New Engl. J. Med.* 250: 679–87.

Sitwell, E. 1962. *The Queens and the Hive*. London: Reprint Society.

Slatin, R. C. 1896. *Fire and Sword in the Sudan*. London: Edward Arnold and Co.

Slaton, W. F. 1881–82. "Smallpox and the Public Schools of Atlanta." *Atlanta Med. Reg.* 1: 581–83.

Sleeman, W. H. 1915. *Rambles and Recollections of an Indian Official*. Karachi: Oxford University Press.

Smart, C. 1879. "Report on Smallpox in the District of Columbia." *Nat. Bd. of Hlth. Bull.* (Washington) 1: 242–43.

———. 1888. *The Medical and Surgical History of the War of the Rebellion*. Part 3: *Medical History*. Washington: U.S. Government Medical Office.

"Smallpox in Brazil." 1879. *Med. Times and Gaz.* (London) 1: 156.

"Smallpox in Hindoostan." 1851. *Med. Times.* (London) n.s., 2: 375–76.

"Smallpox before Jenner." 1896. *Brit. Med. J.* 1: 1261–64.

"Small-pox in Massachusetts: A Review of its Prevalence." 1894. *Boston Med. Surg. J.* 131: 42–44.

"Smallpox at Milan." 1888. *Lancet* (London) 2: 88–89.

"Smallpox in New Zealand." 1872. *Med. Times and Gaz.* (London) 2: 334.

"Smallpox in the Soudan." 1898. *Brit. Med. J.* 2: 1003–4.

"Smallpox in the United States and Canada." 1932. *Med. Ann. Distr. Columbia* 1: 176.

Smith, A. H. 1894. *Chinese Characteristics*. New York: Fleming H. Revell Co.

Smith, F. P. 1871. "Smallpox in China." *Med. Times and Gazette* (London) 2: 277.

Smith, G. E. 1912. *The Royal Mummies*. Cairo: Imprimerie de l'Institut Français d' Archeologie Orientale.

Smith, H. H. 1880. *Brazil*. London: Sampson Low, Marston, Searle, and Rivington.

Smith, J. L. 1854. "A Review of Epidemic Smallpox as It Has Prevailed in New York City." *N.Y. J. Med.*, n.s. 13: 59–68.

Smith, Malcolm. 1947. *A Physician at the Court of Siam*. London: Country Life.

Smith, Michael M. 1974. "The 'Real Expedición Marítima de la Vacuna' in New Spain and Guatemala." *Trans. Amer. Phil. Soc.*, n.s., 64, part 1: 1–74.

"Some Royal Death Beds: Mary II." 1910. *Brit. Med. J.* 2: 148–49.

Soper, F. L. 1966. "Smallpox-World Changes and Implications for Eradication." *Amer. J. Publ. Hlth.*, 56: 1652–56.

Sorrenson, M. P. K. 1967. *Land Reform in the Kikuyu Country*. Nairobi: Oxford University Press.

Souter, G. 1966. *New Guinea: The Last Unknown*. New York: Taplinger Publishing Co.

Southey, R. 1817. *History of Brazil*. London: Longman, Hurst, Rees, Orme, and Brown, Paternaster Row.

Spence, J. D. 1975. *Emperor of China*. New York: Random House.

Spence, J. M. 1878. *The Land of Bolivar*. London: Sampson Low, Marston, Searle and Rivington.

Sprengel, K. 1794. *Beiträge zur Geschichte der Medicin*. Halle: Rengerschen Buchhandlung.

Spry, W. J. J. 1895. *Life on the Bosphorus*. London: H. S. Nichols.

St. John, H. 1853. *The Indian Archipelago*. London: Longman, Brown, Green and Longmans.

Stanley, H. M. 1872. *How I Found Livingstone*. New York: Scribner, Armstrong and Co.

———. 1878. *Through the Dark Continent*. New York: Harper and Brothers.

Stark, R. B. 1977. "Immunization Saves Washington's Army." *Surg. Gyn. Obst.* 144: 425–31.

Starkey, O. P. 1939. *The Economic Geography of Barbados*. New York: Columbia University Press.

Statham, J. C. B. 1922. *Through Angola*. London: William Blackwood and Sons.

"Statistisch: Ubersicht über 1872–3." 1873–74. *St. Petersb. Med. Ztschr.*, n.s. 4: 381.

Stearn, E. W., and Stearn, A. E. 1943. "Smallpox Immunization of the Amerindian." *Bull. Hist. Med.* 13: 601–13.

———. 1945. *The Effect of Smallpox on the Destiny of the Amerindian*. Boston: Bruce Humphries.

Stearns, R. P. 1950. "Remarks upon the Introduction of Inoculation for Smallpox in England." *Bull. Hist. Med.* 24: 103–22.

Stepp, J. W., and Hill, I. W., eds. 1961. *Mirror of War*. Englewood Cliffs: Prentice-Hall.

Stevenson, S. 1915. *The Heart of Jainism*. London: Oxford University Press.

Stewart, R. C. "Early Vaccinations in British North America." *Canad. Med. Ass. J.* 39: 181–83.

Stoddard, W. D. 1890. *Inside the White House in War Time*. New York: Charles L. Webster and Co.

"The Story of Gloucester." 1897–98. *Nature* 57: 221–23.

Strayer, J. R.; Gatzke, H. W.; and Harbison, E. H. 1961. "India, China, and Japan during the European Middle Ages." In *The Course of Civilization*. New York: Harcourt Brace and World.

Strickland, A. 1885. *Lives of the Queens of England*. London: George Bell and Sons.

Stromberg, A. A. 1931. *A History of Sweden*. New York: Macmillan Co.

Struik. D. J. 1948. *Yankee Science in the Making*. Boston: Little, Brown and Co.

Svanstromi, R., and Palmstierna, C. F. 1934. *A Short History of Sweden*. Oxford: Clarendon Press.

Swan, R. 1968. "The History of Medicine in Canada." *Med. Hist.* 12: 42–51.

Tandy, E. C. 1923. "Local Quarantine and Inoculation for Smallpox in the American Colonies (1620–1775)." *Amer. J. Publ. Hlth.* 13: 203–7.

Tannenbaum, F. 1963. *Slave and Citizen*. New York: Vintage Books.

Tao, C. S. 1936. "A Study of the Smallpox Prevalance and Inoculation Data in Some Districts of Kiangsu Province." *J. Shanghai Sci. Inst.*, sect. 4, 2: 185–224.

Tarling, N. 1971. *Britain: The Brookes and Brunei*. Kuala Lumpur: Oxford University Press.

Taylor, C. E. 1970. "Gaining Public Acceptance and Maintaining Regular Programs in the Developing Countries." In *Proceedings International Conference on Application of Vaccines Against Viral, Rickettsial, and Bacterial Diseases of Man*, 14–18 December, Scientific Publication no. 226. Washington: Pan American Health Organization.

Taylor, M. 1870. *Student's Manual of the History of India*. London: Longmans, Green and Co.

Tekeste, A. T., et. al. 1979. "Smallpox Eradication in Ethiopia." WHO/SE/79.144.

Theal, G. M. 1892. *History of South Africa From 1795 to 1872*. London: George Allen and Unwin.

———. [1897] 1969. *History of South Africa Under the Dutch East India Company*. Reprint. New York: Negro Universities Press.

———. 1903. *Records of Southeastern Africa*. London: Government of the Cape Colony.

Thapar, R. 1966. *A History of India*. Harmondsworth: Penguin Books.

Thompson, S. J. 1913. *The Silent India*. Edinburgh: Williams Blackwood and Sons.

Thomson, J. C. 1887. "The Heavenly Flowers." *China Medical Missionary Journal* 1, no. 4: 157–161.

Thorwald, J. 1962. *Macht und Geheimnis der Frühen Ärzte*. London: Thames and Hudson.

Thucydides. 1977. *History of the Peloponnesian War*. Translated by Rex Warner. Harmondsworth: Penguin Books.

Thursfield, H. 1940. "Smallpox in the American War of Independence." *Ann. Med. Hist.* 3d series, 2: 312–8.

Thurston, H., and Attwater, D. 1956. *Butler's Lives of the Saints*. New York: P. J. Kennedy and Sons.

Tomkins, H. 1886. "Small-Pox Epidemics in London." *Lancet* 1: 827–28.

Tooke, W. 1800. *View of the Russian Empire during the Reign of Catherine the Second*. 2d ed. London: Longman and Rees.

Tormo, M. 1949. *La Armada en el Reinado de los Borbones*. Barcelona: Libreria Editorial Argos.

Tregonning, K. G. 1958. *Under Chartered Company Rule*. Singapore: University of Malaya Press.

Trent, J. C. 1946a. "Benjamin Waterhouse (1754–1846)." *J. Hist. Med.* 1: 357–64.

———. 1946b. "The London Years of Benjamin Waterhouse." *J. Hist. Med.* 1: 25–40.

Trevelyan, G. O. 1912. *George the Third and Charles Fox*. London: Longmans, Green and Co.

Truax, R. 1968. *The Doctors Warren of Boston*. Boston: Houghton Mifflin Co.

Tulloch, J. L. 1980. "The Last 50 Years of Smallpox in Africa." *WHO Chronicle* 34: 407–12.

Tupp, A. C. 1877. *Imperial Gazetteer, Northwest Province*. Agra.

Tyson, J. 1901. "Historical Note on Smallpox." *Phila. Med. J.* 8: 901.

United Kingdom. Dept. of Health and Social Security. 1980. *Report of the Investigation into the Cause of the 1978 Birmingham Smallpox Occurrence*. London. Her Majesty's Stationery Office, 22 July.

United Kingdom. H. M. Secretary of State for India. 1908. *Imperial Gazetteer of India*. New ed. Oxford: Clarendon Press.

———. 1909. *Imperial Gazetteer of India*. New ed. Oxford: Clarendon Press.

U.S. Congress. 1961. *Biographical Directory of the American Congress, 1774–1961*. Washington, D.C.: U.S. Government Printing Office.

"Vaccination against Smallpox in the United States: A Re-evaluation of the Risks and Benefits." 1971. *Morbidity and Mortal. Wkly Rept.* 20: 339–45.

Van der Zee, H., and Van der Zee, B. 1973. *William and Mary*. London: Macmillan and Co.

Van Rooyen, C. E., and Scott, G. D. 1948. "Smallpox Diagnosis with Special Reference to Electron Microscopy." *Canad. J. Publ. Hlth.* 39: 467–77.

Varavarn, Prince Sakol. 1930. "Public Health and Medical Service." In *Siam: General and Medical Features*, edited by the Executive Committee of the Eighth Congress of the Far Eastern Association of Tropical Medicine. Bangkok: His Majesty's Government.

Vasselli, J. A. 1951. "A Pestilence Census Taker in New Jersey." *Bull. Hist. Med.* 25: 380–83.

Vaughn, J. C. 1907. "On the Incidence of Smallpox in Calcutta." *Ind. Med. Gaz.* 42: 241–50.

Vaughn, V. C. 1923. "Smallpox before and after Edward Jenner." *Hygeia* 1: 205–11.

Vedder, H. 1938. *South West Africa in Early Times*. London: Oxford University Press.

Vega, J. 1943. *Luis I de España*. Madrid: Afrodisio Aquado.

Verger, P. 1954. *Dieux d'Afrique*. (Translated by E. Hopkins.) Paris: Paul Hartman.

———. 1957. "Notes sur le culte des orisa et vodun." (Translated by E. Hopkins.) *Memoires de L'Institut Française d'Afrique Noire* (Ifan Dakar). 51: 236–69.

———. 1964. *Bahia and the West African Trade, 1549–1851*. Ibadan: Ibadan University Press.

———. 1976. *Trade Relations between the Bight of Benin and Bahia from the Seventeenth to the Nineteenth Century*. Translated by E. Crawford. Ibadan: Ibadan University Press.

Von Hebra, F. 1866. *On Diseases of the Skin, Including the Exanthemata*. Edited and translated by C. H. Fagge. London: New Sydenham Society.

Von Höhnel, L. 1894. *Discovery of Lakes Rudolf and Stephanie*. London: Longmans, Green and Co.

Von Richter, W. M. 1817. *Geschichte der Medicin in Russland*. Moscow: N. S. Wsewolojsky.

Wack, H. W. 1905. *The Story of the Congo Free State*. New York: Knickerbocker Press.

Waddell, L. A. 1906. *Lhasa and Its Mysteries*, 3d ed. London: Methuen and Co.

Wadhams, S. H. 1899–90. "Smallpox in Puerto Rico." *Yale Med. J.* 6: 279–85.

Wagner, H. R. 1944. *The Rise of Fernando Cortez*. Berkeley: Cortes Society.

Wahl, M. 1883. "Statistische Mittheilungen über 3 Pockenepidemien in Essen Während der Jahre 1866–7, 1871–2, u. 1881–2." *Deutsche Med. Wchnschr. Berl.* 9: 684–702.

Walker, E. A. 1928. *A History of South Africa*. London: Longmans, Green and Co.

Walsh, R. 1836. *A Residence at Constantinople*. London: Frederick Westley and A. H. Davis.

Wanderings of a Pilgrim in Search of the Picturesque. 1850. London: Pelham Richardson.

Wandruszka, A. 1965. *The House of Habsburg*. Garden City: Doubleday and Co.

Wang, C.-Y. 1972. *Loves and Lives of Chinese Emperors*. Taipei: Mei Ya Publications.

Warburton, W. 1755. *An Account of the Rise, Progress and State of the Hospital for Relieving Poor People Afflicted with the Small-Pox, and for Inoculation*. London: Paternaster Row.

Ward, A. M. 1960. "Smallpox and Vaccination in the Armed Forces." *St. Bartholomew's Hosp. J.* 64: 197–99.

Ward, A. W., et al., eds. "The Eighteenth Century." In *The Cambridge Modern History*, vol. 6, p. 376. Cambridge: At the University Press.

Ware, R. 1861. "The Epidemic of Smallpox in 1859–60." *Boston Med. Surg. J.* 64: 85–90.

Waring, J. I. 1964. *A History of Medicine in South Carolina.* Columbia: South Carolina Medical Association.

Warner, B. H. n.d. "Political and Social Conditions during the War." In *Washington During War Time*, edited by M. Benjamin. Washington: National Tribune Co.

Webb, M. E. 1873. "On the Smallpox Epidemic in Boston in 1872–3." *Bost. Med. Surg. J.* 89: 201–5, 225–33.

Webster, N. [1799] 1970. *A Brief History of Epidemic and Pestilential Diseases.* Reprint. New York: Burt Franklin.

Weeks, J. H. 1913. *Among Congo Cannibals.* London: Seeley, Service and Co.

Weinstein, I. 1947. "An Outbreak of Smallpox in New York City." *Amer. J. Publ. Hlth.* 37: 1376–84.

Weithaler, K. L., and de Quadros, C. A. 1973. "Zur Epidemologie der Pocken in Aethiopien." *Aertzl. Praxis* 25: 841–44.

Welch, W. M. 1885. "The Jenner of America." *Proc. Philadelphia Cty. Med. Soc.* 7: 172–201.

Wells, W. L. 1872. "Report on Climatology and Epidemics of Pennsylvania for 1871." *Trans. Amer. Med. Ass. Philadelphia* 23: 437–58.

Werner, E. T. C. 1932. *A Dictionary of Chinese Mythology.* Shanghai: Kelly and Walsh.

Wessels, C. 1924. *Early Jesuit Travels in Central Asia.* Hague: Martinus Nijhoff.

Wheeler, Douglas L. 1964. "A Note on Smallpox in Angola, 1670–1875." *Studia* 13–14: 351–62.

White, C. B. 1881–82. "Review of Smallpox in New Orleans." *New Orleans Med. Surg. J.*, n.s., 9: 739–47.

Wiedner, D. L. 1962. *A History of Africa.* New York: Vintage Books.

Wienerisches Diarium, no. 797, 21–24 March, 1711.

Wienerisches Diarium, no. 803, 11–14 April, 1711.

Wilkins, W. J. 1972. *Hindu Mythology.* Delhi: Delhi Book Store.

Wilkinson, H. C. 1958. *The Adventurers of Bermuda*, 2d ed. London: Oxford University Press.

Wilkinson, L. 1979. "The Development of the Virus Concept as Reflected in Corpora of Studies on Individual Pathogens. 5: Smallpox and the Evolution of Ideas on Acute (Viral) Infections." *Med. Hist.* 23: 1–28.

Wilks, I. 1975. *Asante in the Nineteenth Century.* London: Cambridge University Press.

Willan, R. 1821. *Miscellaneous Works of the Late Robert Willan, M. D.* Edited by Ashby Smith. London.

Willcocks, J. 1904. *From Kabul to Kumasi.* London: John Murray.

"William Hillary, M.D., in the Barbadoes." 1964. *New Engl. J. Med.* 270: 153.

Williams, H. 1950. *Ceylon, Pearl of the East.* London: Robert Hale.

Williams, H. S. 1963. *Foreigners in Mikadoland.* Tokyo: Charles E. Tuttle Co.

Williams, H. U. 1909. "The Epidemic of the Indians of New England, 1616–1620." *Johns Hopkins Hosp. Bull.* 20:340–49.

Williams, L. R. 1915. "The Smallpox Epidemic at Niagara Falls." *Amer. J. Publ. Hlth.* 5: 423–37.

Willis, J. R. 1971. "The Spread of Islam." In *The Horizon History of Africa,* edited by A. M. Josephy, Jr. New York: American Heritage Publishing Co.

Wilmot, A. 1889. *The History of Our Own Times in South Africa.* London: J. C. Juta and Co.

Windley, A. T. 1903. "Leicester and Smallpox: Thirty Year's Experience." *J. of State Med.* 2: 21–30.

Windley, L. n.d. "Dwight Baldwin and the Smallpox Epidemic of 1853." *Lahaina Jottings.* Vol. 1, no. 2. Lahaina, Maui, Hawaii: Lahaina Restoration Foundation.

Wingate, F. R. 1893. *Ten Years Captivity in the Mahdi's Camp.* 10th ed. New York: Charles Scribner's Sons.

Winslow, O. E. 1974. *A Destroying Angel.* Boston: Houghton Mifflin Co.

Wise, T. A. 1845. *Commentary on the Hindu System of Medicine.* Calcutta: Baptist Mission Press.

Wolman, R. S. 1978. "A Tale of Two Colonial Cities: Inoculation against Smallpox in Philadelphia and in Boston." *Trans. Stud. Coll. Physicians Philad.* 45: 338–47.

Wong, K. C., and Wu, L.-T. 1936. *History of Chinese Medicine.* 2d ed. Shanghai: National Quarantine Service.

Wood, W. A. R. 1926. *A History of Siam.* London: T. F. Unwin. Ltd., Reprinted Bangkok, 1959.

Woodson, R. S. 1898. "Smallpox in Cuba." *J. Amer. Med. Assoc.* 31: 1466–68.

Woodward, S. B. 1925. "Smallpox in the United States, Insular Possessions, New England and Massachusetts, 1913–1923." *Boston Med. and Sur. J.* 192: 60–64.

———. 1932. "The Story of Smallpox in Massachusetts." *New Engl. J. Med.* 206: 1181–91.

Woodward, S. B., and Feemster, R. F. 1933. "The Relation of Smallpox Morbidity to Vaccination Laws." *New Engl. J. Med.* 208: 317–18.

Worcester, D. C. 1914. *Philippines: Past and Present.* New York: MacMillan Co.

Worcester, D. E., and Schaeffer, W. G. 1956. *The Growth and Culture of Latin America.* New York: Oxford University Press.

World Health Organization. 1969. "Recent Outbreak—Dahomey." *Wkly. Epidem. Rec.* 44: 649.

———. 1970. "Smallpox Surveillance." *Wkly. Epidem. Rec.* 45: 66.

———. 1971. "Smallpox Surveillance: Brazil." *Wkly. Epidem. Rec.* 46: 160.

———. 1972. "Smallpox: Yugoslavia." *Wkly. Epidem. Rec.* 47: 161–62.

———. 1973. "Smallpox: United Kingdom." *Wkly. Epidem. Rec.* 48: 146, 161, 186.

———. 1974a. "Smallpox: Japan." *Wkly. Epidem. Rec.* 49: 45.

———. 1974b. "Smallpox Surveillance." *Wkly. Epidem. Rec.* 49: 12.

———. 1975. "Smallpox Surveillance." *Wkly. Epidem. Rec.* 50: 14.

———. 1976. "Smallpox Surveillance." *Wkly. Epidem. Rec.* 51: 11.

———. 1977. "Eradication of Smallpox in Burma." SEA/Smallpox/83.

———. 1978. "Smallpox Surveillance: United Kingdom." *Wkly. Epidem. Rec.* 53: 265; 279, 283, 295.

———. 1979a. "Smallpox Eradication in China." WHO/SE/79.142.

———. 1979b. "Smallpox Surveillance." *Wkly. Epidem. Rec.* 54: 3.

———. 1979c. "Special Report on Smallpox and Its Eradication in Yunnan Province; China." WHO/SME/79.10.

———. 1979d. "Supplement to the Report to the International Commission for the Certification of Smallpox Eradication in the Republic of Djibouti." WHO/SE/79.143, addendum 1.

———. 1980. *The Global Eradication of Smallpox.* Geneva: World Health Organization.

World Health Organization and Ministry of Health, Family Planning, and Population Control. 1977. *Smallpox Eradication in Bangladesh.* Report to the International Assessment Commission on the Smallpox Eradication Programme in Bangladesh. SEA/Smallpox/82.

Wright, D. 1877. In *History of Nepal.* edited by S. S. Singh and S. Gunanaud. Cambridge: University Press.

Wunderlich, C. A. 1873. "Mittheilungen über die Gegenwartige Pockenepidemie in Leipzig." *Arch. d. Heilk. Leipzig.* 14: 97–106.

Yonge, C. D. 1867. *The History of France under the Bourbons.* London: Tinsley Brothers.

Zetterberg, E., et. al. 1966. "Epidemiology of Smallpox in Stockholm in 1963." *Acta Med. Scand.* Suppl. no. 464, pp. 9–42.

Zinsser, H. 1960. *Rats, Lice and History.* New York: Bantam Books.

Zwanenberg, D. Van. 1978. "The Suttons and the Business of Inoculation." *Med. Hist.* 22: 71–82.

Index